Pediatric Infectious Disease: Part I

Editors

MARY ANNE JACKSON
ANGELA L. MYERS

INFECTIOUS DISEASE CLINICS OF NORTH AMERICA

www.id.theclinics.com

Consulting Editor
HELEN W. BOUCHER

September 2015 • Volume 29 • Number 3

ELSEVIER

1600 John F. Kennedy Boulevard • Suite 1800 • Philadelphia, Pennsylvania, 19103-2899.
http://www.theclinics.com

INFECTIOUS DISEASE CLINICS OF NORTH AMERICA Volume 29, Number 3
September 2015 ISSN 0891–5520, ISBN-13: 978-0-323-39567-0

Editor: Kerry Holland
Developmental Editor: Donald Mumford

Infectious Disease Clinics of North America (ISSN 0891–5520) is published in March, June, September, and December by Elsevier Inc., 360 Park Avenue South, New York, NY 10010-1710. Periodicals postage paid at New York, NY and additional mailing offices. Subscription prices are $295.00 per year for US individuals, $510.00 per year for US institutions, $145.00 per year for US students, $350.00 per year for Canadian individuals, $638.00 per year for Canadian institutions, $420.00 per year for international individuals, $638.00 per year for international institutions, and $200.00 per year for Canadian and international students. To receive student rate, orders must be accompanied by name of affiliated institution, date of term, and the *signature* of program/ residency coordinator on institution letterhead. Orders will be billed at individual rate until proof of status is received. Foreign air speed delivery is included in all *Clinics* subscription prices. All prices are subject to change without notice. **POSTMASTER**: Send address changes to *Infectious Disease Clinics of North America*, Elsevier Health Sciences Division, Subcription Customer Service, 3251 Riverport Lane, Maryland Heights, MO 63043. **Customer Service: 1-800-654-2452 (US). From outside of the US and Canada, call 1-314-447-8871. Fax: 1-314-447-8029. E-mail: JournalsCustomerService-usa@elsevier.com (print support) or JournalsOnlineSupport-usa@elsevier.com (online support).**

Infectious Disease Clinics of North America is also published in Spanish by Editorial Inter-Médica, Junin 917, 1er A 1113, Buenos Aires, Argentina.

Reprints. For copies of 100 or more, of articles in this publication, please contact the Commercial Reprints Department, Elsevier Inc., 360 Park Avenue South, New York, New York 10010-1710. Tel. 212-633-3874, Fax: 212-633-3820, E-mail: reprints@elsevier.com.

Infectious Disease Clinics of North America is covered in *MEDLINE/PubMed (Index Medicus), Current Contents/ Clinical Medicine, Science Citation Alert, SCISEARCH,* and *Research Alert.*

Printed in the United States of America.

Contributors

CONSULTING EDITOR

HELEN W. BOUCHER, MD, FIDSA, FACP
Director, Infectious Diseases Fellowship Program, Division of Geographic Medicine and Infectious Diseases, Tufts Medical Center; Associate Professor of Medicine, Tufts University School of Medicine, Boston, Massachusetts

EDITORS

MARY ANNE JACKSON, MD, FAAP, FIDSA, FPIDS
Division Director, Infectious Diseases, Children's Mercy Hospital Professor of Pediatrics; University of Missouri-Kansas City School of Medicine, Kansas City, Missouri

ANGELA L. MYERS, MD, MPH, FAAP, FPIDS
Pediatric Infectious Diseases Fellowship Program Director, Children's Mercy Hospital; Associate Professor of Pediatrics, University of Missouri-Kansas City School of Medicine, Kansas City, Missouri

AUTHORS

DUHA N. AL-ZUBEIDI, MD
Assistant Professor of Pediatrics, Division of Infectious Diseases and Associate Medical Director, Department of Pediatrics, Children's Mercy Hospital, Infection Prevention and Control, University of Missouri-Kansas City, Kansas City, Missouri

RAVIT ARAV-BOGER, MD
Associate Professor, Pediatric Infectious Diseases, Johns Hopkins University School of Medicine, Baltimore, Maryland

JOHN C. ARNOLD, MD
Chairman of Pediatrics, Pediatrics and Infectious Diseases, Naval Medical Center San Diego, San Diego, California

ROBERT S. BALTIMORE, MD
Professor of Pediatrics and Epidemiology, Section of Pediatric Infectious Disease, Department of Pediatrics, School of Public Health, Yale School of Medicine, New Haven, Connecticut

ERIC A. BIONDI, MD, MS
Assistant Professor, Department of Pediatrics, University of Rochester Medical Center, Rochester, New York

JOHN S. BRADLEY, MD
Professor and Chief, Director, Division of Infectious Diseases, Department of Pediatrics, Rady Children's Hospital San Diego, University of California San Diego School of Medicine, San Diego, California

STEVEN C. BUCKINGHAM, MD, MA
Associate Professor, Department of Pediatrics, Le Bonheur Children's Hospital, University of Tennessee College of Medicine, Memphis, Tennessee

CARRIE L. BYINGTON, MD
H.A. and Edna Benning Presidential Professor, Department of Pediatrics, University of Utah, Salt Lake City, Utah

SILVIA S. CHIANG, MD
Clinical Postdoctoral Fellow, Section of Infectious Diseases, Department of Pediatrics, Baylor College of Medicine, Houston, Texas; Visiting Fellow, Department of Global Health and Social Medicine, Harvard Medical School, Boston, Massachusetts

C. BUDDY CREECH, MD, MPH
Associate Professor of Pediatrics, Vanderbilt Vaccine Research Program, Division of Pediatric Infectious Diseases, Department of Pediatrics, Vanderbilt University School of Medicine, Nashville, Tennessee

ROBERT W. ELDER, MD
Assistant Professor of Pediatrics and Internal Medicine, Section of Pediatric Cardiology, Yale School of Medicine, New Haven, Connecticut

STEPHANIE A. FRITZ, MD, MSCI
Assistant Professor of Pediatrics, Division of Pediatric Infectious Diseases, Department of Pediatrics, Washington University School of Medicine, St Louis, Missouri

JENNIFER L. GOLDMAN, MD, MS
Divisions of Pediatric Infectious Diseases and Clinical Pharmacology, Department of Pediatrics, Children's Mercy Hospitals and Clinics, University of Missouri-Kansas City School of Medicine, Kansas City, Missouri

CHRISTOPHER J. HARRISON, MD, FAAP, FPIDS
Director of Infectious Diseases Research Laboratory, Director of Pediatric VTEU KC Unit, Children's Mercy Hospitals at Kansas City, and Professor of Pediatrics, University of Missouri-Kansas City School of Medicine, Kansas City, Missouri

SCOTT H. JAMES, MD
Assistant Professor of Pediatrics, Division of Infectious Diseases, Department of Pediatrics, University of Alabama at Birmingham, Birmingham, Alabama

DAVID W. KIMBERLIN, MD
Professor of Pediatrics, Division of Infectious Diseases, Department of Pediatrics, University of Alabama at Birmingham, Birmingham, Alabama

SHEENA MUKKADA, MD
Fellow in Pediatric Infectious Disease, Department of Pediatrics, Le Bonheur Children's Hospital, University of Tennessee College of Medicine; Department of Infectious Diseases, St. Jude Children's Research Hospital, Memphis, Tennessee

JASON G. NEWLAND, MD, MEd
Division of Pediatric Infectious Diseases, Department of Pediatrics, Children's Mercy Hospitals and Clinics, University of Missouri-Kansas City School of Medicine, Kansas City, Missouri

CHRISTIAN RENAUD, MD, MSc, FRCPC
Medical Director of Virology Laboratory CHU Sainte-Justine, Associate Professor of Microbiology, Immunology and Infectious Diseases, Medical Microbiologist, Pediatric

Infectious Diseases, Centre Hospitalier Universitaire Sainte-Justine, Université de Montréal, Montréal, Québec, Canada

ANNE H. ROWLEY, MD
Professor of Pediatrics, Northwestern University Feinberg School of Medicine, and Attending Physician, Division of Pediatric Infectious Diseases, The Ann and Robert H. Lurie Children's Hospital of Chicago, Chicago, Illinois

JULIA S. SAMMONS, MD, MSCE
Department of Infection Prevention and Control, The Children's Hospital of Philadelphia, Division of Infectious Diseases, Perelman School of Medicine at the University of Pennsylvania, Philadelphia, Pennsylvania

JEFFREY R. STARKE, MD
Professor of Pediatrics, Section of Infectious Diseases, Department of Pediatrics, Baylor College of Medicine, Houston, Texas

DOUGLAS S. SWANSON, MD
Associate Professor of Pediatrics, Division of Infectious Diseases, Department of Pediatrics, University of Missouri-Kansas City School of Medicine, Kansas City, Missouri

PHILIP TOLTZIS, MD
Division of Pediatric Critical Care, Rainbow Babies and Children's Hospital, Case Western Reserve University School of Medicine, Cleveland, Ohio

Contents

> Herpes simplex virus (HSV) 1 and HSV-2 infections are highly prevalent worldwide and are characterized by establishing lifelong infection with periods of latency interspersed with periodic episodes of reactivation. Acquisition of HSV by an infant during the peripartum or postpartum period results in neonatal HSV disease, a rare but significant infection that can be associated with severe morbidity and mortality, especially if there is dissemination or central nervous system involvement. Diagnostic and therapeutic advances have led to improvements in mortality and, to a lesser extent, neurodevelopmental outcomes, but room exists for further improvement.

> The wide spectrum of congenital cytomegalovirus (CMV) disease and known differences in the biology and in vitro growth of CMV strains continue to drive studies in search for specific viral genetic determinants that may predict severity of congenital CMV disease. Several CMV genes have been studied in detail in congenitally infected children, but the complexity of the viral genome and differences in the definition of symptomatic disease versus asymptomatic CMV infection continue to raise questions related to what constitutes a pathogenic CMV strain.

> Human parechoviruses (HPeVs) were initially classified as echoviruses. HPeVs occur worldwide, comprising up to 17 genotypes. HPeV1 and HPeV3 are most common. Clinical disease varies somewhat among genotypes. HPeV1 causes mostly gastrointestinal infections. HPeV3's prominence is due to its causing sepsis syndromes and central nervous system (CNS) infections in young infants. Currently, HPeV3 is the most common single cause of aseptic meningitis/meningoencephalitis in infants less than 90 days old in North America, usually with biannual summer-fall seasonality. HPeV3 CNS infections usually lack cerebrospinal fluid pleocytosis. Mortality and sequelae are uncommon, usually accompanying initially severe or neurologically complicated acute illnesses.

Staphylococcus aureus infections pose a significant health burden. The emergence of community-associated methicillin-resistant *S aureus* has resulted in an epidemic of skin and soft tissue infections (SSTI), and many patients experience recurrent SSTI. As *S aureus* colonization is associated with subsequent infection, decolonization is recommended for patients with recurrent SSTI or in settings of ongoing transmission. *S aureus* infections often cluster within households, and asymptomatic carriers serve as reservoirs for transmission; therefore, a household approach to decolonization is more effective than measures performed by individuals alone. Novel strategies for the prevention of recurrent SSTI are needed.

The incidence of *Clostridium difficile* infection (CDI) has risen among children and *C difficile* is increasingly recognized as an important cause of healthcare-associated diarrhea among pediatric patients. Still, increased identification of CDI in healthy children in the community and increased testing among infants requires cautious interpretation, given the high prevalence of asymptomatic colonization in young infants and frequent detection of viruses and other co-pathogens in stool specimens in these age groups. The significance of CDI among infants and the implications of positive *C difficile* testing among healthy children in the community are areas in need of further study.

The challenge of diagnosing childhood tuberculosis (TB) results from its paucibacillary nature and the difficulties of sputum collection in children. Mycobacterial culture, the diagnostic gold standard, provides microbiological confirmation in only 30% to 40% of childhood pulmonary TB cases and takes up to 6 weeks to result. Conventional drug susceptibility testing requires an additional 2 to 4 weeks after culture confirmation. In response to the low sensitivity and long wait time of the traditional diagnostic approach, many new assays have been developed. These new tools have shortened time to result; however, none of them offer greater sensitivity than culture.

Antibiotic resistance remains a major health threat and the overuse of antimicrobials contributes to this serious problem. Antimicrobial stewardship programs (ASPs) are effective in decreasing the inappropriate use of antimicrobials. The development of pediatric ASPs is increasing and these programs have proven effective in optimizing antimicrobial use in children. The value of ASPs is gaining recognition and the expansion of stewardship into additional health care settings is expected. Collaborative efforts are underway among pediatric ASPs to enhance best practices and develop efficient and effective strategies to minimize unnecessary antimicrobial use in children.

Robert W. Elder and Robert S. Baltimore

The epidemiology of infective endocarditis (IE) appears to be related to changes in the management of children with congenital heart disease (CHD) and the virtual disappearance of rheumatic heart disease. To better understand these changes, we divide the history into: I. The pre-surgical era, II. The early years of CHD surgical intervention, correlated with introduction of antibiotics, III. The modern era of cardiac interventions. Microbiologic changes include an early predominance of viridans streptococci and an overtaking by staphylococci. Additionally, there have been advances in imaging that allow earlier detection of IE and a reduction in IE-related mortality.

Anne H. Rowley

Kawasaki disease (KD) must be considered in the differential diagnosis of any child with fever for 4 to 5 days and compatible clinical and laboratory features, and in any infant with prolonged fever and compatible laboratory features, even in the absence of the classic clinical signs. Prompt therapy is required, because delayed or unrecognized KD can lead to lifelong heart disease or death in previously healthy children. Most children with KD respond to a single 2 g/kg dose of intravenous gammaglobulin with oral aspirin, but a small subset require additional therapies to resolve the clinical illness.

Sheena Mukkada and Steven C. Buckingham

Tick-borne infections create diagnostic challenges because they tend to present with nonspecific findings. Because clinicians often fail to recognize tick-borne illnesses in early stages, therapy is frequently delayed or omitted. This is especially problematic for rickettsial infections (Rocky Mountain spotted fever, ehrlichiosis, and anaplasmosis), because the risk of long-term morbidity and mortality increases with delayed treatment. We emphasize the need for clinicians to maintain a high index of suspicion for tick-borne infections; to diagnose these illnesses presumptively, without waiting for confirmatory laboratory test results; and to promptly start therapy with doxycycline, even in young children, when rickettsial infections are suspected.

John C. Arnold and John S. Bradley

For a child with a suspected bone or joint infection, knowledge of the workup and initial therapy is important to provide quality care. Fever and pain are hallmarks of a pediatric osteoarticular infection, although occasionally the signs and symptoms can be more subtle. The use of C-reactive protein to diagnose and validate effective management of treatment has become standard. Multiple reports confirm the success of much shorter intravenous (IV) courses than traditionally taught. The ideal IV and oral antibiotic duration, as well as defining the markers indicating need for surgical intervention, are questions yet to be answered.

The evaluation and management of well-appearing febrile infants less than 3 months of age has presented a decades-long clinical conundrum for providers. This article reviews the epidemiology of bacterial and viral infections in these infants. It discusses evidence-based diagnostic and treatment strategies, including appropriate use of testing, admission to the hospital, use of antibiotics, and hospital discharge. It also highlights the substantial variation in care for febrile infants and provides strategies to standardize practice.

INFECTIOUS DISEASE CLINICS
OF NORTH AMERICA

Preface

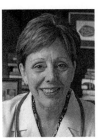 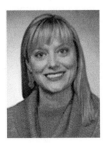

Mary Anne Jackson, MD, FAAP, FIDSA, FPIDS   Angela L. Myers, MD, MPH, FAAP, FPIDS
Editors

We are delighted to present this issue of *Infectious Disease Clinics of North America*, the first of a two-part series that addresses pediatric infections.

Several of the topics for the first issue are pathogen-specific with an emphasis on clinical focus, practical guidance, and emerging science in the field. Additional articles tackle subject matter related to cutting-edge topics in pediatric ID.

A state-of-the-art review of neonatal herpes simplex virus infection is presented by Drs James and Kimberlin, and Dr Arav-Boger tackles the topic of strain-specific cytomegalovirus and its role in defining clinical disease severity. A comprehensive review of human parechovirus 3, which has emerged as an important cause of meningoencephalitis in young infants, is beautifully written by Drs Renaud and Harrison. Drs Creech, Fritz, and Al-Zubeidi spotlight *Staphylococcus aureus*, with an emphasis on managing the child with recurrent infection, and Drs Sammon and Toltzis outline the pitfalls in diagnosing *Clostridium difficile* in children. Dr Starke anchors the review of *Mycobacterial tuberculosis*, and with Drs Chiang and Swanson, authors an all-inclusive article that emphasizes newer techniques for diagnosis.

Cutting-edge topics are provided with articles on pediatric antibiotic stewardship, written by Drs Goldman and Newland, and Drs Elder and Baltimore summarize the changing epidemiology of pediatric endocarditis. Dr Rowley has written a stand-alone article that emphasizes the complexities of diagnosing and treating Kawasaki disease, and Drs Buckingham and Mukkada review the importance of prompt recognition and treatment of tick-borne infections. Last of all, Dr Bradley and Arnold provide a state-of-the-art look at the approach to diagnosis and treatment of osteoarticular infection, and Drs Byington and Biondi summarize the contemporary strategies to evaluate and manage the febrile young infant.

When we undertook this labor of love, our goal was to enlist as authors the key experts in pediatric ID and to ensure for the reader that every contributor provided an extraordinary review. We can safely say that the list of authors is extraordinary, representing the top clinicians and researchers of our field. We feel this issue offers comprehensive, state-of-the-art summaries focused on some of the most important pediatric pathogens that have evolved or emerged over the last decade. We thank the editors, especially Donald Mumford, for helping us keep the issue on track, and

Infect Dis Clin N Am 29 (2015) xiii–xiv
http://dx.doi.org/10.1016/j.idc.2015.06.001
0891-5520/15/$ – see front matter © 2015 Published by Elsevier Inc.

Dr Boucher for inviting us to compile it. We hope that pediatric providers, including infectious diseases physicians and others, find this issue helpful to their practice. We look forward to the upcoming second issue, which will focus on vaccine-preventable infections.

Mary Anne Jackson, MD, FAAP, FIDSA, FPIDS
Infectious Diseases
Children's Mercy Hospital
University of Missouri-
Kansas City School of Medicine
2401 Gillham Road
Kansas City, MO 64108, USA

Angela L. Myers, MD, MPH, FAAP, FPIDS
Pediatric Infectious Diseases
Children's Mercy Hospital
University of Missouri-
Kansas City School of Medicine
2401 Gillham Road
Kansas City, MO 64108, USA

E-mail addresses:
mjackson@cmh.edu (M.A. Jackson)
amyers@cmh.edu (A.L. Myers)

Neonatal Herpes Simplex Virus Infection

Scott H. James, MD[a], David W. Kimberlin, MD[b],*

KEYWORDS

- Neonatal herpes • Herpes simplex virus • Genital herpes
- Mother-to-child transmission • Antiviral therapy

KEY POINTS

- Most women who transmit herpes simplex virus (HSV) to their infants have no known history of genital herpes.
- The clinical classifications for neonatal HSV infections (skin, eye, and/or mouth; central nervous system; and disseminated disease) are predictive of morbidity and mortality.
- Intravenous acyclovir, 60 mg/kg/d divided every 8 hours, remains the treatment of choice for the acute management of neonatal HSV infections.
- Six months of suppressive-dose oral acyclovir following the initial treatment course improves neurodevelopmental outcomes and reduces the frequency of skin recurrences, although some patients still have significant morbidity from their disease.

INTRODUCTION

Herpes simplex virus (HSV) infections are extremely common worldwide and account for a large burden of disease, including potentially life-threatening infections, in all age groups. HSV genital infections are particularly common in adolescents and adults, and carry the risk of mother-to-child transmission (MTCT) when occurring in pregnant women. Neonatal HSV infection occurs with less frequently, especially considering the high prevalence of HSV infections in the general population, but it is a serious and often invasive infection of which clinicians must be aware. Although advancing diagnostic and therapeutic modalities have improved clinical outcomes in the past several decades, neonatal HSV infections remain a significant cause of morbidity and mortality in this vulnerable population. This article offers an overview of the disease process, epidemiology, clinical diagnostic and therapeutic considerations,

[a] Department of Pediatrics, University of Alabama at Birmingham, Children's Harbor Building 308, 1600 7th Avenue South, Birmingham, AL 35233-1711, USA; [b] Department of Pediatrics, University of Alabama at Birmingham, Children's Harbor Building 303, 1600 7th Avenue South, Birmingham, AL 35233-1711, USA
* Corresponding author.
E-mail address: dkimberlin@peds.uab.edu

Infect Dis Clin N Am 29 (2015) 391–400
http://dx.doi.org/10.1016/j.idc.2015.05.001
0891-5520/15/$ – see front matter © 2015 Elsevier Inc. All rights reserved.

id.theclinics.com

outcomes, and potential complications. Ongoing and future avenues of investigation designed both to prevent MTCT and optimize therapeutic intervention in affected infants are highlighted.

PATHOGEN DESCRIPTION

HSVs exist as 2 distinct viral types: type 1 (HSV-1) and type 2 (HSV-2), both of which are associated with neonatal disease. HSV-1 and HSV-2 are categorized in the alpha herpesvirus subfamily of the Herpesviridae family of DNA viruses, along with varicella-zoster virus. As a subfamily, alpha herpesviruses are characterized by short replicative cycles, host cell destruction, and the ability to establish lifelong latency in sensory neural ganglia following primary infection.[1]

Both HSV-1 and HSV-2 are large enveloped virions marked by an icosahedral nucleocapsid arranged around a core of linear, double-stranded DNA. The lipid envelope and nucleocapsid are separated by a tightly adherent proteinaceous tegument. The HSV lipid bilayer envelope is embedded with surface glycoproteins that mediate attachment and entry into host cells and are responsible for evoking the host response. The envelope glycoproteins gB, gD, gH, and gL have been shown to be essential to cell entry.[2] Viral replication within an HSV-infected cell occurs through a cascade of steps including cell surface attachment, entry of the viral genome into the nucleus, transcription, DNA synthesis, capsid assembly, DNA packaging, envelopment via passage through the trans-Golgi network, and egress of new virions as the host cell is destroyed.

The genomes of HSV-1 and HSV-2 share approximately 50% homology, resulting in significant antigenic cross reactivity.[3] Type-specific glycoproteins, such as glycoprotein G (gG-1 and gG-2 for HSV-1 and HSV-2, respectively), allow differentiation of the 2 virus types via an antigen-specific antibody response. Differentiation of HSV type can also be achieved by restriction endonuclease fingerprinting, DNA sequencing, and increasingly by real-time polymerase chain reaction (PCR).[4–6]

RISK FACTORS

Neonatal HSV infections are most commonly acquired in the setting of maternal genital herpes infection in which there is viral shedding from the genital tract at or around the time of delivery. Risk factors for acquiring genital herpes include:

- Female gender
- Low family income
- Minority ethnic group
- Longer duration of sexual activity
- Past history of other sexually transmitted infections
- Higher number of sexual partners[7]

Women with no serologic evidence of prior HSV infection have a nearly 4% chance of acquiring HSV-1 or HSV-2 during the course of pregnancy (a first-episode primary infection), whereas women who are seronegative for HSV-2 but seropositive for HSV-1 have a 2% chance of acquiring HSV-2 during pregnancy (a first-episode nonprimary infection).[8] Viral reactivation from latency and subsequent antegrade translocation of virus from sensory neural ganglia to skin and mucosal surfaces can occur during pregnancy as well (a recurrent infection). Recurrent genital lesions pose a significantly lower risk for transmission to an exposed infant than first-episode primary infections (2% vs 57%), likely because of the transplacental passage of protective antibodies as well as lesser amounts of virus for a shorter period of time in the genital tract in recurrent infections.[9]

In seeking to mitigate the risk of MTCT in mothers with first-episode primary or first-episode nonprimary infections, a major limitation is the difficulty in identifying infections that are either completely asymptomatic or so clinically subtle that they are missed or misdiagnosed. One study showed that nearly 80% of women who transmitted HSV to their infants have no known history, previous or at the time of delivery, of genital HSV lesions.[10]

In addition to the differentiated risk of transmission to the neonate seen in primary versus recurrent maternal genital infection, several other risk factors[9,11] for MTCT of HSV infection have been identified:

- Vaginal delivery (vs cesarean delivery)
- Use of a fetal scalp electrode or other invasive instrumentation (disruption of the infant's cutaneous barrier)
- Maternal infection with HSV-1 (vs HSV-2)
- Detection of HSV-1 or HSV-2 from cervix or external genitalia at the time of delivery (via PCR or viral culture)
- Prolonged duration of rupture of membranes

SEROPREVALENCE OF HERPES SIMPLEX VIRUS INFECTION AND INCIDENCE OF NEONATAL DISEASE

Humans are the only known natural reservoir of HSV. Because it is not a reportable disease and is often subclinical, the true incidence of orolabial and genital HSV infections is unknown. However, surveillance of seroprevalence data can give some indication of how common HSV infections are in the general population. The overall prevalence of HSV antibodies increases with age, indicating ongoing exposure to these viruses within the population. More than 90% of adults have acquired HSV-1 infection by their fifth decade of life, although only a small fraction of infected persons develop clinically apparent disease at the time of acquisition.[12] HSV-1 infection is more commonly acquired earlier in life than is HSV-2, although a trend toward early acquisition of both viral types is noted in persons of lower socioeconomic status.[13,14]

Both HSV-1 or HSV-2 can cause genital infection, but HSV-1 traditionally is more associated with orolabial lesions, whereas HSV-2 is more associated with genital lesions. More recent data suggest that HSV-1 has become the more prevalent cause of genital herpes in certain populations of young women, accounting for up to 80% of genital herpes cases.[15,16] Neither HSV-1 nor HSV-2 displays any distinct seasonal variation in their incidence of infection.

Although there had previously been an increasing trend in HSV-2 seroprevalence in developed countries,[17,18] more recent seroepidemiologic studies have shown a plateau of both HSV-1 and HSV-2 in the United States. In adolescents and adults less than 50 years old, the seroprevalences of HSV-1 and HSV-2 were approximately 58% and 17%, respectively, during the period from 1999 to 2004, whereas a follow-up study spanning from 2005 to 2010 showed HSV-1 seroprevalence to have slightly declined (54%), whereas the HSV-2 seroprevalence had not significantly changed (16%).[19,20]

Regarding MTCT of HSV, studies have shown 20% to 30% of pregnant women to be seropositive for HSV-2 and that most women with a known history of genital herpes reactivate at least once during the course of a pregnancy.[21–24] In virologic surveillance of pregnant women with a known history of recurrent genital herpes, the rate of asymptomatic viral shedding at the time of delivery is as high as 1.4%, meaning that perinatal exposure of a newborn to HSV likely occurs more frequently than clinicians are aware.[25] Although the presence of active herpetic genital lesions or asymptomatic shedding of virions are risk factors in themselves, recurrent HSV infection such as this still constitutes less of a risk for transmission of HSV infection to a newborn than does acquiring a new primary or first-episode infection near the time of delivery.

The incidence of neonatal HSV infection in the United States is estimated to be as high as 1 in 3200 deliveries.[9] Based on an approximation of more than 4 million deliveries per year in the United States, this accounts for an estimated 1500 annual cases of neonatal HSV infection; a significant number, but still remarkably low given the overall prevalence of HSV infection. Consistent with the increasing proportion of HSV-1 genital lesions, most neonatal HSV infections in developed countries are caused by HSV-1 as well.[26,27]

GEOGRAPHIC DISTRIBUTION OF DISEASE BURDEN

HSV-1 and HSV-2 infections are common in both developed and less-developed countries worldwide. Global estimates indicate that more than 400 million people between the ages of 15 and 49 years were living with an HSV-2 infection in 2012, more than half of whom were women.[28] Included in this total prevalence is an estimated incidence of 19 million newly infected persons per year. Africa, the Americas, south-east Asia, and the western Pacific regions accounted for the greatest disease burden.

CLINICAL CORRELATION

MTCT of HSV infection can occur during one of 3 time periods:

- Peripartum (85%)
- Postpartum (10%)
- In utero (5%)

In utero HSV transmission, also known as congenital or antepartum transmission, is the least common route of MTCT, with an estimated transmission rate of 1 in 300,000 deliveries in the United States.[29] It presents with distinct symptoms (**Table 1**) already present at the time of birth. Intrauterine HSV infection has been found to occur with both primary and recurrent maternal HSV infections,[30] although the risk from a recurrent infection is less.

Peripartum transmission of HSV is the most common route of MTCT and can occur when there is symptomatic or asymptomatic shedding of virus from the genital tract around the time of delivery. Similar to peripartum transmission, postpartum transmission also occurs as a result of direct contact with infectious HSV virions, although instead of being exposed during passage through the birth canal the exposure typically originates from contact with orolabial or cutaneous lesions on an HSV-infected person.

HSV infections acquired peripartum and postpartum cause the same range of neonatal disease, which is clinically categorized as:

Table 1 Clinical manifestations of congenital HSV infection		
Cutaneous	**Neurologic**	**Ocular**
Active herpetic lesions	Microcephaly	Optic atrophy
Scarring	Intracranial calcifications	Chorioretinitis
Aplasia cutis	Hydranencephaly	Microphthalmia
Hyperpigmentation or hypopigmentation	—	—

- Skin, eye, and/or mouth (SEM) disease
- Central nervous system (CNS) disease
- Disseminated disease

These clinical classifications are predictive of both morbidity and mortality and are helpful in defining the duration of antiviral therapy needed.[9,31–34] By definition, SEM disease does not involve the CNS or other organ systems. Infants with HSV CNS disease may have mucocutaneous involvement, but they do not have evidence of any other organ system involvement. Disseminated HSV infection may involve multiple organ systems, including the CNS; liver; lungs; adrenals; gastrointestinal tract; and/or the skin, eyes, or mouth.[35] Overall, approximately half of all infants with neonatal HSV infection have some form of CNS involvement, whether as a component of disseminated disease or in isolation as CNS disease. Studies of the natural history of neonatal HSV infection have delineated the expected clinical distribution of disease categories.[35] SEM disease accounts for approximately 45% of neonatal HSV infections, CNS disease makes up another 30%, and disseminated disease accounts for the remaining 25%.

PATIENT HISTORY AND PHYSICAL EXAMINATION

In utero, or congenital, HSV infection presents as a distinct clinical entity characterized by the triad of cutaneous, neurologic, and ocular manifestations present at birth (see **Table 1**). Although these findings represent the classic presentation of congenital HSV infections, clinical manifestations occur on a spectrum and the clinician should be aware that more subtle presentations are possible.

Neonatal HSV infections acquired by either peripartum or postpartum MTCT show the same spectrum of disease categories (SEM, CNS, or disseminated disease), with neither route of transition being associated with increased severity of disease compared with the other. Common historical and physical findings for each disease classification of neonatal HSV infection are outlined here.

Skin, Eye, and/or Mouth Disease

- Presents about 9 to 11 days after birth, on average[36]
- More than 80% of the time, presents with characteristic vesicular or ulcerative skin lesions; patients may appear clinically well otherwise
- By definition, does not have evidence of visceral or CNS dysfunction
- If mucocutaneous lesions are not evident initially, may present with nonspecific symptoms such as poor oral intake, temperature instability, and irritability

Disseminated Disease

- Presents about 9 to 11 days after birth, on average[36]
- May present with a septic appearance, most notably respiratory failure, hepatic failure, and disseminated intravascular coagulopathy
- Cutaneous lesions may be present, but up to 40% of infants with disseminated disease never develop a vesicular rash during the course of their illness[35]

Central Nervous System Disease

- Typically presents later than SEM or disseminated disease, on average at about 16 to 17 days after birth[36]
- Presentation commonly involves nonspecific symptoms such as lethargy, irritability, poor oral intake, and temperature instability

- Signs of underlying CNS involvement may also be present, including a bulging fontanelle and focal or generalized seizures
- Cutaneous lesions may be present, but up to 35% of infants with CNS disease never develop a vesicular rash during the course of their illness[35]

DIAGNOSTIC TESTING

Isolation of HSV by viral culture remains the definitive method of diagnosing neonatal HSV infection, although detection of HSV DNA by qualitative PCR from the cerebrospinal fluid (CSF) is a routinely acceptable method for defining CNS involvement in neonatal HSV infection. Serologic studies are not routinely recommended for diagnostic purposes in neonatal HSV infections.

Before initiation of empiric parenteral acyclovir in an infant with suspected neonatal HSV infection, the following diagnostic specimens[37] should be obtained:

1. Swab specimens from the mouth, nasopharynx, conjunctivae, and anus (surface cultures) for HSV culture and, if desired, for HSV PCR
2. Specimens of skin vesicles and CSF for HSV culture and PCR, respectively
3. Whole-blood sample for HSV PCR
4. Whole-blood sample for measuring alanine aminotransferase

Obtaining a blood sample for HSV PCR can be helpful in establishing a diagnosis of neonatal HSV infection, especially in infants who present without cutaneous lesions.[38] Blood HSV PCR is positive in most patients with neonatal HSV infection regardless of their clinical classification[39] and therefore should not be used to determine extent of disease or appropriate duration of treatment. In some instances, blood HSV PCR is the only positive diagnostic test, suggesting that the diagnosis may have been missed or significantly delayed without performing this assay.

A recent report by Melvin and colleagues[39] shed light on the potential utility of assessing quantitative values of blood HSV DNA. It showed that plasma HSV DNA levels at the time of presentation correlated with clinical classification of neonatal HSV disease, with higher HSV DNA concentrations seen in infants classified as having disseminated HSV infection.[40] However, until more data are available, quantitative HSV PCR from blood should not routinely be used to determine disease classification.

Little is known about whether persistence of PCR positivity in the blood correlates clinically with disease resolution or outcome in the setting of neonatal HSV infection. Blood HSV PCR may remain positive throughout the course of antiviral treatment but the clinical significance of this is unknown. At present, serial HSV PCR assays from the blood are not recommended as a means to monitor response to therapy.

TREATMENT

Prompt recognition and timely initiation of empiric antiviral therapy are of great value in the treatment of neonatal HSV infections. The best outcomes are seen when appropriate antiviral therapy is started before the onset of significant viral replication within the CNS or widespread dissemination throughout the body.

Early antiviral agents such as idoxuridine and vidarabine were evaluated and proved to be of limited tolerability and efficacy, but acyclovir was licensed in 1982 and was found to have an improved safety profile that allowed higher doses and, subsequently, increased efficacy. Acyclovir, given intravenously at a dose of 60 mg/kg/d divided every 8 hours, remains the treatment of choice for neonatal HSV infections.

The current treatment recommendations are:

- Begin empiric intravenous acyclovir at a dose of 60 mg/kg/d divided every 8 hours in all cases of suspected or confirmed neonatal HSV infection
- If the diagnostic evaluation is positive, continue intravenous acyclovir for:
  - 14 days in SEM disease
  - At least 21 days in CNS disease or disseminated disease
- When there is CNS involvement, a repeat lumbar puncture should be performed near the end of therapy to document that the CSF is negative for HSV DNA on PCR assay; if the PCR result remains positive near the end of a 21-day treatment course, intravenous acyclovir should be continued for another week, with repeat CSF PCR assay performed near the end of the extended treatment period and another week of parenteral therapy if it remains positive[37]
- After completion of the full course of parenteral therapy, administer a suppressive course of oral acyclovir at a dose of 300 mg/m^2/dose, 3 times a day for 6 months
- Monitor absolute neutrophil count at the second and fourth weeks of suppressive therapy and then monthly throughout the remainder of the oral suppressive treatment period; if the absolute neutrophil count reproducibly decreases to fewer than 500 cells/μL, acyclovir should be held until neutrophil counts recover.

CLINICAL OUTCOMES AND COMPLICATIONS

In the preantiviral era, most neonatal HSV infections resulted in significant morbidity or mortality. As antiviral therapies have been developed, marked improvement in mortality at 1 year and in the rates of long-term neurodevelopmental impairment have been achieved, with the notable exception of neurodevelopmental outcomes in CNS disease.[32,34,41,42] **Table 2** shows the changes in morbidity and mortality as antiviral therapy has progressed over time.

After completion of the appropriate course of intravenous acyclovir for neonatal HSV infection, a 6-month suppressive course of oral acyclovir has been shown to be beneficial. Infants with CNS involvement who received acyclovir at a dose of 300 mg/m^2/dose 3 times a day for 6 months had better neurodevelopmental outcomes

Table 2				
Mortality and neurodevelopmental impairment in neonatal HSV infection				
	Mortality at 1 y (%)		Neurodevelopmental Impairment (%)	
Treatment	Disseminated	CNS	Disseminated	CNS
Preantiviral era[32]	85	50	50	67
Vidarabine[41]	50	14	42	43
Acyclovir (30 mg/kg/d)[41]	61	14	40	71
Acyclovir (60 mg/kg/d)[34]	29	4	17	69
Acyclovir (60 mg/kg/d) followed by 6 mo of oral suppressive acyclovir therapy (300 mg/m^2/dose administered 3 times per day)[42]	Not applicable	Not applicable		31[a]

[a] Includes infants with CNS disease as well as infants with CNS involvement in the setting of disseminated disease.

than the placebo group, and infants with CNS and SEM disease had less frequent recurrences of skin lesions while receiving suppressive therapy.[42]

SUMMARY

HSV infections are highly prevalent worldwide, causing a broad spectrum of disease in all age groups. Acquisition of either HSV-1 or HSV-2 leads to lifelong infection characterized by periodic reactivation. Neonatal exposure to HSV is common, but MTCT remains low. Although rare, neonatal HSV infection can be associated with significant morbidity and mortality, especially if there is dissemination or CNS involvement. Although the past 3 decades have seen substantial improvements in diagnostic and therapeutic capabilities, poor clinical outcomes remain unacceptably common. There is continued need for further investigation into new methodologies for the prevention of acquisition of HSV infection in women of childbearing age, interruption of MTCT, screening for asymptomatic shedding at the time of delivery, and the development of novel antiviral therapies, including combination therapies, with improved efficacy.

REFERENCES

1. Whitley RJ. Herpes simplex virus. In: Scheld MW, Whitley RJ, Marra CM, editors. Infections in the central nervous system. 3rd edition. Philadelphia: Lippincott Williams & Wilkins; 2004. p. 123–44.
2. Akhtar J, Shukla D. Viral entry mechanisms: cellular and viral mediators of herpes simplex virus entry. FEBS J 2009;276(24):7228–36.
3. Roizman B. The structure and isomerization of herpes simplex virus genomes. Cell 1979;16(3):481–94.
4. Buchman TG, Roizman B, Adams G, et al. Restriction endonuclease fingerprinting of herpes simplex virus DNA: a novel epidemiological tool applied to a nosocomial outbreak. J Infect Dis 1978;138(4):488–98.
5. Umene K, Kawana T. Divergence of reiterated sequences in a series of genital isolates of herpes simplex virus type 1 from individual patients. J Gen Virol 2003;84(Pt 4):917–23.
6. Reil H, Bartlime A, Drerup J, et al. Clinical validation of a new triplex real-time polymerase chain reaction assay for the detection and discrimination of Herpes simplex virus types 1 and 2. J Mol Diagn 2008;10(4):361–7.
7. ACOG Committee on Practice Bulletins. ACOG practice bulletin. Clinical management guidelines for obstetrician-gynecologists. No. 82 June 2007. Management of herpes in pregnancy. Obstet Gynecol 2007;109(6):1489–98.
8. Brown ZA, Selke S, Zeh J, et al. The acquisition of herpes simplex virus during pregnancy. N Engl J Med 1997;337(8):509–15.
9. Brown ZA, Wald A, Morrow RA, et al. Effect of serologic status and cesarean delivery on transmission rates of herpes simplex virus from mother to infant. JAMA 2003;289(2):203–9.
10. Whitley RJ, Corey L, Arvin A, et al. Changing presentation of herpes simplex virus infection in neonates. J Infect Dis 1988;158(1):109–16.
11. Pinninti SG, Kimberlin DW. Maternal and neonatal herpes simplex virus infections. Am J Perinatol 2013;30(2):113–9.
12. Corey L. Herpes simplex virus. In: Mandell GL, Bennett JE, Dolin R, editors. Mandell, Douglas, and Bennett's principles and practice of infectious diseases. 6th edition. Philadelphia: Elsevier Churchill Livingstone; 2005. p. 1762–80.

13. Nahmias AJ, Lee FK, Beckman-Nahmias S. Sero-epidemiological and sociological patterns of herpes simplex virus infection in the world. Scand J Infect Dis Suppl 1990;69:19–36.
14. Tunback P, Bergstrom T, Andersson AS, et al. Prevalence of herpes simplex virus antibodies in childhood and adolescence: a cross-sectional study. Scand J Infect Dis 2003;35(8):498–502.
15. Bernstein DI, Bellamy AR, Hook EW 3rd, et al. Epidemiology, clinical presentation, and antibody response to primary infection with herpes simplex virus type 1 and type 2 in young women. Clin Infect Dis 2013;56(3):344–51.
16. Roberts CM, Pfister JR, Spear SJ. Increasing proportion of herpes simplex virus type 1 as a cause of genital herpes infection in college students. Sex Transm Dis 2003;30(10):797–800.
17. Corey L, Wald A, Celum CL, et al. The effects of herpes simplex virus-2 on HIV-1 acquisition and transmission: a review of two overlapping epidemics. J Acquir Immune Defic Syndr 2004;35(5):435–45.
18. Fleming DT, McQuillan GM, Johnson RE, et al. Herpes simplex virus type 2 in the United States, 1976 to 1994. N Engl J Med 1997;337(16):1105–11.
19. Xu F, Sternberg MR, Kottiri BJ, et al. Trends in herpes simplex virus type 1 and type 2 seroprevalence in the United States. JAMA 2006;296(8):964–73.
20. Bradley H, Markowitz LE, Gibson T, et al. Seroprevalence of herpes simplex virus types 1 and 2–United States, 1999-2010. J Infect Dis 2014;209(3):325–33.
21. Kulhanjian JA, Soroush V, Au DS, et al. Identification of women at unsuspected risk of primary infection with herpes simplex virus type 2 during pregnancy. N Engl J Med 1992;326(14):916–20.
22. Kucera P, Gerber S, Marques-Vidal P, et al. Seroepidemiology of herpes simplex virus type 1 and 2 in pregnant women in Switzerland: an obstetric clinic based study. Eur J Obstet Gynecol Reprod Biol 2012;160(1):13–7.
23. Sheffield JS, Hill JB, Hollier LM, et al. Valacyclovir prophylaxis to prevent recurrent herpes at delivery: a randomized clinical trial. Obstet Gynecol 2006; 108(1):141–7.
24. Watts DH, Brown ZA, Money D, et al. A double-blind, randomized, placebo-controlled trial of acyclovir in late pregnancy for the reduction of herpes simplex virus shedding and cesarean delivery. Am J Obstet Gynecol 2003;188(3):836–43.
25. Arvin AM, Hensleigh PA, Prober CG, et al. Failure of antepartum maternal cultures to predict the infant's risk of exposure to herpes simplex virus at delivery. N Engl J Med 1986;315(13):796–800.
26. Kropp RY, Wong T, Cormier L, et al. Neonatal herpes simplex virus infections in Canada: results of a 3-year national prospective study. Pediatrics 2006;117(6): 1955–62.
27. Jones CA, Raynes-Greenow C, Issacs D. Population-based surveillance of neonatal HSV infection in Australia (1997-2011). Clin Infect Dis 2014;59(4): 525–31.
28. Looker KJ, Magaret AS, Turner KM, et al. Global estimates of prevalent and incident herpes simplex virus type 2 infections in 2012. PLoS One 2015;10(1): e114989.
29. Baldwin S, Whitley RJ. Intrauterine herpes simplex virus infection. Teratology 1989;39(1):1–10.
30. Hutto C, Arvin A, Jacobs R, et al. Intrauterine herpes simplex virus infections. J Pediatr 1987;110(1):97–101.
31. Whitley R, Arvin A, Prober C, et al. Predictors of morbidity and mortality in neonates with herpes simplex virus infections. N Engl J Med 1991;324(7):450–4.

32. Whitley RJ, Nahmias AJ, Soong SJ, et al. Vidarabine therapy of neonatal herpes simplex virus infection. Pediatrics 1980;66(4):495–501.
33. Whitley RJ, Yeager A, Kartus P, et al. Neonatal herpes simplex virus infection: follow-up evaluation of vidarabine therapy. Pediatrics 1983;72(6):778–85.
34. Kimberlin DW, Lin CY, Jacobs RF, et al. Safety and efficacy of high-dose intravenous acyclovir in the management of neonatal herpes simplex virus infections. Pediatrics 2001;108(2):230–8.
35. Kimberlin DW, Lin CY, Jacobs RF, et al. Natural history of neonatal herpes simplex virus infections in the acyclovir era. Pediatrics 2001;108(2):223–9.
36. Whitley RJ, Roizman B. Herpes simplex viruses. In: Richman DD, Whitley RJ, Hayden FG, editors. Clinical virology. 2nd edition. Washington, DC: ASM Press; 2004. p. 375–401.
37. American Academy of Pediatrics. Herpes simplex. In: Kimberlin DW, Brady MT, Jackson MA, et al, editors. Red book: 2015 report of the committee on infectious diseases. 30th edition. Elk Grove Village (IL): American Academy of Pediatrics; 2015. p. 432–45.
38. Cantey JB, Mejias A, Wallihan R, et al. Use of blood polymerase chain reaction testing for diagnosis of herpes simplex virus infection. J Pediatr 2012;161(2): 357–61.
39. Melvin AJ, Mohan KM, Schiffer JT, et al. Plasma and cerebrospinal fluid herpes simplex virus levels at diagnosis and outcome of neonatal infection. J Pediatr 2015;166(4):827–33.
40. James SH, Kimberlin DW. Quantitative herpes simplex virus concentrations in neonatal infection. J Pediatr 2015;166(4):793–5.
41. Whitley R, Arvin A, Prober C, et al. A controlled trial comparing vidarabine with acyclovir in neonatal herpes simplex virus infection. N Engl J Med 1991;324(7): 444–9.
42. Kimberlin DW, Whitley RJ, Wan W, et al. Oral acyclovir suppression and neurodevelopment after neonatal herpes. N Engl J Med 2011;365(14):1284–92.

Strain Variation and Disease Severity in Congenital Cytomegalovirus Infection: In Search of a Viral Marker

Ravit Arav-Boger, MD

KEYWORDS

- Cytomegalovirus • Congenital infection • Strains • Genotypes • Multiple strains
- Immune evasion genes • Population-based sequencing
- Next-generation sequencing

KEY POINTS

- Genetic diversity of cytomegalovirus (CMV) strains has been reported in children and adults.
- Sequence variability exists in CMV genes that may affect immune responses and viral dissemination.
- Viruses transmitted from mother to child share the same genetic content. Placental transmission appears to be independent of a specific virus strain.
- Sequencing of several hypervariable genes from original samples or low-passage virus isolates has generally yielded the same genetic information.
- Overall, there is no linkage between the different variable CMV genes, resulting in a very large number of CMV strains circulating in the population.
- Next-generation sequencing may allow better classification of strains once standardization of sequencing between laboratories is accomplished.

INTRODUCTION

Infection with cytomegalovirus (CMV) is the leading cause of congenital infection and the most common infectious source of central nervous system (CNS) damage and sensorineural hearing loss (SNHL) in the United States.[1,2] The outcome of

---

Division of Infectious Diseases, Department of Pediatrics, Johns Hopkins University School of Medicine, 200 North Wolfe Street, Baltimore, MD 21287, USA
E-mail address: boger@jhmi.edu

Infect Dis Clin N Am 29 (2015) 401–414
http://dx.doi.org/10.1016/j.idc.2015.05.009
0891-5520/15/$ – see front matter
id.theclinics.com

congenital CMV infection is highly variable. Of infected infants, around 10% to 15% exhibit severe symptoms at birth. Of the 85% to 90% who are asymptomatic at birth, 10% to 15% will later develop hearing loss and other neurologic deficits.[3,4] It is not clear why some infants have fatal or multisystem disease while others have no clinical evidence of abnormalities in the neonatal period or later.[5] The severity of fetal disease varies widely, ranging from stillbirth due to multisystem disease to no abnormalities. Similarly, the long-term outcome of congenital CMV infection ranges from no apparent impairments to significant CNS damage manifested as global developmental delay, cerebral palsy, hearing loss, or impaired vision, appearing alone or in combination.

Interest in the identification of pathogenic CMV strains originated from this wide spectrum of disease manifestations along with laboratory findings of genetic variability and differences in growth characteristics of the very distinctive CMV strains.[6,7] Vaccine studies have also contributed to the hypothesis that CMV strains have different pathogenic potential. The laboratory-adapted strains AD169 and Towne, which have been passaged multiple times in human fibroblasts, were found to be attenuated when administered as vaccine candidates. However, the Toledo strain, which had only been passaged several times in tissue culture, caused disease when administered to seropositive individuals.[8] Identification of CMV strains, that when acquired can lead to severe disease outcome, would allow for early diagnosis and outcome prediction and may direct vaccine development targeted to specific viral products. In the era before availability of sensitive high-throughput sequencing, only selected genes have been sequenced from the CMV genome, which ranges from 220 to 240 kB in length. These genes, some of which were discovered to be hypervariable, were selected based on data supporting their potential role in pathogenicity and dissemination of CMV. The more recent introduction of sensitive high-throughput sequencing techniques provides new information on sequence variation among CMV strains and may lead to better categorization of strains, but requires standardization and stringent criteria for strain definition.

This review addresses the following topics, among others:

1. Genetic variability of CMV strains—genotypic analysis
2. Next-generation sequencing (NGS) and its implications for identification of a genetic marker
3. The role of multiple CMV strains in outcome of congenital CMV infection.

GENETIC DEFINITIONS

Locus: a specific location of DNA sequence (**Box 1**)

Clade: a grouping that includes a common ancestor and all its descendants. Phylogeny is used to define a clade.

Open reading frame (ORF): a DNA sequence that, when translated into amino acids, contains no stop codons.

Linkage: linked genes are adjacent to each other on a chromosome; thus, they are likely to be transmitted or inherited together.

Molecular mimicry: a strategy used by many viruses to subvert and regulate antiviral immunity. Identical or similar amino acid sequences shared between pathogens and the host are responsible for molecular mimicry.

NGS: non-Sanger-based high-throughput DNA sequencing technologies. Millions or billions of DNA strands are sequenced in parallel, yielding substantially more throughput and minimizing the need for the fragment-cloning methods that are often used in Sanger sequencing of genomes.

> **Box 1**
> **Definitions**
>
> The following definitions were used to describe the genetic content of CMV[9]:
>
> Strain
>
> Overall description of viral genomic structure based on the sum of all loci tested. Strains can be distinguished from one another by differences in one locus or multiple loci.
>
> Genotype
>
> A combination of subtype designations based on sequence data obtained from 2 or more gene loci.
>
> Subtype
>
> Cluster pattern based on sequence data at any one gene locus.
>
> Variant
>
> Minor nucleotide changes observed within a subtype.
>
> Isolate
>
> CMV recovered from a human specimen and passaged in culture a limited number of times.
>
> Clustering
>
> Represents a clade of closely related genomes.
>
> Linkage
>
> A pair or group of genes being tightly held together during DNA replication so that they are more likely than not to be found together in any CMV in which any one of them is found.

GENERAL INFORMATION—THE CYTOMEGALOVIRUS GENOME AND CYTOMEGALOVIRUS STRAINS

The double-stranded DNA genome of wild-type CMV strains consists of 2 each unique long (UL) and unique short (US) regions, connected at their ends by identical small amino acid sequences (internal repeat sequences) that are arranged in opposite directions (inverted) (**Fig. 1**). The UL and US regions can flip around from right to left during replication, resulting in 4 possible isomers of the viral genome.[10] CMV has evolved with the human host, and the origin of the most recent common root for the α- (eg, herpes simplex), β- (eg, CMV), and γ- (eg, Epstein-Barr virus) herpesviruses is estimated to have occurred about 400 million years ago.[11] Under the selection of the host immune response, each herpesvirus developed solutions to allow for its survival. In addition to enzymes and proteins involved in DNA replication and structural proteins, CMV encodes for proteins that can affect virulence through immune evasion and molecular

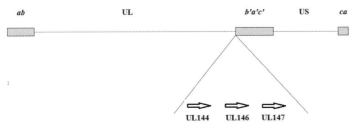

Fig. 1. Structural organization of the double stranded CMV genome of wild-type clinical isolates. *ab*, *ca* and *b'a'c'* represent inverted repeat sequences.

mimicry.[12] These functions, which can potentially limit host defenses against lytic or latent infection, are encoded by CMV genes that play immunomodulatory roles, resulting in more efficient virus replication. Genes affecting virulence have been identified in both UL and US regions of the CMV genome (**Table 1**). The first instance of molecular mimicry in CMV was identified as a major histocompatibility complex (MHC)-I homolog and is designated UL18. UL18 encodes a protein with 20% similarity to classical human MHC-I proteins.[13] MHC-I molecules present peptides derived from pathogens and cell proteins on the cell surface. Cytotoxic T cells (CTLs) recognize and lyse virus-infected cells through engagement of the T-cell receptor with MHC-I molecules presenting viral antigens at the surface of infected cells. The prevention of MHC-I expression allows these cells to escape CTL detection. Viral proteins can interfere with class I antigen presentation. Interference in antigen presentation and consequent MHC-I downregulation on the cell surface might allow infected cells to evade virus-specific CTLs, but downregulation of MHC-I molecules makes these cells susceptible to lysis by natural killer (NK) cells. UL18, MHC-I homolog acts as a decoy to block NK cell cytotoxicity.

Sequencing of clinical CMV isolates obtained from different cohorts of CMV-infected patients reveals that several CMV genes have highly different areas of sequences within apparently important genes. These areas of difference within a gene are called variable regions or polymorphisms. When multiple variable sequences are found in a given gene, it is designated as a hypervariable region.

Table 1
Potential virulence factors in the cytomegalovirus genome

Gene/Homology	Function	Number of Genotypes (Reference)
US3/none	Interferes with MHC-I/II processing so CMV antigen not presented efficiently to host immune system	11[14]
UL40/HLA-E homolog	Protects infected cells against NK cytotoxicity	12[14,15]
US28/G-protein coupled receptor	Promotes chemotaxis	5[16]
US27/G-protein coupled receptor	Extracellular virus spread	N/A
UL33, UL78/chemokine receptors	Regulation of cellular chemokine receptors (CXCR4 and CCL5)	4[17]
UL144/cytokine receptor	Inhibition of T-cell proliferation, induction of chemokines via NF-KB	3[18]
α-Chemokine	Neutrophil chemotaxis	14[19,20]
UL147/α-chemokine	Unknown	11[19,20]
UL36/[a]	Antiapoptotic	N/A
UL37/[a]	Viral mitochondria inhibitor of apoptosis	N/A
UL18/MHC-1 homolog	NK cell decoy	10[14]
UL111A/IL10 homolog	Inhibits MHC class II expression	12[14]

Abbreviations: CCL5, chemokine (C-C motif) ligand 5; CXCR4, C-X-C, chemokine receptor type 4; N/A, not reported from clinical isolates; NF-kB, nuclear factor kappa-light-chain-enhancer of activated B cells.
[a] Functional (not sequence) homology to host antiapoptotic genes.

The first complete sequence of a CMV genome was published in 1990,[21] and differences between the laboratory-adapted strains, known as AD169 and Towne, and the closer-to-wild-type Toledo strain were later localized to ORFs located in the UL/b' region of the genome (see **Fig. 1**).[6] These ORFs are thought to play a role in CMV replication or disease in vivo because they were lost on extensive passage in vitro. Although most genetic loci within the UL and US regions are highly conserved, proteins produced by genes in the UL/b' region are among those associated with immune evasion. These proteins include cytokine and chemokine homologs that can have remarkable sequence variability (hypervariable).

However, these areas did not change much if at all during ongoing replication in any given patient nor did they seem to change much when spreading from patient to patient, which means that known genotypes are mostly stable.[19,22] In addition, linkage between specific genes was rare, but there were exceptions. For example, the UL16 and UL147 genes were linked.[9,23]

WHAT IS THE BEST SOURCE FOR GENOTYPIC STUDIES?

CMV replicates in multiple cells and tissues in vivo. In organ and bone marrow transplant recipients, serial viral load testing from whole blood or plasma guides decisions for initiation of anti-CMV therapy and duration of therapy.[24] However, in congenitally infected children, viral loads from blood may increase or decrease in the same patient unpredictably, and the duration of viremia may be short.[25] Generally, saliva and urine samples provide the most reliable and informative sources for CMV genotyping. Saliva was reported to have slightly better yield for CMV detection by polymerase chain reaction (PCR) in congenitally infected children compared with urine.[26] Multiple passages of virus replication in cell culture can induce mutations in genes or complete loss of some genes that might slowdown or be unnecessary for growth in human fibroblasts (the cell line in which CMV is usually grown in the laboratory). Therefore, the question was whether mutations discovered during sequencing were really present in the originally sampled body fluid, or might they represent an artifact after passing in tissue culture?

Sequences of CMV genes have been compared from CMV-infected original samples and tissue-culture isolates from the same original sample to determine whether growth in culture could select for mutations. In general, isolates collected from the same patient showed excellent correlation for several genetic loci between the original and multiple passaged isolates.[9] However, in a study of 4 clinical strains passed in several cell lines in tissue culture, CMV genes RL13 and the UL128 locus (consisting of genes UL128, UL130, and UL131A) mutated quickly during passage in human cells during standard sequencing. Mutations in RL13 occurred in fibroblast, epithelial, and endothelial cells, and those in the UL128 locus were limited to fibroblasts and detected later than RL13.[27] Several clinical isolates analyzed directly by NGS did not reveal mutations in these genes,[28] but mutations in several gene loci were present in CMV isolated from original body fluids. Mutations were identified in CMV genes RL5A, UL9, UL111A, and UL150 that were culture-independent (ie, spontaneous mutations in vivo). Future analysis of multiple clinical samples by NGS will assist in defining mutations across the CMV genome and their potential role as markers for disease outcome.

The Era Before High-Throughput/Next-Generation Sequencing

Two main classes of CMV genes have been studied in detail in samples collected from congenitally infected children: (1) the surface glycoprotein-B (gB), -H (gH), -N (gN), and -O (gO); and (2) the cytokine/chemokine homologs of human cellular genes that had been hijacked into the CMV genome. The underlying hypothesis was that polymorphisms in CMV genes that encode for proteins targeted by host immune response, such as envelope glycoproteins, as well as virus-captured human homologs of cytokines and chemokines could be associated with variability in controlling CMV infection.

Genotypes for CMV could be defined by differences in a single gene or some combination of linked genes. There is currently no consensus on what constitutes a clinically relevant genotype. Conflicting data exist for the single-gene genotypes investigated to date.

GENETIC VARIABILITY IN THE TUMOR NECROSIS FACTOR RECEPTOR–LIKE GENE, UL144

A truncated tumor necrosis factor-α-like receptor gene (UL144) was discovered in a region of the CMV genome deleted in highly passaged laboratory strains, but present in all fresh clinical isolates.[6] Sequence variability of UL144 was originally reported from 45 low-passage clinical isolates, revealing 3 major UL144 genotypes that were genetically unlinked with the 4 previously described major genotypes of the UL55 gene encoding for gB.[29] Similar variability was demonstrated in low-passage isolates collected from children attending daycare centers and congenitally infected infants in both Texas and Iowa. No linkage of UL144 genotype with gB subtypes was found,[30] meaning that any gB genotype could be present with any UL144 genotype. Children from the 2 different geographic locations were found to shed the same gB and or UL144.

Whether more severe outcomes of congenital CMV are related to specific UL144 genotypes remains controversial. For example, the author showed an association with UL144 genotypes A and C, and recombinants (A/B and A/C) ($P = .04$)[31] using isolates retrospectively collected from congenitally infected children who were school-aged and whose outcome was definitively known. This is important because some children who appear asymptomatic early in life may develop progressive hearing loss (symptomatic congenital CMV) that is diagnosed later (eg, near school entry). It was also found that UL144 genotype C was associated with other severe outcomes; for example, pregnancy termination was associated with genotype C from amniotic fluids collected in Italy ($P = .03$),[18] and genotype C was marginally associated with symptomatic disease in newborns (odds ratio, 8.81 [95% confidence interval, 0.48–164.02]; $P = .05$). Note the wide confidence interval encompassing 1.0.

Despite this, it was found that overall UL144 genotype C was not necessarily associated with higher viral loads in amniotic fluids. This finding was unexpected, given that higher viral loads are thought to predict worse outcomes in congenital CMV infection. In fact, genotype B (the most common UL144 genotype found in congenitally infected children) seemed more predictive of higher viral loads in symptomatic newborns than asymptomatic infants ($P = .003$).

Another study of UL144 genotypes in congenitally infected children had clinical follow-up at ages 12 to 18 months. It revealed that UL144 genotypes A and C were associated with a high-plasma viral load ($P<.04$) and both genotypes A and C were significantly associated with worse developmental outcome.[32] Further follow-up of this cohort for outcome of congenital CMV infection should assist in confirming these genotype data.

Genotyping during the CMV and Hearing Multicenter Screening (CHIMES) study also revealed that UL144 genotype C was more common in symptomatic children, but interestingly not specifically associated with SNHL.[16]

Despite these studies implicating UL144 genotype C with more severe outcomes, several other reports did not support an association between specific UL144 genotypes and outcome of congenital CMV infection.[16,33–36]

A large sample collection from multicenter trials of congenitally infected infants that has several years of follow-up, strict definition of symptomatic versus asymptomatic CMV disease, and outcome measures, in conjunction with whole genome sequencing, might clarify the role of UL144 genotypes or CMV proteins that may interact with UL144 genotypes as potential diagnostic markers.

GENETIC VARIABILITY IN UL146 AND UL147

Two α-chemokine genes, UL146 and UL147, are physically adjacent in the CMV genome. They have consistently shown extreme hypervariability (polymorphism) in all tested CMV isolates regardless of the patient population or geographic location from which the CMV isolates were obtained.[19,20,36–43] The 12 to 14 distinct UL146 and UL147 genotypes differ by more than 60% at the amino acid level.[19,40] Despite there being many described genotypes of UL146 and UL147, new genotypes did not arise over the time frame analyzed to date[19,36]; this indicates that rapid sequence drift in UL146 and 147 is not the underlying mechanism of this gene variability.

Polymorphisms have been noted throughout UL146, and also within a small region of UL147 corresponding to a possible signal peptide.[19,37] CMV isolates obtained from multiple members of families with a congenitally infected infant were sequenced. The UL146 genotype from different isolates cultured from any given family was the same within that family.[41] In each family, an older sibling of the congenitally infected infant rather than the father was the virus source for most pregnant women.

Extreme hypervariability of UL146 and UL147 in 23 congenially infected children was reported.[20] Because of the small sample size and large number of genotypes for these genes, no specific UL146 or UL147 genotype was associated with disease outcome. In a study of 121 infants from Poland (32 of whom were congenitally infected newborns), genotype G1 was more prevalent in symptomatic infants; an association between UL146 genotype and viruria was identified.[38] Nevertheless, much larger studies with hundreds of isolates will be required to identify a correlation between UL146/UL147 genotypes and outcome of congenital infection.

US28

CMV encodes for a functional β-chemokine receptor (US28) that binds and sequesters extracellular chemokines and may alter protective host immune responses.[44] Although there are much fewer (only 5) US28 genotypes compared with UL144, UL146/UL147, no association between a specific US28 genotype and outcome of congenital CMV infection is apparent.[16,18]

GLYCOPROTEIN N (UL73)

In Italian cohorts, 4 genotypes gN (UL73) have been identified, and all were transmitted from mother to child. Glycoprotein N-1 (gN-1) was associated with improved long-term outcome.[45] In a later study from the same group, gN-1 and gN-3a genotypes were associated with no symptoms at birth and a favorable long-term outcome, whereas gN-4 genotype was associated with symptoms at birth, abnormal imaging results, and sequelae ($P<.05$).[46] However, in the CHIMES study, the 7 gN genotypes did not correlate with symptomatic CMV disease.[16]

GLYCOPROTEIN O (UL74)

Four genotypes of UL74 have been identified, with a high level of sequence variability among the genotypes. Sequence variability among clinical strains was up to 46% in amino acids, including deletions and amino acid changes.[47] Similar genotypes were found in HIV and non-HIV-infected individuals. Genetic linkage between gN and gO has been reported.[48]

GLYCOPROTEIN H (UL75)

The gH gene was sequenced in the CHIMES study along with gN and gB. No particular genotype (5 for UL55, 2 for UL75, and 7 for UL73) was associated with symptomatic infection or SNHL.[16]

GLYCOPROTEIN B (UL55)

gB mediates virus attachment and entry into infected cells, cell-to-cell transmission, and syncytium formation.[49] A significant proportion of neutralizing antibody to CMV in human serum is specific for epitopes on gB, and essentially all CMV-infected individuals have antibody to gB.[50] Thus, it is not surprising that the gB gene has been commonly sequenced from both adults and children. Despite some suggested correlation, it appears that none of the 5 major gB genotypes are predictors of congenital CMV outcome,[16,18,51] although genotype 3 was more common in congenitally infected neonates with SNHL ($P = .009$).[35]

MIXED INFECTION WITH MULTIPLE CYTOMEGALOVIRUS STRAINS

Mixed infections have traditionally been reported from immunocompromised hosts. Multiple strains were detected in AIDS patients[52] and transplant recipients.[53,54] Previously, CMV-seropositive transplant recipients became infected with new CMV strains from their donors.[54] Multiple CMV strains were detected in blood from 5 of 11 CMV-infected renal transplant patients,[22] all of whom were seronegative before transplantation. Thus, infection with multiple strains in these patients could have occurred through acquisition of strains from normal seropositive donors who harbored and transmitted multiple CMV strains or the transplant recipients were susceptible to multiple exposures at different time points. In addition to acquisition of new strains over time, replacement of strains can occur.[23] Immunocompromised hosts can become a reservoir for generation of new CMV strains in vivo through recombination.[55]

Multiple CMV strains have been reported far less commonly in normal hosts and usually when repeated exposures to new sources of CMV would be expected. For example, 4 of 8 women attending a sexually transmitted disease clinic excreted distinct CMV strains simultaneously at different sites or shed new strains when studied serially.[56] Infection with new CMV strains has also been reported in children attending daycare centers.[57,58] Previously, immune mothers were reported to acquire a new CMV strain during pregnancy and transmit it to their offspring.[59] Multiple CMV strains were identified in autopsy tissues after in utero death as a result of disseminated CMV infection.[18] One recent report on strain diversity in healthy CMV-seropositive women suggested that 15 of 16 women who tested PCR positive (total 2.9% PCR positivity in that cohort) were infected with more than one strain based on genotyping gN and gB from blood or urine samples.[60] However, the time of primary infection was unknown in these women, so it is not possible to draw conclusions as to diversity of CMV strains acquired around seroconversion. In addition, the detection of multiple genotypes from blood samples in that cohort may suggest that this specific population was at risk for infection with multiple strains. However, information on potential risks or immunodeficiency was not available. The detection of a single strain or multiple CMV strains was investigated in a cohort of healthy seronegative women who participated in a

CMV gB vaccine clinical trial, followed until they acquired CMV, and then for up to 3 years afterward.[9] CMV genotyping was based on direct PCR sequencing at several distinct gene loci, including UL55, UL144, UL146, and UL9, from different body fluids collected at intervals after infection. CMV genotypes were also compared between original body fluids and after cell culture isolation, to address whether growth in culture might select for strains that grow more efficiently and therefore mask the detection of multiple strains. In 53 of 55 women, one CMV strain was detected, based on sequencing of UL55 and UL144. There was no evidence for acquisition of new strains or of sequence changes based on testing of multiple genetic loci. All known genotypes of gB, UL144, and UL146 were identified, similar to those reported from other studies.[19,61] DNA sequence data obtained from cultured isolates matched the sequences obtained from original fluids, suggesting that original urine or saliva samples in which high virus load is achieved may provide the most useful or efficacious source for genotyping without the need for culturing. Although most women had their own unique strain, 25% of women enrolled in the study at different times and with no known epidemiologic links shed the same CMV strain based on sequencing of 4 variable genetic loci. Because this CMV strain was found to be shared based on comparison of hypervariable genotypes (UL55, UL144, UL146, UL9), it is unlikely that sequencing of additional loci would have further distinguished the strains. These data suggest that a common CMV strain can be shed and circulate in a specific geographic region during a short time.

Despite these data in young women with recent primary CMV infection, results from the CHIMES study have shown that congenitally infected children may be infected with more than one CMV strain. In that study, mixed infections were detected in 45% of infants, both symptomatic and asymptomatic. These data need additional confirmation and interlaboratory validation.[16] It is also possible that the women from the gB vaccine trial could acquire new CMV strains in longer follow-up studies. Altogether, the identification of multiple CMV strains from seemingly normal asymptomatic hosts raises questions about the clinical significance of infection with multiple strains.

THE ERA OF NEXT-GENERATION SEQUENCING

The NGS era is marked by a massive increase in the throughput and resolution of the genomics field. The NGS approach analyzes the total DNA present in an isolate; thus, it is not only targeting viral DNA. DNA extracted from cells grown in culture contains mainly cellular DNA and low DNA copies of viral DNA. In one study, only 3% of sequence reads collected directly from the sample were of viral origin, but it was possible to reconstruct the complete genome using these 3% of reads.[28] This approach may be relevant to situations in which CMV DNA is abundant in original samples. DNA amplification steps may assist in sequencing the CMV genome from samples low in CMV DNA.

A study using 454 GS FLX (Roche, Branford, CT) technology analyzed CMV populations by sequencing PCR amplicons of the hypervariable genes UL73, UL74, and UL139 from lung transplant recipients.[62] Viral populations were identified with mixtures of up to 6 genotypes. Usually, 1 or 2 genotypes represented most of the population, whereas the other genotypes were present at frequencies less than 10%. Testing of serial samples collected from the patients revealed fluctuation in the genotype abundance, although the sequence itself did not change, again confirming the stability of CMV genes. The authors appropriately noted that PCR amplification may result in artificial recombinants and cautioned about problems in interpretation of deep sequencing experiments.[63,64]

The complete CMV genome was assembled using overlapping PCR amplicons.[65,66] BAC clones of AD169 and Toledo were resequenced to establish a quality filtering

---

Box 2
The genetics of congenital cytomegalovirus

- The strain detected from mother is the same strain transmitted to her child.
- Transmission has not been reported to depend on a specific strain.
- The same strains are detected in the same human family.
- In most congenital infections one strain is detected.
- Mixed infections have been reported with unclear relevance to disease progression.
- Urine or saliva isolates that have been minimally passaged in cell culture can provide a good source for CMV genotyping.
- NGS can be used in the future for genotype classification in large cohorts.

---

threshold for distinguishing real intrahost variants from PCR errors. In a first study, the viral populations of 3 congenitally infected infants were characterized. The genetic diversity of viral populations was comparable to quasispecies RNA viruses such as HIV. Variants present at high frequencies ($\geq$90%) accounted for 20% of reads, whereas low-frequency variants ($\leq$10%) represented 73% of reads, which corroborated with the study of UL73, UL74, and UL139 amplicons in lung transplant recipients.[62] Compared with the diversity found in the congenitally infected infants, intrahost diversity was lower in malignant gliomas.[67] One might suggest that during early life there might be higher replication capacity of CMV, which might lead de novo mutations. However, this is not supported by other studies showing stability of hypervariable CMV genes in immunocompromised hosts. It is also important to distinguish between the finding of random variants and subtype variants, the latter being the subject of investigation for a genetic marker for disease severity. The concept of intrahost diversity requires testing of additional samples from other patient populations as well as development of criteria for sequence standardization of viral genomes. In another study, serial urine and plasma isolates were collected from 5 congenitally infected infants.[59] In the same compartment, the consensus sequences differed only by 0.2% at the nucleotide level, indicating stability of the viral populations. However, in one child, comparison of isolates collected concurrently from urine and plasma revealed a 1% variability. The observed dynamics were modeled using demographic variables (population size and structure) and selective pressures. Although the effects of positive selection in a specific compartment were small, evidence for positive selection was found when comparing different compartments. It is possible that this child was infected with 2 different strains, but additional studies may provide data related to the importance of sequencing samples from different compartments using NGS.

The ability to analyze outcomes from a large data set of genetic polymorphisms was demonstrated by use of artificial neural network. Using sequence data from the hypervariable genes UL144, UL146, UL147, and US28, the network was trained and correctly predicted congenitally infected infants to be symptomatic or asymptomatic at birth in 90% of cases.[68] This technique can be applied to analyze outcomes from whole-genome sequences.

SUMMARY

Studies for the identification of a viral marker of CMV disease outcome have generated more debates than consensus, bur several themes have been reproducible (**Box 2**). There is no doubt that investigations should continue involving well-controlled populations, interlaboratory validation, and standardization of both genotypes and strains. NGS can be useful for subtype categorization and may assist in clear definitions of strains.

ACKNOWLEDGMENTS

The author thanks her mentor, Dr Gary Hayward, for ongoing teaching and wonderful advice and support over the years.

REFERENCES

1. Yow MD, Demmler GJ. Congenital cytomegalovirus disease–20 years is long enough. N Engl J Med 1992;326:702–3.
2. Manicklal S, Emery VC, Lazzarotto T, et al. The "silent" global burden of congenital cytomegalovirus. Clin Microbiol Rev 2013;26:86–102.
3. Demmler GJ. Infectious Diseases Society of America and Centers for Disease Control. Summary of a workshop on surveillance for congenital cytomegalovirus disease. Rev Infect Dis 1991;13:315–29.
4. Stagno S. Cytomegalovirus. In: Klein J, Remington JS, editors. Infectious disease of the fetus and newborn infant. 4th edition. Philadelphia: Saunders WB; 1995. p. 312–53.
5. Stagno S, Pass RF, Dworsky ME, et al. Congenital cytomegalovirus infection: the relative importance of primary and recurrent maternal infection. N Engl J Med 1982;306:945–9.
6. Cha TA, Tom E, Kemble GW, et al. Human cytomegalovirus clinical isolates carry at least 19 genes not found in laboratory strains. J Virol 1996;70:78–83.
7. Brown JM, Kaneshima H, Mocarski ES. Dramatic interstrain differences in the replication of human cytomegalovirus in SCID-hu mice. J Infect Dis 1995;171:1599–603.
8. Quinnan GV Jr, Delery M, Rook AH, et al. Comparative virulence and immunogenicity of the Towne strain and a nonattenuated strain of cytomegalovirus. Ann Intern Med 1984;101:478–83.
9. Murthy S, Hayward GS, Wheelan S, et al. Detection of a single identical cytomegalovirus (CMV) strain in recently seroconverted young women. PLoS One 2011;6:e15949.
10. Mocarski ES. Cytomegaloviruses and their replication. In: Fields BN, Knipe DM, Howley PM, editors. Fields virology. 3rd edition. Philadelphia: Lippincott Williams & Wilkins; 1996. p. 2447–92.
11. McGeoch DJ, Gatherer D, Dolan A. On phylogenetic relationships among major lineages of the Gammaherpesvirinae. J Gen Virol 2005;86:307–16.
12. Prichard MN, Penfold ME, Duke GM, et al. A review of genetic differences between limited and extensively passaged human cytomegalovirus strains. Rev Med Virol 2001;11:191–200.
13. Beck S, Barrell BG. Human cytomegalovirus encodes a glycoprotein homologous to MHC class-I antigens. Nature 1988;331:269–72.
14. Garrigue I, Faure-Della CM, Magnin N, et al. UL40 human cytomegalovirus variability evolution patterns over time in renal transplant recipients. Transplantation 2008;86:826–35.
15. Heatley SL, Pietra G, Lin J, et al. Polymorphism in human cytomegalovirus UL40 impacts on recognition of human leukocyte antigen-E (HLA-E) by natural killer cells. J Biol Chem 2013;288:8679–90.

16. Pati SK, Pinninti S, Novak Z, et al. Genotypic diversity and mixed infection in newborn disease and hearing loss in congenital cytomegalovirus infection. Pediatr Infect Dis J 2013;32:1050–4.

17. Deckers M, Hofmann J, Kreuzer KA, et al. High genotypic diversity and a novel variant of human cytomegalovirus revealed by combined UL33/UL55 genotyping with broad-range PCR. Virol J 2009;6:210.

18. Arav-Boger R, Willoughby RE, Pass RF, et al. Polymorphisms of the cytomegalovirus (CMV)-encoded tumor necrosis factor-alpha and beta-chemokine receptors in congenital CMV disease. J Infect Dis 2002;186:1057–64.

19. Lurain NS, Fox AM, Lichy HM, et al. Analysis of the human cytomegalovirus genomic region from UL146 through UL147A reveals sequence hypervariability, genotypic stability, and overlapping transcripts. Virol J 2006;3:4.

20. Arav-Boger R, Foster CB, Zong JC, et al. Human cytomegalovirus-encoded alpha-chemokines exhibit high sequence variability in congenitally infected newborns. J Infect Dis 2006;193:788–91.

21. Chee MS, Bankier AT, Beck S, et al. Analysis of the protein-coding content of the sequence of human cytomegalovirus strain AD169. Curr Top Microbiol Immunol 1990;154:125–69.

22. Stanton R, Westmoreland D, Fox JD, et al. Stability of human cytomegalovirus genotypes in persistently infected renal transplant recipients. J Med Virol 2005;75: 42–6.

23. Rasmussen L, Geissler A, Winters M. Inter- and intragenic variations complicate the molecular epidemiology of human cytomegalovirus. J Infect Dis 2003;187: 809–19.

24. Kotton CN, Kumar D, Caliendo AM, et al. Updated international consensus guidelines on the management of cytomegalovirus in solid-organ transplantation. Transplantation 2013;96:333–60.

25. Arav-Boger R, Pass RF. Diagnosis and management of cytomegalovirus infection in the newborn. Pediatr Ann 2002;31:719–25.

26. Ross SA, Ahmed A, Palmer AL, et al. Detection of congenital cytomegalovirus infection by real-time polymerase chain reaction analysis of saliva or urine specimens. J Infect Dis 2014;210:1415–8.

27. Dargan DJ, Douglas E, Cunningham C, et al. Sequential mutations associated with adaptation of human cytomegalovirus to growth in cell culture. J Gen Virol 2010;91:1535–46.

28. Cunningham C, Gatherer D, Hilfrich B, et al. Sequences of complete human cytomegalovirus genomes from infected cell cultures and clinical specimens. J Gen Virol 2010;91:605–15.

29. Lurain NS, Kapell KS, Huang DD, et al. Human cytomegalovirus UL144 open reading frame: sequence hypervariability in low-passage clinical isolates. J Virol 1999;73:10040–50.

30. Bale JF Jr, Petheram SJ, Robertson M, et al. Human cytomegalovirus a sequence and UL144 variability in strains from infected children. J Med Virol 2001;65:90–6.

31. Arav-Boger R, Battaglia CA, Lazzarotto T, et al. Cytomegalovirus (CMV)-encoded UL144 (truncated tumor necrosis factor receptor) and outcome of congenital CMV infection. J Infect Dis 2006;194:464–73.

32. Waters A, Hassan J, De GC, et al. Human cytomegalovirus UL144 is associated with viremia and infant development sequelae in congenital infection. J Clin Microbiol 2010;48:3956–62.

33. Picone O, Costa JM, Chaix ML, et al. Human cytomegalovirus UL144 gene polymorphisms in congenital infections. J Clin Microbiol 2005;43:25–9.

34. Nijman J, Mandemaker FS, Verboon-Maciolek MA, et al. Genotype distribution, viral load and clinical characteristics of infants with postnatal or congenital cytomegalovirus infection. PLoS One 2014;9:e108018.

35. Yan H, Koyano S, Inami Y, et al. Genetic variations in the gB, UL144 and UL149 genes of human cytomegalovirus strains collected from congenitally and postnatally infected Japanese children. Arch Virol 2008;153:667–74.

36. Heo J, Petheram S, Demmler G, et al. Polymorphisms within human cytomegalovirus chemokine (UL146/UL147) and cytokine receptor genes (UL144) are not predictive of sequelae in congenitally infected children. Virology 2008;378: 86–96.

37. Arav-Boger R, Zong JC, Foster CB. Loss of linkage disequilibrium and accelerated protein divergence in duplicated cytomegalovirus chemokine genes. Virus Genes 2005;31:65–72.

38. Paradowska E, Jablonska A, Plociennikowska A, et al. Cytomegalovirus alpha-chemokine genotypes are associated with clinical manifestations in children with congenital or postnatal infections. Virology 2014;462–463:207–17.

39. Aguayo F, Murayama T, Eizuru Y. UL146 variability among clinical isolates of human cytomegalovirus from Japan. Biol Res 2010;43:475–80.

40. Bradley AJ, Kovacs IJ, Gatherer D, et al. Genotypic analysis of two hypervariable human cytomegalovirus genes. J Med Virol 2008;80:1615–23.

41. Revello MG, Campanini G, Piralla A, et al. Molecular epidemiology of primary human cytomegalovirus infection in pregnant women and their families. J Med Virol 2008;80:1415–25.

42. Hassan-Walker AF, Okwuadi S, Lee L, et al. Sequence variability of the alpha-chemokine UL146 from clinical strains of human cytomegalovirus. J Med Virol 2004;74:573–9.

43. He R, Ruan Q, Qi Y, et al. Sequence variability of human cytomegalovirus UL146 and UL147 genes in low-passage clinical isolates. Intervirology 2006;49:215–23.

44. Pleskoff O, Casarosa P, Verneuil L, et al. The human cytomegalovirus-encoded chemokine receptor US28 induces caspase-dependent apoptosis. FEBS J 2005;272:4163–77.

45. Pignatelli S, Dal Monte P, Rossini G, et al. Intrauterine cytomegalovirus infection and glycoprotein N (gN) genotypes. J Clin Virol 2003;28:38–43.

46. Pignatelli S, Lazzarotto T, Gatto MR, et al. Cytomegalovirus gN genotypes distribution among congenitally infected newborns and their relationship with symptoms at birth and sequelae. Clin Infect Dis 2010;51:33–41.

47. Rasmussen L, Geissler A, Cowan C, et al. The genes encoding the gCIII complex of human cytomegalovirus exist in highly diverse combinations in clinical isolates. J Virol 2002;76:10841–8.

48. Yan H, Koyano S, Inami Y, et al. Genetic linkage among human cytomegalovirus glycoprotein N (gN) and gO genes, with evidence for recombination from congenitally and post-natally infected Japanese infants. J Gen Virol 2008;89: 2275–9.

49. Navarro D, Paz P, Tugizov S, et al. Glycoprotein B of human cytomegalovirus promotes virion penetration into cells, transmission of infection from cell to cell, and fusion of infected cells. Virology 1993;197:143–58.

50. Pass RF, Zhang C, Evans A, et al. Vaccine prevention of maternal cytomegalovirus infection. N Engl J Med 2009;360:1191–9.

51. Yamamoto AY, Mussi-Pinhata MM, de Deus Wagatsuma VM, et al. Human cytomegalovirus glycoprotein B genotypes in Brazilian mothers and their congenitally infected infants. J Med Virol 2007;79:1164–8.

52. Baldanti F, Sarasini A, Furione M, et al. Coinfection of the immunocompromised but not the immunocompetent host by multiple human cytomegalovirus strains. Arch Virol 1998;143:1701–9.

53. Puchhammer-Stockl E, Gorzer I, Zoufaly A, et al. Emergence of multiple cytomegalovirus strains in blood and lung of lung transplant recipients. Transplantation 2006;81:187–94.

54. Chou SW. Acquisition of donor strains of cytomegalovirus by renal-transplant recipients. N Engl J Med 1986;314:1418–23.

55. Chou SW. Reactivation and recombination of multiple cytomegalovirus strains from individual organ donors. J Infect Dis 1989;160:11–5.

56. Chandler SH, Handsfield HH, McDougall JK. Isolation of multiple strains of cytomegalovirus from women attending a clinic for sexually transmitted disease. J Infect Dis 1987;155:655–60.

57. Bale JF Jr, Petheram SJ, Souza IE, et al. Cytomegalovirus reinfection in young children. J Pediatr 1996;128:347–52.

58. Bale JF Jr, O'Neil ME, Fowler SS, et al. Analysis of acquired human cytomegalovirus infections by polymerase chain reaction. J Clin Microbiol 1993;31:2433–8.

59. Boppana SB, Rivera LB, Fowler KB, et al. Intrauterine transmission of cytomegalovirus to infants of women with preconceptional immunity. N Engl J Med 2001; 344:1366–71.

60. Novak Z, Ross SA, Patro RK, et al. Cytomegalovirus strain diversity in seropositive women. J Clin Microbiol 2008;46:882–6.

61. Dolan A, Cunningham C, Hector RD, et al. Genetic content of wild-type human cytomegalovirus. J Gen Virol 2004;85:1301–12.

62. Gorzer I, Guelly C, Trajanoski S, et al. Deep sequencing reveals highly complex dynamics of human cytomegalovirus genotypes in transplant patients over time. J Virol 2010;84:7195–203.

63. Gorzer I, Guelly C, Trajanoski S, et al. The impact of PCR-generated recombination on diversity estimation of mixed viral populations by deep sequencing. J Virol Methods 2010;169:248–52.

64. Zong JC, Arav-Boger R, Alcendor DJ, et al. Reflections on the interpretation of heterogeneity and strain differences based on very limited PCR sequence data from Kaposi's sarcoma-associated herpesvirus genomes. J Clin Virol 2007;40:1–8.

65. Renzette N, Bhattacharjee B, Jensen JD, et al. Extensive genome-wide variability of human cytomegalovirus in congenitally infected infants. PLoS Pathog 2011;7: e1001344.

66. Renzette N, Gibson L, Bhattacharjee B, et al. Rapid intrahost evolution of human cytomegalovirus is shaped by demography and positive selection. PLoS Genet 2013;9:e1003735.

67. Bhattacharjee B, Renzette N, Kowalik TF. Genetic analysis of cytomegalovirus in malignant gliomas. J Virol 2012;86:6815–24.

68. Arav-Boger R, Boger YS, Foster CB, et al. The use of artificial neural networks in prediction of congenital CMV outcome from sequence data. Bioinform Biol Insights 2008;2:281–9.

Human Parechovirus 3
The Most Common Viral Cause of Meningoencephalitis in Young Infants

Christian Renaud, MD, MSc, FRCPC[a], Christopher J. Harrison, MD[b],*

KEYWORDS

• Neonate • Meningitis • Encephalitis • HPeV • Seizure • White matter

KEY POINTS

• Human parechovirus 3 (HPeV3), the most common viral cause of infant central nervous system infection, has cyclic (every 2–3 years) and seasonal (summer through early autumn) outbreaks.

• HPeV3 disease presents somewhat like enterovirus disease; mostly as an irritable infant less than 90 days old with high fever for 3 to 5 days without focus (ie, sepsis/meningitis presentation).

• HPeV3 confirmation is by reverse transcription polymerase chain reaction (RT-PCR) of cerebrospinal fluid (CSF) or, less often, serum, but RT-PCR–positive CSF usually lacks pleocytosis.

• Peripheral leukopenia/lymphopenia and modestly increased C-reactive protein levels are common, but liver dysfunction or other laboratory abnormalities are uncommon.

• Mortality/sequelae are rare and can follow difficult–to-control seizures.

• Treatment is supportive, although anecdotal data suggest a potential effect of early intravenous immunoglobulin therapy in some cases.

INTRODUCTION

Human parechoviruses (HPeV) are in the picornavirus family, a group of important, highly diverse human pathogens. Other picornaviruses include enteroviruses (EVs), hepatoviruses, and rhinoviruses. Specific picornaviruses have been classically associated with specific clinical presentations (eg, polioviruses with spastic paralysis;

Conflicts of Interest: Neither C. Renaud nor C.J. Harrison has any conflicts of interest to declare for this article.
[a] Pediatric Infectious Diseases, Centre Hospitalier Universitaire Sainte-Justine, Université de Montréal, 3175 Ch de la Côte-Sainte-Catherine, Montréal, Québec, Canada; [b] Department of Pediatrics, Children's Mercy Hospitals at Kansas City, University of Missouri-Kansas City School of Medicine, 2401 Gillham Road, Kansas City, MO 64108, USA
* Corresponding author.
E-mail address: cjharrison@cmh.edu

Infect Dis Clin N Am 29 (2015) 415–428
http://dx.doi.org/10.1016/j.idc.2015.05.005
id.theclinics.com

coxsackievirus A16 with hand, foot and mouth disease; coxsackievirus B2 with myocarditis; and hepatitis A virus with hepatocyte injury). Recently, other picornaviruses have been found to cause unusual outbreaks, including EV71 causing severe central nervous system (CNS) infection in Asia, rhinovirus C causing severe pneumonia, coxsackievirus A4 causing Kawasaki disease–like syndrome, and EVD68 causing severe asthma-like presentations. Initially, HPeV genotype 3 was associated with sepsis-like episodes and CNS infection. Further surveillance showed that HPeV3 CNS infections occurred mostly in infants less than 90 days of age. This article describes the current status of HPeV3.

VIROLOGY

- There are 16 to 17 HPeV genotypes
- HPeV has diverged into many strains, likely because of lack of self-correcting processes for the genome
- CNS infections are mainly caused by HPeV3
- Differences in human cell attachment structures (eg, virus protein-1 [VP1]), among HPeV genotypes may affect clinical expression of disease

HPeV, like other picornaviruses, is a small, nonenveloped, positive-sense RNA virus.[1,2] Two HPeVs were discovered during a summer diarrhea outbreak in children in Ohio in 1956 but originally were classified as echovirus 22 and echovirus 23 within the EV genus.[3] They were renamed HPeV genotypes 1 and 2 in 1999 based on newly described differences compared with other picornaviruses in their genome, proteins, and biological properties.[4–7]

HPeV are genotyped based on the major structural protein gene, VP1 (**Fig. 1**).[8] Although 16 to 17 genotypes have been described, most data concern genotypes 1 to 8, with HPeV1 and HPeV3 being the most prevalent strains. HPeV1's wide genetic variability led to further division into 2 clades (subsets): HPeV1A and HPeV1B.[8] Frequent nucleic acid recombination events between the same or differing genotypes seem to be responsible for HPeV's genetic diversity, including the presence of mosaic genomes (mixtures of genetic parts from more than one strain).[9–12]

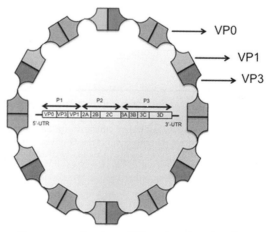

Fig. 1. HPeV virion with genome structure. UTR, untranslated region.

VP1 is an outer capsid protein playing a crucial role for HPeV entry into host cells. VP1 usually possesses a specific docking sequence that interacts with integrins on human cell surfaces.[13] However, HPeV3, HPeV7, and HPeV8, and some strains of HPeV1 and HPeV5, lack this specific docking sequence. Whether the absence of docking sequence has any specific impact on the disease produced by these genotypes is unknown.[14] HPeV can undergo point mutations because of error-prone RNA polymerase protein and because HPeVs have no proofreading mechanism (ie, no self-correcting of RNA errors), which contributes to antigenic drift (similar to the drift seen in seasonal influenza strains). Statistical genomic analysis of these mutations shows that currently circulating HPeV genotypes shared a common ancestor from around 4 centuries ago. Since then, HPeV has evolved into different lineages that have spread widely.[15]

TROPISM

- HPeV can be detected in many body sites
- HPeV can be shed for weeks to months after active disease has ceased

The primary replication site for HPeV is thought to be the respiratory and/or gastrointestinal tracts, although it has also been detected in blood, cerebrospinal fluid (CSF), and middle ear fluid.[16] Transmission occurs by contact with infected respiratory secretions or the fecal-oral route. Congenital HPeV has not been described to date. Like EV, HPeVs seem to be shed for weeks to months in feces, with one estimate of 51 days.[17] Although data are scant on shedding duration from the respiratory tract, estimates suggest 1 to 3 weeks. HPeV3 has a particular ability to affect brain and be detected in CSF (and blood). There is 1 report of HPeV detection in breast milk.[18]

EPIDEMIOLOGY

- HPeV is found worldwide, with HPeV1B and HPeV3 being most common.
- Disease caused by HPeV, particularly HPeV3, occurs mostly in young infants.
- HPeV3 has a summer-autumn season with outbreaks mostly every other year.
- HPeV3 is the most common single virus causing CNS infections in young infants in the United States, compared with multiple types of EV that generally circulate during a season.

Among the 16 to 17 genotypes, the most common type has been HPeV1B subtype, followed by HPeV3. The next in prevalence are HPeV1A subtype, HPeV2, HPeV5, and HPeV6.[18–21] HPeV3 was detected mostly in infants less than the age of 3 months, whereas HPeV1B was detected in children up to 3 years of age and HPeV6 seemed to infect even older patients.[22–24] Few patients infected with HPeV after the age of 10 years have been reported,[17,25–27] although recent data indicate that mothers of infants infected with HPeV3 are sometimes concurrently infected and may be the source of the infant infection (Klatte and colleagues, unpublished, 2014). HPeV overall seropositive rates range from 22% to 88% in children between 2 and 24 months old, 70% in children 5 years old, and 95% in adults.[23]

Differences in seasonality have been reported for different HPeV genotypes. Types found mostly in stool may have peaks in winter (December to February), whereas those causing sepsis-like illnesses and CNS infections in young infants peak from summer to autumn (June–October).[28–31]

HPeV3 outbreaks occur in temporal clusters on a seasonal basis generally with a similar season as that of EVs (ie, summer-autumn season [July–October for HPeV3 vs June–November for EV]). Several reports have documented a biennial pattern of HPeV3 infection,[28–30] whereas 1 or more EV serotypes can be detected each year in the United States. Reports have specifically failed to support a biennial pattern with non-HPeV3 genotypes. Cocirculation of multiple HPeV genotypes within a community or geographic region is common. Nevertheless, HPeV3 has been the most frequent single viral agent causing neonatal sepsis/meningitis in summer-autumn seasons since 2005 (**Fig. 2**).

In addition to pediatric community outbreaks, HPeVs have been associated with nosocomial outbreaks in pediatric and neonatal units.[29] HPeV, like other Picornaviridae, spreads easily in childcare settings.[32,33] Various HPeV genotypes have been reported in stools from asymptomatic patients, indicating that HPeV detection in stool does not necessarily confirm active disease.[17,31] Some HPeV genotypes (HPeV8–HPeV16) have been detected only in stools so far. Recently, HPeV10, HPeV13, and HPeV15 were detected in stools from Pakistani children,[34] whereas a possible new genotype (HPeV17) was described in a child from Thailand.[35] HPeVs have also been described as possible zoonotic pathogens because strains that are known to infect human were cultured from primates in Bangladesh (genotypes 1, 4, 5, 12, 14, 15)[36] and from pigs in Bolivia (genotype 4).[37]

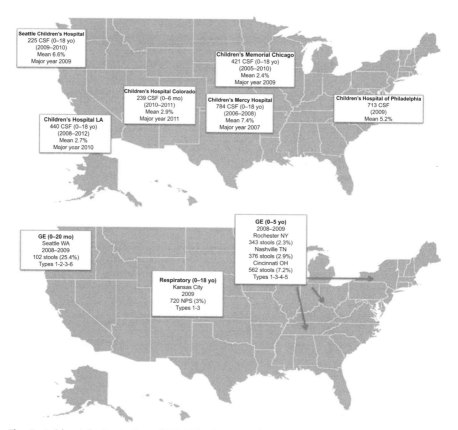

Fig. 2. Epidemiologic studies of HPeV in the United States. (*Top*) Identified from CSF and (*Bottom*) identified from stools in patients with gastroenteritis (GE) or respiratory samples. LA, Los Angeles; mo, months old; yo, years old. (*Data from* Refs.[28,30,32,69–74])

CLINICAL PRESENTATION, DIFFERENTIAL DIAGNOSIS, AND EMPIRIC APPROACH

- HPeV types other than HPeV3 most often present as less severe respiratory or gastrointestinal disease, often at ages greater than 90 days.
- HPeV3 causes disease most often in young infants (ie, <90 days of age).
- HPeV3's clinical presentations mimic EV; neonatal systemic herpes simplex virus (HSV) disease; or serious bacterial infections, including sepsis/meningitis.
- Consider HPeV3 infection in young infants who present with either fever and no focus or as sepsis/meningitis but also with a normal CSF (ie, no pleocytosis).
- Consider HPeV3 in febrile young infants with seizures, particularly when seizures are difficult to control.

Clinical manifestations of HPeV infections in infants and young children are diverse. HPeV of different genotypes can present differently; for example, HPeV1 is most often associated with gastrointestinal disease and other HPeV genotypes with respiratory illnesses. However, HPeV3 most often causes systemic/CNS disease in young infants less than 90 days of age. Presenting symptoms are consistent with sepsis-like illness, meningitis, or a nonspecific febrile illness.[27] Presentations in which HPeV3 should be suspected include neonatal seizure and neonatal sepsis (**Table 1**).

Neonatal seizures plus fever or hypothermia within the first months of life should trigger a complete sepsis work-up, including lumbar puncture.[38] Lumbar puncture in young febrile infants and any febrile infant with new-onset seizures, is important to rule out bacterial infection by standard cultures and HSV infection by HSV polymerase chain reaction (PCR) on blood and CSF. If those are negative, other infectious agents (eg, systemic viruses) should be sought. Antimicrobial therapy, including antibiotics and acyclovir, can be started while waiting for results. EV and HPeV reverse transcription (RT) PCR on CSF, and blood if possible, are indicated, particularly in

Table 1
Differential diagnosis of neonatal seizures and neonatal sepsis

Neonatal Seizure	Neonatal Sepsis
Infectious	Infectious
• HSV	• HSV
• HPeV3	• HPeV3
• EVs	• EVs
• HHV6	• HHV6
• CMV	• CMV
• Bacterial meningitis or ventriculitis (*Listeria monocytogenes*, *Streptococcus agalactiae*, *Escherichia coli*, *Citrobacter koseri*)	• Respiratory viruses
	• EVs or, more rarely, rotavirus
• Bacterial intracranial abscess	• Bacterial sepsis (*L monocytogenes*, *S agalactiae*, *E coli*)
• Congenital toxoplasmosis	• Acute pyelonephritis
	• Necrotizing enterocolitis
Noninfectious	Noninfectious
• Cerebral thrombosis or hemorrhage	• Metabolic disorders
• Electrolyte disorders	• Genetic disorders
• Metabolic disorders	• Hematologic disorders
• Genetic disorders	
• Epilepsy	
• Hypoxic ischemic encephalopathy	
• Malformations of cortical development	

Abbreviations: CMV, cytomegalovirus; HHV, human herpes virus.

summer and autumn months in North America. Seizures suggest encephalitis with potential CNS injury and should trigger electroencephalogram and MRI evaluations. Neonatal seizures, usually without fever or hypothermia, may be the presenting feature of inherited genetic and metabolic diseases, which must also be ruled out if this initial work-up is unrevealing.

In febrile infants less than 3 month old presenting without seizures but with sepsis-like symptoms or some signs suggesting meningoencephalitis (lethargy or bulged anterior fontanel), evaluation should be similar to that noted earlier for febrile seizure work-ups. Testing should include routine bacterial cultures on blood, urine, and CSF plus blood and CSF testing by a molecular assay, which could include PCR or RT-PCR for HSV and for EV. Further generic viral cultures (conjunctiva, throat, anus or stool, and urine) seeking EV and HSV are warranted. More rarely, sepsislike syndrome as well as meningoencephalitis could be related to acute or congenital cytomegalovirus (CMV) or acute human herpes virus-6 (HHV6) infections. PCR for those two viruses can be performed on the CSF, blood, throat, or urine (specifically for CMV). Respiratory viruses such as adenovirus[39] or influenza, and enteric virus infections, mainly rotavirus,[40] have also been associated with sepsis-like syndrome in neonates. The presence of concurrent upper respiratory tract infection/myalgia/gastroenteritis among the family contacts can point to a viral cause.

There are other less common presentations for HPeV. HPeV infections can mimic or complicate other syndromes. Hemophagocytic lymphohistiocytosis (HLH) can be either familial or induced by a wide array of infectious agents, including HPeV.[41–43] Note that HPeV3 sepsis is capable of causing increased blood ferritin level, cholesterol level, C-reactive protein level, liver enzyme levels, and pancytopenia in the absence of bone marrow confirmation of HLH. HPeV3 sepsis can also be associated with coagulopathy and severe hepatitis.[30,44] Prolonged prothrombin and partial thromboplastin time with thrombocytopenia and progressive hepatic failure have been described in this scenario. Reye syndrome, characterized by encephalopathy and liver dysfunction with fatty infiltration, was associated with a lethal HPeV6 infection in a 1-year-old girl.[27] Rarely, HPeV3 causes myocarditis,[45] myositis syndrome, or death in infants.[46]

CLINICAL DIFFERENTIATION FROM ENTEROVIRUS

- There are no consistent reliable clinical clues that differentiate HPeV from EV in young infants.

The clinical presentations and seasonality in infants infected with EV or HPeV3 during the first months of life have a fair amount of overlap.[47] Both EV and HPeV3 present with high fevers (often >38.9°C), irritability, decreased activity, and some sense from the parents that the child is experiencing abdominal discomfort. Neither HPeV3 nor EV (the exception is EVD68) produces notable respiratory symptoms or wheezing. Clinical clues to differentiate HPeV3 from EV are limited, the major one being less frequent facial rash in HPeV, although both produce truncal/extremity rashes. Tachycardia out of proportion to tachypnea also has been observed more frequently in HPeV3 than in EV. Seizures can occur with either virus but seizures can be particularly difficult to control with HPeV3.

USEFUL ROUTINE LABORATORY TOOLS

- A complete blood count with differential can be helpful.

The most useful tools to distinguish HPeV3 from EV, short of PCR testing on blood or CSF, are laboratory based (**Table 2**). The peripheral leukocyte count

Table 2
HPeV3 presentations: outcome

(A) Sepsis-like Syndrome <90 d of Age	(B) Clinical Infant Encephalitis	(C) Febrile Coagulopathy	(D) Myocarditis
Clinical			
Fever Irritability Decreased activity	Fever Irritability Decreased activity plus Seizures; may be difficult to control	Same as (A) plus Ecchymoses or purpura	Same as (A) plus Dilated myocardium and pulmonary edema
General laboratory			
Peripheral leukopenia or lymphopenia Modestly increased C-reactive protein level	Same as (A)	Same as (A) plus Abnormal clotting studies Increased liver function studies	Peripheral leukopenia or lymphopenia Modestly increased C-reactive protein level
CSF			
No pleocytosis Mildly increased protein levels (+) RT-PCR for HPeV3	No pleocytosis Modestly increased protein levels (+) RT-PCR for HPeV3	Same as (B)	Same as (A)
MRI brain			
In general not performed	White matter changes	Data not available	Data not available
Outcome			
In general no sequelae	Subset with cognitive or motor sequelae	May be lethal	May be lethal

and peripheral lymphocyte count are more often decreased with HPeV3.[48] In contrast, EV is associated with absolute leukocyte and lymphocyte counts that are normal to somewhat increased.[30,48,49] Although not common in either group, increased liver function studies are more frequently seen with EV. Levels of inflammatory markers (eg, C-reactive protein) are modestly increased with both HPeV3 and EV.

THE KEY IS CEREBROSPINAL FLUID TESTING

- CSF pleocytosis from HPeV3 CNS infection is uncommon.
- HPeV-specific RT-PCR is diagnostic and does not detect EVs.

CSF abnormalities are less common with HPeV3 than other viral CNS infections in which the pathogen is detectable in the CSF. The absence of CSF pleocytosis is virtually universal (up to 90%) in patients with HPeV3. Although 30% of infants less than 2 months old do not show pleocytosis with EV, most show CSF leukocyte counts in the 50 to 250 cells per mm³ range.[50,51] Abnormal CSF glucose concentrations are not expected with either EV or HPeV, although hypoglycorrhachia can be seen (rarely) with echoviruses. CSF protein levels may be modestly increased in less than 50% of patients with HPeV3, and somewhat more frequently with EVs. In neonatal HSV CNS infections, pleocytosis is expected, as are increased protein concentrations.[52]

HPeV3 does not grow well on routine cell culture in clinical laboratories and results require 5 to 7 days of incubation. The most specific identification for HPeV3 is by RT-PCR (discussed later). Molecular assays currently used for EV detection do not detect HPeV3, and vice versa, although a duplex assay designed to detect both has been described.[53]

MRI CHANGES WITH HUMAN PARECHOVIRUS 3

- MRI is useful in HPeV infection in which neurologic signs/symptoms (eg, seizures) occur.
- MRI findings are mostly in white matter.

Although CNS infections were first noted with HPeV1, the CNS seems to be a more frequent and particular target of HPeV3, possibly because of its having a different receptor on human cells than several other HPeV genotypes. Patients with HPeV3 with seizures, or less frequently with altered mental status, may show white matter inflammatory changes on MRI (**Fig. 3**). These changes can be temporary, although long-term sequelae, including paralysis, have been reported rarely.

When white matter injury occurs with HPeV3, the changes can involve subcortical white matter and complete fiber tracts (eg, gray matter regions in the posterior thalamus, optic radiations, and corpus callosum).[49] A subset of children with MRI abnormalities can have sequelae such as cognitive defects or cerebral palsy–like symptoms. Although not identical, HPeV3's MRI pattern is reminiscent of that with HHV6 encephalitis, another virus associated with seizures and absence of pleocytosis.[54] Local CNS innate immune response (eg, toll-like receptor [TLR]-8) activation has been suggested as a key element in the white matter changes.[55] The trigger for TLR-8 activation is single-stranded RNA, which is the configuration for the HPeV3 genome.

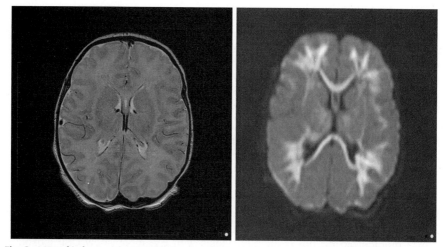

Fig. 3. MRI of infant with HPeV3 infection. Left panel represents MRI with contrast showing altered signal in white matter. This change is difficult to see because most white matter at this age is unmyelinated. The changes are more visible in the diffusion-weighted image on the right as intense white color (image on right is supposed to be less sharp than that on left). The axial diffusion-weighted image shows abnormal signal in the cerebral white matter, basal ganglia, and corpus callosum (bright areas). Apparent diffusion coefficient map images (not shown) confirm restricted diffusion consistent with extensive cytotoxic edema.

DIAGNOSIS

- Viral culture for HPeV is slow and not sufficiently sensitive.
- HPeV serology is rarely used to confirm HPeV active infection because antibody develops late in the course and ~90% of people more than 1 year of age are seropositive.
- HPeV-specific RT-PCR on blood and CSF samples can confirm active HPeV infection.
- As of mid-2015, no commercial kits exist for HPeV detection.
- HPeV can be detected in stools of asymptomatic patients because of prolonged shedding after illness has ceased.

The initially described strains of HPeV (HPeV1 and HPeV2) were isolated by cell culture because of their EV-like cytopathic effect. However, not all HPeV genotypes replicate equally on the same cell lines. Benschop and colleagues[8] documented that HT29 (primary colorectal adenocarcinoma) cells recovered 75% of all cultivatable HPeV from genotypes 1, 4, and 6 in stool specimens. HPeV1 and HPeV4 could also be cultured using tMK (tertiary cynomolgus monkey kidney), Vero (African green monkey kidney), A549 (human lung adenocarcinoma), and rhabdomyosarcoma cells.[8,56] In contrast, HPeV3 is more fastidious and grows slowly and only on Vero and A549 cells. The availability of cell culture facilities is now limited to research and reference laboratories.

Research-only enzyme immunoassays using synthetic peptides derived from capsid proteins VP0 and VP3 have been developed[57,58] for antibody testing. However, interpretation of such serologic results is complicated by the high seroprevalence rate observed in the general population by age 2 years. No commercial serology reagents are available and therefore their use has been limited to research prevalence studies.

Because of the inherent limitations of cell culture and serology, diagnosis of HPeV infection has predominantly relied on molecular methods. In 2008, 2 major real-time RT-PCR protocols were published. Since then, a few others (including minor modifications of the initial protocols) have been reported.[59,60] Almost all PCR protocols identify aspects of a specific sequence that overall is conserved among all EV and HPeV genotypes: the 5' untranslated region (UTR). However, there are sufficient differences within this conserved genomic region between EV and HPeV that primers have been developed to detect any EV but not detect any HPeV. EV primers therefore do not detect HPeV and vice versa. Further, within HPeV genera, genotype-specific sequencing is available in research laboratories to distinguish HPev3 from other HPeV genotypes.

No HPeV-specific commercial reagents are currently approved by the US Food and Drug Administration (FDA) but some have been CE (Conformité Européenne) approved and offer good performance. Several in-house developed protocols have shown good sensitivity and specificity. Some of them have been compared with culture and have shown much higher sensitivity. However, no head-to-head comparison between differing RT-PCR protocols has been published so far.

Because EV clinical presentations overlap with HPeV, testing is often desirable for both EV and HPeV on the same limited quantity of CSF in the same patient. Therefore, a few research protocols have combined primers from both targets in a biplexed assay so a single PCR run can detect either or both without losing sensitivity.

Similar to EV detection, CSF and blood are the preferred samples to prove active HPeV infection. PCR detection can also be performed in respiratory samples, including throat and nasopharyngeal swabs, or stool samples. Detection of HPeV in blood or CSF proves active infection. PCR of stool or respiratory samples can be misleading because shedding can occur for weeks to months after active disease has ceased. Because HPeV is an RNA virus, it is more susceptible to degradation during transport. Consequently, it is important to transport specimens rapidly to the laboratory and to keep samples refrigerated until the PCR is performed. If it is anticipated that PCR will not be performed within a day, freezing the sample at −80°C may be warranted.

Only a few clinical laboratories perform HPeV testing because of the absence of FDA-approved reagents. Nonetheless, 2 editorials from North American journals have emphasized the necessity to diagnose HPeV infections.[61,62] A recent international consortium working group on encephalitis diagnosis has also included HPeV testing in its recommendations for cases occurring in children less than 3 years old.[63] In order to make the diagnosis rapidly, more laboratories should be able to perform HPeV RT-PCR testing in the coming years.

MANAGEMENT

- No specific anti-HPeV treatment is available as of 2015.
- Intravenous immunoglobulin (IGIV) has been used anecdotally.

Management of HPeV disease, like EV disease, is supportive. Specific supportive protocols should be implemented for seizures, coagulopathy/hepatitis syndrome, or myocarditis presentations. These protocols are beyond the scope of this article.

There are no specific antiviral drugs for HPeV3. Pleconaril was available on a compassionate basis until 2012 and was shown to have an impact on severe EV disease in small numbers of patients. However, it is no longer available. Other drugs are under investigation for treatment of EV, particularly EV71. Speculation exists that some may have anti-HPeV activity.

As alternatives to specific antivirals, speculation arose over the utility of IGIV for treatment of HPeV3 because potential benefit has been reported for early IGIV treatment of severe EV disease. This speculation led to an anecdotal report of success in treating myocarditis.[45] It is therefore possible to extrapolate from that experience that IGIV might be useful if used early in the course of severe HPeV3 liver or heart inflammatory disease.[64]

IGIV has also been used successfully for decades to suppress chronic CNS enteroviral infections in children with agammaglobulinemia.[65,66] From that experience, it could be postulated that IGIV treatment might also affect CNS infections caused by HPeV3, although there are no data in early 2015.

Up to 70% of the adult population is seropositive to HPeV3,[67] so it is possible that IGIV contains some neutralizing antibody to HPeV3. However, titers are likely to vary from lot to lot, so there is no assurance that adequate titers would be found in any given lot.[68] It is unclear whether treatment with IGIV is a useful strategy for HPeV3 disease.

OUTCOME

- The outcomes of HPeV3 CNS infections are mostly benign.
- Cognitive and motor deficits can occur, mostly following illnesses that have neurologic findings during acute disease.

Permanent paralysis and CNS sequelae have been reported in small numbers of patients. However, most HPeV3 CNS infections documented in the United States have had apparently normal short-term outcomes. Long-term follow-up is not available.

Patients presenting with seizures and MRI white matter changes seem to be more likely to have sequelae related to cognitive defects or motor issues, but such outcomes seem uncommon in the North American experience.

In many ways the outcome of HPeV3 infections seems to be similar to that of EV, with most being benign, but there remains a small subset of patients who may have severe disease or sequelae. Whether these patients with severe sequelae have a genetic predisposition or there is some variation in strains of HPeV3 producing more severe disease has not been determined to date.

REFERENCES

1. Boivin G, Abed Y, Boucher FD. Human parechovirus 3 and neonatal infections. Emerg Infect Dis 2005;11(1):103–5.
2. Harvala H, Simmonds P. Human parechoviruses: biology, epidemiology and clinical significance. J Clin Virol 2009;45(1):1–9.
3. Wigand R, Sabin AB. Properties of ECHO types 22, 23 and 24 viruses. Arch Gesamte Virusforsch 1961;11:224–47.
4. Coller BA, Chapman NM, Beck MA, et al. Echovirus 22 is an atypical enterovirus. J Virol 1990;64(6):2692–701.
5. Hyypiä T, Horsnell C, Maaronen M, et al. A distinct picornavirus group identified by sequence analysis. Proc Natl Acad Sci U S A 1992;89(18):8847–51.
6. Oberste MS, Maher K, Pallansch MA. Complete sequence of echovirus 23 and its relationship to echovirus 22 and other human enteroviruses. Virus Res 1998; 56(2):217–23.
7. Ghazi F, Hughes PJ, Hyypiä T, et al. Molecular analysis of human parechovirus type 2 (formerly echovirus 23). J Gen Virol 1998;79(Pt 11):2641–50.
8. Benschop K, Minnaar R, Koen G, et al. Detection of human enterovirus and human parechovirus (HPeV) genotypes from clinical stool samples: polymerase chain reaction and direct molecular typing, culture characteristics, and serotyping. Diagn Microbiol Infect Dis 2010;68(2):166–73.
9. Benschop KS, Williams CH, Wolthers KC, et al. Widespread recombination within human parechoviruses: analysis of temporal dynamics and constraints. J Gen Virol 2008;89(Pt 4):1030–5.
10. Ito M, Yamashita T, Tsuzuki H, et al. Isolation and identification of a novel human parechovirus. J Gen Virol 2004;85(Pt 2):391–8.
11. Thoi TC, Than VT, Kim W. Whole genomic characterization of a Korean human parechovirus type 1 (HPeV1) identifies recombination events. J Med Virol 2014; 86(12):2084–91.
12. Zhu R, Luo L, Zhao L, et al. Characteristics of the mosaic genome of a human parechovirus type 1 strain isolated from an infant with pneumonia in China. Infect Genet Evol 2015;29:91–8.
13. Joki-Korpela P, Marjomäki V, Krogerus C, et al. Entry of human parechovirus 1. J Virol 2001;75(4):1958–67.
14. Williams CH, Panayiotou M, Girling GD, et al. Evolution and conservation in human parechovirus genomes. J Gen Virol 2009;90(Pt 7):1702–12.
15. Faria NR, de Vries M, van Hemert FJ, et al. Rooting human parechovirus evolution in time. BMC Evol Biol 2009;9:164.
16. Sillanpää S, Oikarinen S, Sipilä M, et al. Human parechovirus as a minor cause of acute otitis media in children. J Clin Virol 2015;62:106–9.
17. Tapia G, Cinek O, Witsø E, et al. Longitudinal observation of parechovirus in stool samples from Norwegian infants. J Med Virol 2008;80(10):1835–42.

18. Klatte LM, Kallemuchikkal U, Harrison CJ, et al. Two year prospective evaluation of human parechovirus and enterovirus CNS infections in infants less than 90 days of age. Boston (MA): IDSA; 2012. Poster 941.

19. Benschop K, Thomas X, Serpenti C, et al. High prevalence of human Parechovirus (HPeV) genotypes in the Amsterdam region and identification of specific HPeV variants by direct genotyping of stool samples. J Clin Microbiol 2008; 46(12):3965–70.

20. Ito M, Yamashita T, Tsuzuki H, et al. Detection of human parechoviruses from clinical stool samples in Aichi, Japan. J Clin Microbiol 2010;48(8):2683–8.

21. Pham NT, Trinh QD, Khamrin P, et al. Diversity of human parechoviruses isolated from stool samples collected from Thai children with acute gastroenteritis. J Clin Microbiol 2010;48(1):115–9.

22. Benschop KS, Schinkel J, Minnaar RP, et al. Human parechovirus infections in Dutch children and the association between serotype and disease severity. Clin Infect Dis 2006;42(2):204–10.

23. Tauriainen S, Martiskainen M, Oikarinen S, et al. Human parechovirus 1 infections in young children–no association with type 1 diabetes. J Med Virol 2007;79(4):457–62.

24. Verboon-Maciolek MA, Krediet TG, Gerards LJ, et al. Clinical and epidemiologic characteristics of viral infections in a neonatal intensive care unit during a 12-year period. Pediatr Infect Dis J 2005;24(10):901–4.

25. Abed Y, Boivin G. Human parechovirus types 1, 2 and 3 infections in Canada. Emerg Infect Dis 2006;12(6):969–75.

26. Figueroa JP, Ashley D, King D, et al. An outbreak of acute flaccid paralysis in Jamaica associated with echovirus type 22. J Med Virol 1989;29(4):315–9.

27. Watanabe K, Oie M, Higuchi M, et al. Isolation and characterization of novel human parechovirus from clinical samples. Emerg Infect Dis 2007;13(6):889–95.

28. Selvarangan R, Nzabi M, Selvaraju SB, et al. Human parechovirus 3 causing sepsis-like illness in children from midwestern United States. Pediatr Infect Dis J 2011;30(3):238–42.

29. Harvala H, Robertson I, McWilliam Leitch EC, et al. Epidemiology and clinical associations of human parechovirus respiratory infections. J Clin Microbiol 2008; 46(10):3446–53.

30. Renaud C, Kuypers J, Ficken E, et al. Introduction of a novel parechovirus RT-PCR clinical test in a regional medical center. J Clin Virol 2011;51(1):50–3.

31. Kolehmainen P, Oikarinen S, Koskiniemi M, et al. Human parechoviruses are frequently detected in stool of healthy Finnish children. J Clin Virol 2012;54(2): 156–61.

32. Braun LE, Renaud C, Fairchok MP, et al. Human parechovirus and other enteric viruses in childcare attendees in the era of rotavirus vaccines. J Ped Infect Dis 2012;1(2):136–43.

33. Moore NE, Wang J, Hewitt J, et al. Metagenomic analysis of viruses in feces from unsolved outbreaks of gastroenteritis in humans. J Clin Microbiol 2015;53(1):15–21.

34. Alam MM, Khurshid A, Shaukat S, et al. Human parechovirus genotypes -10, -13 and -15 in Pakistani children with acute dehydrating gastroenteritis. PLoS One 2013;8(11):e78377.

35. Chuchaona W, Khamrin P, Yodmeeklin A, et al. Detection and characterization of a novel human parechovirus genotype in Thailand. Infect Genet Evol 2015;31: 300–4.

36. Oberste MS, Feeroz MM, Maher K, et al. Characterizing the picornavirus landscape among synanthropic nonhuman primates in Bangladesh, 2007 to 2008. J Virol 2013;87(1):558–71.

37. Nix WA, Khetsuriani N, Peñaranda S, et al. Diversity of picornaviruses in rural Bolivia. J Gen Virol 2013;94(Pt 9):2017–28.
38. Vasudevan C, Levene M. Epidemiology and aetiology of neonatal seizures. Semin Fetal Neonatal Med 2013;18(4):185–91.
39. Ronchi A, Doern C, Brock E, et al. Neonatal adenoviral infection: a seventeen year experience and review of the literature. J Pediatr 2014;164(3):529–35.e1–4.
40. Oh KW, Moon CH, Lee KY. Association of rotavirus with seizures accompanied by cerebral white matter injury in neonates. J Child Neurol 2015;1:1–7.
41. Hara S, Kawada J, Kawano Y, et al. Hyperferritinemia in neonatal and infantile human parechovirus-3 infection in comparison with other infectious diseases. J Infect Chemother 2014;20(1):15–9.
42. Aviner S, Sofer D, Shulman LM, et al. Hemophagocytic lymphohistiocytosis associated with parechovirus 3 infection. J Pediatr Hematol Oncol 2014;36(4): e251–3.
43. Yuzurihara SS, Ao K, Hara T, et al. Human parechovirus-3 infection in nine neonates and infants presenting symptoms of hemophagocytic lymphohistiocytosis. J Infect Chemother 2013;19(1):144–8.
44. Levorson RE, Jantausch BA, Wiedermann BL, et al. Human parechovirus-3 infection: emerging pathogen in neonatal sepsis. Pediatr Infect Dis J 2009;28(6):545–7.
45. Wildenbeest JG, Wolthers KC, Straver B, et al. Successful IVIG treatment of human parechovirus-associated dilated cardiomyopathy in an infant. Pediatrics 2013;132(1):e243–3247.
46. Sedmak G, Nix WA, Jentzen J, et al. Infant deaths associated with human parechovirus infection in Wisconsin. Clin Infect Dis 2010;50(3):357–61.
47. Verboon-Maciolek MA, Krediet TG, Gerards LJ, et al. Severe neonatal parechovirus infection and similarity with enterovirus infection. Pediatr Infect Dis J 2008; 27(3):241.
48. Sharp J, Harrison CJ, Puckett K, et al. Characteristics of young infants in whom human parechovirus, enterovirus or neither were detected in cerebrospinal fluid during sepsis evaluations. Pediatr Infect Dis J 2013;32(3):213–6.
49. Verboon-Maciolek MA, Groenendaal F, Hahn CD, et al. Human Parechovirus causes encephalitis with white matter injury in neonates. Ann Neurol 2008; 64(3):266–73.
50. Mulford WS, Buller RS, Arens MQ, et al. Correlation of cerebrospinal fluid (CSF) cell counts and elevated CSF protein levels with enterovirus reverse transcription-PCR results in pediatric and adult patients. J Clin Microbiol 2004;42:4199–203.
51. Seiden JA, Zorc JJ, Hodinka RL, et al. Lack of CSF pleocytosis in young infants with enterovirus infections of CNS. Pediatr Emerg Care 2010;26(2):77–81.
52. Caviness AC, Demmler GJ, Selwyn BJ. Clinical and laboratory features of neonatal HSV infection: a case-control study. Pediatr Infect Dis J 2008;27(5):425–30.
53. Selvarajua SB, Nix WA, Oberste MS, et al. Optimization of a combined human parechovirus-enterovirus real-time reverse transcription-PCR assay and evaluation of a new parechovirus 3-specific assay for cerebrospinal fluid specimen testing. J Clin Microbiol 2013;51(2):452–8.
54. Akasaka M, Sasaki M, Ehara S, et al. Transient decrease in cerebral white matter diffusivity on MR imaging in human herpes virus-6 encephalopathy. Brain Dev 2005;27(1):30–3.
55. Volpe JJ. Neonatal encephalitis and white matter injury — more than just inflammation? Ann Neurol 2008;64(3):232–6.
56. Westerhuis BM, Jonker SC, Mattao S, et al. Growth characteristics of human parechovirus 1 to 6 on different cell lines and cross- neutralization of human

parechovirus antibodies: a comparison of the cytopathic effect and real time PCR. Virol J 2013;10:146.

57. Abed Y, Wolf D, Dagan R, et al. Development of a serological assay based on a synthetic peptide selected from the VP0 capsid protein for detection of human parechoviruses. J Clin Microbiol 2007;45(6):2037–9.

58. Alho A, Marttila J, Ilonen J, et al. Diagnostic potential of parechovirus capsid proteins. J Clin Microbiol 2003;41(6):2294–9.

59. Nix WA, Maher K, Johansson ES, et al. Detection of all known parechoviruses by real-time PCR. J Clin Microbiol 2008;46(8):2519–24.

60. Benschop K, Molenkamp R, van der Ham A, et al. Rapid detection of human parechoviruses in clinical samples by real-time PCR. J Clin Virol 2008;41(2):69–74.

61. Landry ML. The molecular diagnosis of parechovirus infection: has the time come? Clin Infect Dis 2010;50(3):362–3.

62. Shah G, Robinson JL. The particulars on parechovirus. Can J Infect Dis Med Microbiol 2014;25(4):186–8.

63. Venkatesan A, Tunkel AR, Bloch KC, et al, International Encephalitis Consortium. Case definitions, diagnostic algorithms, and priorities in encephalitis: consensus statement of the international encephalitis consortium. Clin Infect Dis 2013;57(8):1114–28.

64. Robinson JL, Hartling L, Crumley E, et al. A systematic review of intravenous gamma globulin for therapy of acute myocarditis. BMC Cardiovasc Disord 2005;5(1):12.

65. Keller MA, Stiehm RE. Passive immunity in prevention and treatment of infectious diseases. Clin Microbiol Rev 2000;13(4):602–14.

66. McKinney RE Jr, Katz SL, Wilfert CM. Chronic enteroviral meningoencephalitis in agammaglobulinemic patients. Rev Infect Dis 1987;9(2):334–56.

67. Pallansch M, Weldon WC, Peñaranda S, et al. Human parechovirus 3 seroprevalence amongst mothers of young infants in the United States. Abstract S77, 29th Clinical Virology Symposium. Daytona Beach, Florida, USA, April 26–May 1, 2013.

68. Westerhuis BM, Koen G, Wildenbeest JG, et al. Specific cell tropism and neutralization of human parechovirus types 1 and 3: implications for pathogenesis and therapy development. J Gen Virol 2012;93(Pt 11):2363–70.

69. Felsenstein S, Yang S, Eubanks N, et al. Human parechovirus central nervous system infections in southern California children. Pediatr Infect Dis J 2014;33(4):e87–91.

70. Messacar K, Breazeale G, Wei Q, et al. Epidemiology and clinical characteristics of infants with human parechovirus or human herpes virus-6 detected in cerebrospinal fluid tested for enterovirus or HSV. J Med Virol 2015;87(5):829–35.

71. Walters B, Peñaranda S, Nix WA, Oberste MS, et al. Detection of human parechovirus (HPeV)-3 in spinal fluid specimens from pediatric patients in the Chicago area. J Clin Virol 2011;52(3):187–91.

72. Elkan M, Graf EH, Hodinka RL. Real-time Taqman RT-PCR for detection of human parechoviruses in infants and young children. Daytona beach (FL): PASCV; 2010. poster session T48.

73. Sharp J1 Bell J, Harrison CJ, Nix WA, et al. Human parechovirus in respiratory specimens from children in Kansas City, Missouri. J Clin Microbiol 2012;50(12):4111–3.

74. Chhabra P, Payne DC, Szilagyi PG, et al. Etiology of viral gastroenteritis in children <5 years of age in the United States, 2008-2009. J Infect Dis 2013;208(5):790–800.

Prevention of Recurrent Staphylococcal Skin Infections

C. Buddy Creech, MD, MPH[a], Duha N. Al-Zubeidi, MD[b], Stephanie A. Fritz, MD, MSCI[c],*

KEYWORDS

- *Staphylococcus aureus* • MRSA • Skin infection • Prevention • Decolonization
- Staphylococcal vaccine • Pediatrics

KEY POINTS

- Most children with a *Staphylococcus aureus* skin and soft tissue infection (SSTI) will experience a recurrent infection within 1 year.
- *S aureus* infections cluster within households, likely because of colonization of family members and household environmental surfaces.
- A combined approach of nasal and skin decolonization is often effective in temporarily eradicating staphylococcal colonization and reducing subsequent SSTI.
- A household approach to decolonization is more effective in reducing SSTI occurrence than decolonization efforts aimed at individual patients alone.

INTRODUCTION

"Once the organisms gain a foothold, they may be very difficult to eradicate; sometimes boil after boil appears and these lesions may continue to develop in crops for months. The scalp, face, and shoulders are favorite sites but any part of the body

Disclosure statement: This work was supported by grants from the National Institutes of Health (K23-AI091690, KL2-RR024994, and UL1-TR000448), the Agency for Healthcare Research and Quality (R01-HS021736), and the Children's Discovery Institute of Washington University and St. Louis Children's Hospital (to S.A. Fritz). The content is solely the responsibility of the authors and does not necessarily represent the official views of the National Institutes of Health or the Agency for Healthcare Research and Quality.

[a] Vanderbilt Vaccine Research Program, Division of Pediatric Infectious Diseases, Department of Pediatrics, Vanderbilt University School of Medicine and the Monroe Carell, Jr. Children's Hospital at Vanderbilt, S2323 MCN, 1161 21st Avenue South, Nashville, TN 37232, USA; [b] Department of Pediatrics, Children's Mercy Hospital Infection Prevention and Control, University of Missouri-Kansas City School of Medicine, 2401 Gillham Road, Kansas City, MO 64108, USA; [c] Division of Pediatric Infectious Diseases, Department of Pediatrics, Washington University School of Medicine, 660 South Euclid Avenue, Campus Box 8116, St Louis, MO 63110, USA
* Corresponding author.
E-mail address: fritz_s@kids.wustl.edu

Infect Dis Clin N Am 29 (2015) 429–464
http://dx.doi.org/10.1016/j.idc.2015.05.007
0891-5520/15/$ – see front matter © 2015 Elsevier Inc. All rights reserved.

may be involved; in some instances, the entire body is covered with furuncles."[1] These prescient words, found in the article on skin infections from the eleventh edition (1940) of *Holt's Diseases of Infancy and Childhood*,[1] are as true today of *Staphylococcus aureus* skin and soft tissue infections (SSTI) as they were in the preantibiotic era. SSTI are among the most common reasons for health care visits in the United States, accounting for more than 14 million outpatient and emergency department visits annually.[2] Moreover, these infections frequently recur, leading to substantial morbidity in the pediatric population and provoking frustration for both patients and clinicians. In this review, the authors describe the epidemiology of *S aureus* SSTI, with a focus on recurrent SSTI; delineate the current paradigm of SSTI pathogenesis; and provide evidence-based recommendations for treatment and prevention of these infections.

THE EMERGENCE OF COMMUNITY-ASSOCIATED METHICILLIN-RESISTANT *STAPHYLOCOCCUS AUREUS*

Staphylococcus aureus is a Gram-positive commensal bacterium that colonizes the anterior nares, as well as other anatomic sites, of approximately one-third of the human population.[3-7] On leaving the site of colonization, *S aureus* can infect virtually any body site, making it the most prevalent pathogen isolated from SSTIs, a leading cause of food-borne illness, the second leading cause of infectious endocarditis,[8] and an important cause (~2%) of all hospital admissions.[9] With an estimated incidence of 32 infections per 100,000 persons, *S aureus* has surpassed *Streptococcus pneumoniae* and *Haemophilus influenzae* to become the most common invasive bacterial pathogen in the United States.[10]

A major challenge posed by *S aureus* is antimicrobial resistance. Soon after the β-lactam antibiotics penicillin and methicillin were introduced into clinical practice, strains of antibiotic-resistant *S aureus* were identified.[11] Over the next several decades, methicillin-resistant *S aureus* (MRSA) became an important health care–associated (HA) pathogen, complicating the care of postsurgical and dialysis patients and the chronically ill.[12-15] Treatment was challenging, owing to resistance to multiple antibiotics; by the turn of the century, MRSA accounted for nearly 60% of all *S aureus* isolates recovered from hospital intensive care units.[16] At present, it is projected that MRSA infections account for greater than 100,000 hospitalizations each year in the United States.[17]

In the late 1990s, a shift in MRSA epidemiology occurred. After the alarming deaths of 4 previously healthy Midwestern children following infection with MRSA,[18] it was realized that MRSA infections were no longer restricted to those with chronic illnesses or frequent hospitalizations; instead MRSA had emerged as a community pathogen, capable of infecting healthy hosts and, thus, was termed *community-associated* (CA) MRSA. Initially thought to represent a feral strain of HA MRSA that had escaped into the community, it was soon determined that CA-MRSA strains were fundamentally different from traditional HA-MRSA strains. Compared with HA-MRSA strains, CA-MRSA strains exhibit a faster bacterial doubling time in vitro,[19] possess a smaller gene cluster (staphylococcal cassette chromosome *mec*) conferring resistance mainly to β-lactam antibiotics (although resistance to other antimicrobials has recently emerged),[20-36] and exhibit altered regulation of exotoxins and other virulence factors,[37-41] characteristics that are thought to correlate with the aggressive clinical behavior and transmissibility of CA-MRSA. CA-MRSA causes a broad spectrum of disease entities, ranging from asymptomatic colonization to SSTI (particularly purulent abscesses) to invasive infections (eg, fulminant necrotizing pneumonia, musculoskeletal infections, fatal bacteremia).[37,42-47] The host and bacterial determinants driving this spectrum are not well understood. Recently, highly virulent strains of methicillin-susceptible *S aureus* (MSSA) belonging to the same genetic lineage as the current CA-MRSA epidemic strains (USA300) have been described.[48,49] These strains share phenotypic similarities with MRSA USA300 strains, leading to SSTI, recurrent abscesses, and invasive, necrotizing infections.

EPIDEMIOLOGY OF PEDIATRIC *STAPHYLOCOCCUS AUREUS* SKIN AND SOFT TISSUE INFECTIONS

The most common manifestation of CA-MRSA infection is SSTI. Although many SSTIs are superficial, they carry significant morbidity, including pain and subsequent scarring caused by drainage procedures and time lost from school and work by patients and their families. Although many patients with CA-MRSA SSTIs are treated as outpatients, patients with moderate to severe SSTI often require hospitalization. SSTI now ranks among the top 10 reasons for pediatric hospital admission.[50]

The epidemiology of staphylococcal SSTI changes rapidly; in the past 15 years, the landscape has been dominated by CA-MRSA. In 2005, Purcell and Fergie[51] demonstrated a substantial increase in MRSA infection incidence in South Texas, increasing from less than 10 cases annually in the 1990s to nearly 500 cases annually by 2003. By 2005, several centers across the United States reported that CA-MRSA accounted for nearly 75% of all staphylococcal infections.[43] These high rates of CA-MRSA necessitated changes in empirical antibiotic therapy when MRSA was suspected,[52] particularly for SSTI in which well more than 50% of infections in most centers were caused by CA-MRSA.[43,44,51,53,54] More recently, Gerber and colleagues[55] performed a retrospective, observational study using the Pediatric Health Information System, a database of clinical and financial data from greater than 40 tertiary care children's hospitals in the United States. Over the 6-year study period, the investigators identified nearly 60,000 children with *S aureus* infections, 51% of whom had infection with MRSA; SSTI comprised 61% of these infections.

MRSA colonizes the anterior nares, throat, rectum, and skin (axilla, inguinal area, and perineum).[4–7,56–59] MRSA carriage is a risk factor for the development of subsequent infections.[3,6,60–64] Colonized individuals are also important sources for transmission.[65] Up to 10% of healthy individuals in the United States are colonized with MRSA.[45,46] The prevalence of MRSA colonization has significantly increased over the past decade,[46,47] accompanied by an increase in MRSA infection incidence. Two studies, using data from the National Ambulatory Medical Care Survey and a large integrated health plan in northern California, have identified children and African Americans as being disproportionally affected by the current CA-MRSA epidemic.[2,66,67] In addition to race and age, there are specific populations who have experienced a substantial increase in SSTI caused by CA-MRSA (**Box 1**). These populations include military personnel, in whom MRSA colonization significantly increases the risk of developing SSTI (compared with MSSA colonization)[63]; prisoners[68–70]; and athletes, in whom colonization can be detected frequently within sports teams, though outbreaks are sporadic.[71–74] In each of these high-risk groups, risk factors for infection include close contact, compromised skin integrity, and increased prevalence of colonization; in addition, outbreaks are often linked to periods of increased colonization or exposure to specific strains of *S aureus* (eg, USA300 CA-MRSA).

PATHOGENESIS OF *STAPHYLOCOCCUS AUREUS* SKIN AND SOFT TISSUE INFECTIONS

In the development of SSTI in an otherwise healthy individual, the site of symptomatic infection is first colonized with a relatively low number of bacteria. Staphylococci

---

Box 1
Risk factors for *S aureus* SSTI

- *S aureus* colonization
- Injection drug use
- Diabetes mellitus
- Chronic dermatologic conditions (eg, eczema)
- Recent use of antimicrobial agents
- African American race
- Previous SSTI
- Close contact with a patient with SSTI
- Participation in contact sports
- Military personnel
- Prisoners

---

easily accomplish this, because more than 80% of humans are intermittently colonized at some point with *S aureus*, including 10% to 15% of humans who are persistently colonized.[3,75,76] Because colonization alone is insufficient to initiate disease, *S aureus* must then reach the deeper portions of the epidermis and dermis through microabrasions of the skin, traumatic injury, or skin disruption caused by inflammatory lesions (eg, eczema). *S aureus* possess several virulence determinants responsible for initiation and maintenance of infection,[77–90] representatives of which are listed in **Table 1**. On invasion, the host inflammatory response leads to microvascular leak, production of inflammatory cytokines/chemokines, and recruitment of leukocytes (in particular, neutrophils).

SKIN AND SOFT TISSUE INFECTION CHARACTERISTICS AND INITIAL MANAGEMENT

SSTI are best characterized by the depth of infection and associated skin structures as described in **Box 2**. The Infectious Diseases Society of America (IDSA) asserts that incision and drainage (I/D) represents the primary treatment of purulent

Table 1
***Staphylococcus aureus* virulence determinants involved in SSTI pathogenesis**

Activity	Mechanism	Virulence Determinant
Adherence to host tissue	—	MSCRAMMs[77]
Tissue destruction	—	Alpha toxin[78]
Nutrient acquisition	Essential metal acquisition	Isd system[79]
Disruption of host defense	Impaired chemotaxis	ChIPS, Eap[80,81]
—	Phagocyte destruction	Leukocidins (LukAB, LukDE, PVL), PSM[82–84]
—	Impaired opsonization	Protein A, polysaccharide capsule[85]
—	Impaired intracellular killing	Staphyloxanthin, catalase, superoxide dismutase[86–90]

Abbreviations: ChIPS, Chemotaxis inhibiting protein of *S aureus*; Isd, iron-regulated surface determinant; MSCRAMM, microbial surface components recognizing adhesive matrix molecules; PSM, phenol-soluble modulin; PVL, Panton Valentine leukocidin.

Box 2
Manifestations of skin infections

Erysipelas

Superficial skin infection characterized by well-demarcated, intensely erythematous lesions; nearly universally caused by *S pyogenes*

Cellulitis

Painful infection of the dermis and subcutaneous tissues, often occurring near breaks in the skin

Impetigo

Relatively superficial infection leading to bullous or nonbullous lesions

Folliculitis

Superficial or deep inflammation of the hair follicle leading to papulopustular lesions

Furuncle

Extension of suppurative infection from the hair follicle, leading to infection of the deeper skin structures (typical abscess)

Carbuncle

An aggregate of infected follicles leading to a deep, painful mass

---

staphylococcal skin abscesses.[91] The procedural approach to abscess drainage has been recently reviewed.[92] It is important to note that sufficient drainage, with disruption of loculations and facilitation of ongoing drainage, is challenging in the pediatric population, often requiring sedation and postprocedural pain management. What is gained by this approach, however, is nearly immediate pain relief from large abscesses, faster wound healing, and access to material for bacterial culture.

Traditionally, drainage has been the mainstay of therapy for most staphylococcal abscesses[93]; this has held true in the contemporary era of CA-MRSA in several studies. In a prospective cohort study by Lee and colleagues[94] of children presenting to a large emergency department with SSTI, greater than 75% of children experienced clinical cure following I/D, even if prescribed an antibiotic that was ineffective (based on eventual susceptibility results). Similarly, Chen and colleagues[95] determined that among children with SSTI who experienced spontaneous drainage or had I/D performed, despite MRSA being the causative agent in 69%, no differences were evident in clinical cure between those receiving cephalexin versus clindamycin. Two randomized trials, one in adults[96] and one in children,[97] have compared trimethoprim-sulfamethoxazole (TMP/SMX) to placebo after I/D of suspected staphylococcal abscesses. Although both trials showed that the clinical cure rate did not differ between treatment groups, receipt of antimicrobial therapy resulted in a lower incidence of early recurrent disease. Although current data are reassuring that antimicrobial agents are not required in all children, definitive data are not yet available in this population. A National Institutes of Health–sponsored clinical trial[98] is expected to answer this question more completely, comparing the effectiveness of clindamycin, TMP/SMX, or placebo, in conjunction with I/D, in the treatment of limited abscesses in adults and children.

Patients for whom antibiotics are currently recommended include patients at the extremes of age and those with severe or extensive disease, rapidly progressing cellulitis, abscess in an anatomic location that precludes adequate drainage, systemic illness or hemodynamic instability, associated septic phlebitis, or failure to improve after I/D alone.[91] As antimicrobial resistance has increased, choices of orally effective antimicrobials have diminished. Agents with in vitro activity against MRSA are provided in **Table 2**. Although antibiotic selection should be directed by one's regional antibiogram, for many communities, clindamycin and TMP/SMX remain good first-line therapeutic agents for suspected CA-MRSA SSTI. However, in a large retrospective study of Tennessee children, Williams and colleagues[99] found that TMP/SMX was less effective than clindamycin in both treating an initial abscess and preventing recurrences of disease. Among 6407 children who underwent drainage, 9% experienced treatment failures within 14 days, and 23% had recurrence within 1 year; both of these outcomes were more likely in children receiving TMP/SMX, compared with clindamycin. Among 41,000 children who did not undergo a drainage procedure, TMP/SMX remained significantly less effective than clindamycin for the initial treatment of SSTI. Despite these observed differences, however, the overall success of TMP/SMX was high; given its availability, tolerability, and low cost, TMP/SMX remains a first-line SSTI agent targeting MSSA and MRSA alike.

EPIDEMIOLOGY OF RECURRENT SKIN AND SOFT TISSUE INFECTION

As many as 70% of patients with CA-MRSA SSTI will experience recurrent SSTI over 1 year (**Table 3**), even after successful initial treatment.[59,97,99–105] These recurrent

Table 2
Systemic antimicrobial agents for the treatment of *Staphylococcus aureus* SSTI

Antimicrobial Agent	Recommended Pediatric Dosage Range (Oral)	Comments
Clindamycin	30–40 mg/kg/d divided q6–8h	• Excellent bioavailability • Noxious smell and taste of oral suspension • Often effective to instruct families to open capsules and sprinkle onto pudding/ice cream • Inducible and constitutive resistance is highly variable between geographic regions (>20% in some areas)
Trimethoprim-sulfamethoxazole	10–20 mg/kg/d divided q12h	• High susceptibility rates • Clinical data confirm effectiveness • May have reduced activity against *S pyogenes*, though data are not clear
Doxycycline	2.2 mg/kg/d divided q12h	• High susceptibility rates • Inappropriate for children <8 y of age • Photosensitivity
Linezolid	30 mg/kg/d divided q8h	• High susceptibility rates • Excellent bioavailability • Expensive compared with other agents
Fluoroquinolones	(Varies by individual quinolone)	• Excellent bioavailability • Overly broad spectrum • Resistance can occur quickly while on therapy because of mutations in DNA gyrase
Rifampin	10 mg/kg/d	• Excellent bioavailability and tissue penetration • Can never be given as single agent as resistance quickly emerges

Table 3
Incidence and risk factors associated with recurrent skin and soft tissue infection

Study Reference	Population; Years Study Performed	Study Design	Treatment or Intervention	Longitudinal Time Frame	Proportion of Patients with Recurrent SSTI	Factors Associated with Recurrent SSTI
Bocchini et al,[104] 2013	12,836 Children presenting to TCH (Houston, TX) with community-associated S aureus infection; 2001–2009	Retrospective cohort study	N/A	76 mo	5% Presented to TCH with documented recurrent S aureus infection (694 with recurrent S aureus infection of any cause, 637 with recurrent S aureus SSTI)	• Age ≤36 mo
Williams et al,[99] 2011	47,501 Children with incident SSTI enrolled in Tennessee Medicaid; 2004–2007	Retrospective cohort study	Treatment with clindamycin, TMP/SMX, or a β-lactam antibiotic	365 d	14% Overall had a documented recurrent SSTI (23% in patients undergoing drainage, 18% of those without drainage)	• In patients undergoing drainage, recurrent SSTI was higher among patients prescribed TMP/SMX or a β-lactam antibiotic • In patients without drainage, prescription of TMP/SMX was associated with recurrent SSTI

(continued on next page)

Table 3
(continued)

Study Reference	Population; Years Study Performed	Study Design	Treatment or Intervention	Longitudinal Time Frame	Proportion of Patients with Recurrent SSTI	Factors Associated with Recurrent SSTI
Chen et al,[100] 2009	95 Children with purulent SSTI in Baltimore, MD; 2006–2007	Subgroup analysis of a double-blind, randomized, controlled trial comparing cephalexin with clindamycin	Treatment with cephalexin or clindamycin (assignment not specified)	3 mo	22% Reported recurrent SSTI	• Baseline MRSA SSTI (compared with baseline MSSA SSTI)
Fritz et al,[103] 2012 (and Fritz unpublished data, 2012)	183 Children with acute CA–S aureus SSTI and concurrent S aureus colonization in St Louis, MO; 2008–2009	Randomized, controlled trial comparing individual vs household decolonization	All patients were assigned a 5-d decolonization regimen of enhanced personal and household hygiene, intranasal 2% mupirocin ointment application twice daily, and daily 4% chlorhexidine body washes	12 mo	63% Reported recurrent SSTI (72% in index decolonization group, 52% in household decolonization group)	• Multiple sites of S aureus colonization at baseline • History of SSTI in year before study enrollment • Younger age • Baseline MSSA SSTI (compared with baseline MRSA SSTI) • Participants prescribed clindamycin for their baseline SSTI were less likely to have a recurrent infection

Study	Population	Study design	Intervention	Duration	Recurrence	Risk factors/notes
Miller et al,[105] 2015	330 Adults and children treated for S aureus SSTI in Los Angeles, CA and Chicago, IL; 2008–2010	Prospective cohort study	N/A	6 mo	51% Reported recurrent SSTI	• Hospitalization in the prior 3 mo • Household fomite contamination with MRSA • Lack of participation in contact sports
Kaplan et al,[59] 2014	987 Children with suspected S aureus SSTI or invasive infection in Houston, TX; 2009–2012	Randomized, controlled trial comparing hygienic measures alone vs hygienic measures plus bleach baths	Participants in the intervention arm bathed in dilute bleach water twice weekly for 3 mo	12 mo	19% Reported medically attended recurrent SSTI (21% hygiene group, 17% bleach bath group)	• Multiple sites of S aureus colonization at baseline • Age ≤1.86 y • White race (compared with African American and Hispanic) • Incidence of recurrence did not differ between children with MRSA vs MSSA baseline infections

Abbreviations: N/A, not applicable; TCH, Texas Children's Hospital.

infections may necessitate repeated courses of antibiotic therapy, further driving development of antibiotic resistance.[106,107] The risk factors governing these recurrent infections are not yet clear, though there are certainly pathogen-level, host-level, and environmental-level variables that contribute to CA-MRSA transmission and risk of recurrence.[108–110] As described earlier, the prescription of systemic antibiotics for SSTI treatment,[96,97] as well as the choice of antibiotic prescribed,[99] may reduce the incidence of recurrent infection. This reduction may be caused by the elimination of staphylococcal colonization, and thus, the endogenous source for infection. Indeed, several prospective studies have demonstrated eradication of MRSA carriage following treatment of SSTI with clindamycin.[111,112]

Clustering of S aureus infections occurs in households.[113–124] Additionally, a high proportion of household members of patients with MRSA infection are colonized with MRSA, frequently with strains identical to those recovered from index patients.[119,125] Although these colonized contacts are often asymptomatic, they serve as important sources for ongoing transmission within households,[5,65,106,125–129] leading to reacquisition and recurrent infection. Households with young children may have a greater risk of transmission through close personal contact.[111,119,130]

PREVENTION STRATEGIES: DECOLONIZATION

S aureus carriage is a risk factor for the development of subsequent infection,[3,6,60–64] and recurrent S aureus SSTI are frequently caused by the same strain type.[104,131,132] Thus, decolonization (ie, "the use of antimicrobial or antiseptic agents to suppress or eliminate S. aureus carriage"[91]) is often prescribed in an attempt to prevent recurrent infections. Such therapies have traditionally been implemented in health care settings to prevent nosocomial S aureus and MRSA infections.[133–144] During the ongoing CA-MRSA epidemic, these measures have been extrapolated to patients in community settings.[91,145,146] Although application of these therapies for a discrete period is effective for MRSA eradication, their effectiveness in infection prevention varies by study; maintenance of eradication often diminishes over time.[101,103,133–136,141–144,147–149] Thus, the optimal preventive strategy for recurrent S aureus SSTI remains elusive; a wide variety of treatment and decolonization practices exist.[91,145,150]

Who Should Undergo Decolonization?

Prior history of SSTI is a risk factor for recurrent SSTI.[64,105] This association, coupled with the pursuit of judicious use of topical antimicrobials, suggests that decolonization is likely not necessary for patients experiencing a first SSTI. Indeed, the IDSA MRSA clinical practice guidelines state that decolonization may be considered after optimizing wound care and hygiene (see later discussion), for patients experiencing recurrent SSTI, and for households in which there is ongoing transmission.[91]

S aureus transmission frequently leads to infections in multiple household members; thus, when decolonization is prescribed, it should be performed by all household members. A randomized trial of 183 households conducted by Fritz and colleagues[103] compared the effectiveness of decolonization of the index patient alone (index group) to decolonization of all household members (household group). The 5-day decolonization regimen included hygiene education, twice-daily application of 2% intranasal mupirocin, and daily body washes with 4% chlorhexidine. Three months following randomization, the incidence of SSTI was significantly lower in index patients assigned to the household decolonization group compared with those in the index group (28% vs 47%, respectively, $P = .02$). This benefit was also demonstrated for household contacts (at 3 months: 4% incidence in household group vs 10% in index group, $P = .01$).

Hygiene Strategies

Before staphylococcal eradication measures are prescribed, attention to basic wound care and personal hygiene should be addressed. Education should be provided to patients and their families regarding the transmissibility of S aureus, particularly through contact with open wounds and contaminated surfaces. Patients should be encouraged to adopt enhanced hygiene practices, including regular bathing and frequent hand washing with soap and water or alcohol-based hand sanitizers. Patients and their contacts should avoid sharing personal hygiene items (eg, towels, deodorant, cosmetics, brushes, razors, toothbrushes, or other items that come into contact with the skin). Additional measures that may reduce transmission and infection risk include using pump or pour lotions (rather than those in jars), keeping fingernails clean and trimmed short, avoiding loofas in the bath or shower, and changing underwear, sleepwear, towels, and washcloths daily.[59,91,101,103,119,146,151]

Environmental surfaces serve as reservoirs for MRSA transmission and MRSA strains can persist in the environment for prolonged intervals, posing a risk for the development of recurrent infections.[34,105,106,109,121–123,128,152–155] Thus, a barrier should be used between bare skin and surfaces touched by multiple people (eg, exercise equipment). Additionally, patients with recurrent SSTI may consider performing environmental hygiene measures, focusing on frequently touched surfaces and using commercially available disinfectants.[91,151] Routine laundry procedures, following the label directions on the detergent and the clothing or linens to be washed, are usually sufficient to disinfect items; use of hot water or bleach for all household laundry is not necessary.[151]

Topical Antimicrobial Agents

Although multiple agents and technologies have been proposed or evaluated for S aureus decolonization,[156] this review focuses on those most readily prescribed and available to patients. An important consideration of any decolonization regimen, regardless of efficacy, is the time and financial burden encumbered by patients, which heavily influences adherence and, thus, the effectiveness of these measures.

Mupirocin (pseudomonic acid A) is produced naturally by Pseudomonas fluorescens.[157–159] Mupirocin targets the bacterial isoleucyl-tRNA synthetase, resulting in protein synthesis inhibition.[160] Mupirocin has antimicrobial activity against staphylococcal and streptococcal species and is prescribed for topical treatment of skin infections as well as eradication of S aureus (both MSSA and MRSA) nasal carriage.

Retapamulin (Altabax) is a semisynthetic antimicrobial derived from the natural compound pleuromutilin, produced by the edible mushroom Pleurotus mutilus.[161,162] Retapamulin inhibits S aureus protein synthesis by binding to the 50S ribosomal subunit.[163,164] At present, retapamulin is approved for treatment of impetigo caused by MSSA or Streptococcus pyogenes. Retapamulin has demonstrated activity against S aureus strains exhibiting resistance to methicillin and mupirocin as well as several other systemic antibiotics.[161,162,165] A phase I/IIa randomized, double-blind, placebo-controlled trial evaluated 3- and 5-day regimens of retapamulin (1%) ointment applied to the anterior nares twice daily in patients persistently colonized with S aureus. Both retapamulin regimens demonstrated efficacy in S aureus eradication 28 days following application compared with placebo.[166] An ongoing randomized trial aims to determine the effectiveness of retapamulin in eradication of mupirocin-resistant MRSA from adult carriers.[167]

Chlorhexidine gluconate is a broad-spectrum biguanide cationic bactericidal agent.[168,169] At low concentrations, chlorhexidine disrupts cytoplasmic membrane integrity; at high concentrations, it causes microbial cytoplasmic contents to congeal.[168] Multiple preparations of chlorhexidine exist, including a liquid topical antiseptic available without a prescription (Hibiclens), an oral rinse, and impregnated cloths.[170] Attractive for the purposes of decolonization, chlorhexidine provides residual antibacterial activity on the skin.[148,171] Of note, as chlorhexidine may result in ocular and ototoxicity, patients should be instructed to avoid the eyes and ears when using this agent.

Bleach, or sodium hypochlorite, has antimicrobial activity against S aureus both in vivo and in vitro. Dilute bleach water baths have traditionally been recommended by dermatologists to treat eczema, presumably by suppressing S aureus growth, which is correlated with disease severity.[172–176] The recommended dilution of bleach varies.[91,101,146,172,175] An in vitro assay determined that the hypochlorite concentration necessary for maximal S aureus killing was 2.5 μL of 6% hypochlorite per milliliter of water (equal to approximately one-half cup bleach in one-quarter bathtub full of water), with an exposure time of 15 minutes yielding a greater than 4-log decrease in S aureus.[174] In clinical practice, to minimize skin irritation, a dilution of one-quarter cup household bleach in one-quarter bathtub ($\sim$13 gal) of water is recommended; for nonstandard bathtubs, 1 teaspoon of bleach should be added per gallon of water. Individuals should soak in the dilute bleach water for 15 minutes. As household bleach is readily available and inexpensive, bleach baths are attractive for the purpose of decolonization. Additionally, soaking body areas that are frequently colonized with S aureus (eg, the groin and axillae) likely provides optimal antimicrobial effect. However, in large families, this strategy may be cumbersome and impractical. A recent feasibility study evaluated a body wash gel preparation of sodium hypochlorite (CLn BodyWash) in patients with atopic dermatitis whose eczematous lesions yielded S aureus.[176] Over 12 weeks, patients experienced significant improvement in severity of their atopic dermatitis; parents reported that the body wash was easier to administer than dilute bleach water baths.

Oral Antibiotics for Decolonization

Trials evaluating the effectiveness of systemic antibiotics in eradicating S aureus or MRSA carriage have produced disparate results. Many of these trials have demonstrated emergence of resistant organisms with the use of oral antibiotics. Additionally, systemic antimicrobials traditionally used for decolonization, in particular rifampin, have been associated with toxicities. Thus, oral antibiotics should be reserved for patients with acute infections and are generally not recommended for staphylococcal decolonization alone.[91,143,177]

Effectiveness of Decolonization in Preventing Skin and Soft Tissue Infection

Several trials have evaluated decolonization measures among healthy individuals in community settings (**Table 4**). S aureus colonizes the anterior nares and the skin at multiple anatomic sites,[4–7,56–58,178] and a greater number of colonized sites confers an increased risk of infection.[59] Additionally, the buttocks and lower extremities are frequent sites for S aureus SSTI.[49,104,145,179] Thus, a decolonization approach targeting intranasal and skin carriage has the greatest potential for success. Among recent trials, studies prescribing both intranasal mupirocin and antimicrobial body washes demonstrated significantly reduced incidence of SSTI,[101,103,180] whereas studies using only intranasal mupirocin[147] or only antimicrobial body washes[59,110,179] showed no significant effect on SSTI incidence.

Many trials to date have prescribed a brief decolonization regimen (eg, 5 days)[101,103]; although reduced SSTI incidence was demonstrated in the months

Table 4
Staphylococcus aureus decolonization trials conducted in healthy populations

Study Reference	Population; Years Study Performed	Study Design	Intervention	Length of Follow-up Period Following Randomization	Outcomes
Raz et al,[181] 1996	34 Children and adults with a history of ≥3 staphylococcal SSTI in the prior year who were also colonized with S aureus in Israel	Randomized double-blind placebo-controlled trial	Baseline decolonization performed by all participants: mupirocin 2% ointment applied to the anterior nares twice daily for 5 d Participants were then randomized to 2 groups: 1. Nasal mupirocin application twice daily for 5 d each mo for 1 y 2. Application of placebo in the same fashion	12 mo	• *S aureus eradication* was significantly higher in the mupirocin group vs the placebo group. • *SSTI incidence* was significantly lower in the mupirocin group vs the placebo group.

(continued on next page)

Table 4
(continued)

Study Reference	Population; Years Study Performed	Study Design	Intervention	Length of Follow-up Period Following Randomization	Outcomes
Ellis et al,[147] 2007	134 US Army personnel enrolled in the Health Care Specialist Course colonized with CA-MRSA, Fort Sam Houston, TX; 2005	Cluster randomized, double-blind placebo-controlled trial	Participants were randomized at the class level to perform: 1. Mupirocin 2% ointment applied to the anterior nares twice daily for 5 d 2. Application of placebo in the same fashion	8–10 wk	• CA-MRSA *eradication* was significantly higher in the mupirocin group vs the placebo group. • *SSTI incidence* was not significantly reduced in the mupirocin group. • *Colonization acquisition and SSTI incidence* were not reduced in the contacts of individuals performing mupirocin decolonization.
Whitman et al,[110] 2010	1562 US Marine recruits attending Officer Candidate School, Quantico, VA; 2007	Cluster randomized, double-blind controlled trial	Participants were randomized at the platoon level to perform: 1. Application of 2% chlorhexidine-impregnated cloths (Sage, Cary, IL) applied over the entire body 3 times a wk for 6 wk 2. Application of control cloths (Comfort Bath, Sage Cary, IL) in a similar fashion	6 wk	• *S aureus colonization incidence* was significantly lower in the chlorhexidine group than the control group. • *SSTI incidence* did not significantly differ between intervention groups.

| Fritz et al,[101] 2011 | Randomized, open-label 4-arm controlled trial | 300 Children and adults with acute CA-SSTI with *S aureus* colonization in St Louis, MO; 2007–2009 | Participants were randomized equally to perform 1 of 4, 5-d decolonization protocols:
1. Enhanced personal and household hygiene alone (controls)
2. Enhanced hygiene with intranasal 2% mupirocin ointment application twice daily
3. Enhanced hygiene, twice-daily intranasal 2% mupirocin, and daily 4% chlorhexidine body washes
4. Enhanced hygiene, twice-daily intranasal 2% mupirocin, and daily dilute bleach-water baths | 4–6 mo | • Compared with controls, at 1 mo, all interventions had a significantly higher rate of *eradication*. At 4 mo, only the group performing hygiene, mupirocin, and bleach baths (group 4) had a significantly higher rate of *eradication* compared with controls.
• At 1 mo, the group performing hygiene, mupirocin, and chlorhexidine (group 3) had a significantly lower *SSTI incidence* compared with controls. At 4 and 6 mo, none of the interventions resulted in a decreased SSTI incidence compared with controls. |

(continued on next page)

Table 4
(continued)

Study Reference	Population; Years Study Performed	Study Design	Intervention	Length of Follow-up Period Following Randomization	Outcomes
Fritz et al,[103] 2012	183 Children with acute CA–S aureus SSTI and concurrent S aureus colonization and their household contacts (844 total participants) in St Louis, MO; 2008–2009	Randomized, open-label 2-arm controlled trial	A 5-d decolonization regimen (including enhanced personal and household hygiene, intranasal 2% mupirocin ointment application twice daily, and daily 4% chlorhexidine body washes) was prescribed to 2 randomization groups: 1. Decolonization was performed by the index patient with acute SSTI alone 2. Decolonization was performed by all household members	12 mo	• *Index patient S aureus eradication* did not differ between groups. • *Index patient SSTI incidence* was significantly lower in the household decolonization group vs the index decolonization group. • *Household contact SSTI incidence* was significantly lower in the household decolonization group vs the index decolonization group.
Kaplan et al,[59] 2014	987 Children with suspected S aureus SSTI or invasive infection in Houston, TX; 2009–2012	Randomized, single-blinded controlled trial	Participants were randomized equally to perform 1. Hygienic measures (controls) 2. Hygienic measures plus bleach baths twice a week for 3 mo	12 mo	• *Incidence of medically attended SSTI* did not differ significantly between groups.

| Ellis et al,[179] 2014 | Cluster randomized trial | 30,209 US Army personnel enrolled in Infantry One Station Unit Training, Fort Benning, GA; 2010–2012 | Platoons were randomized to
1. Standard hygiene: Preventive medicine briefing, standardized SSTI treatment, and cleaning of high-touch common surfaces with standard disinfectants
2. Enhanced standard hygiene: Standard hygiene (as described for Group 1), an extra 10-min shower with soap and a washcloth once a week, provision of a first aid kit, and supplemental SSTI education for trainees and drill sergeants
3. Chlorhexidine: Standard and enhanced hygiene components (as described for Groups 1 and 2) plus 4% chlorhexidine body wash (after using their personal soap) for the extra shower once a week | 14 wk | • *Incidence of purulent SSTI* (of any cause) was significantly lower in the chlorhexidine group.
• *Incidence of MRSA SSTI* did not differ significantly between intervention groups. |

immediately following decolonization, many participants experienced recurrent infection over longer intervals. These findings likely reflect ongoing exposure to colonized individuals and environmental reservoirs and suggest that, especially for patients experiencing multiple infection recurrences, a periodic approach to decolonization may provide more effective, sustained protection.[181] A randomized trial of pediatric patients with SSTI by Kaplan and colleagues[59] evaluated daily hygienic measures alone compared with hygienic measures accompanied by twice-weekly dilute bleach water baths performed for 3 months. Over the 12-month study period, the incidence of medically attended recurrent SSTI did not differ significantly between the group performing bleach baths compared with the hygiene-only group (17% vs 21%, respectively, $P = .15$). Of note, as not all patients with recurrent SSTI seek medical attention,[7] the effectiveness of this intervention may have been underestimated.

Based on existing evidence, guidance from the Centers for Disease Control and Prevention and IDSA, and the authors' clinical experience, the authors propose a preventive approach to recurrent staphylococcal SSTI that optimizes hygiene measures, targets nasal and skin colonization, and includes all household members (**Fig. 1**).

A POTENTIAL UNDESIRABLE REPERCUSSION OF DECOLONIZATION: ANTIMICROBIAL RESISTANCE

An important consideration for S aureus decolonization is the emergence of staphylococcal strains resistant to topical antimicrobials, which has been demonstrated in vitro and in vivo (**Table 5**).[157–159,169,182–185] This resistance in turn predicts failure of S aureus decolonization efforts and has led to hospital outbreaks with resistant strains.[158,182,186–194] An additional concern is that the genes conferring resistance to mupirocin (most commonly mupA) and chlorhexidine (most commonly qacA/B or smr) are carried on plasmids that can also harbor genes conferring resistance to other systemic antibiotics.[158,168,182,187,195–198] A challenge to US clinicians is the paucity of commercially available resistance testing for mupirocin and chlorhexidine; at present there are no interpretive break points established by the Food and Drug Administration.[158]

FUTURE DIRECTIONS

Despite the effectiveness of topical antimicrobials in eradicating S aureus carriage, patients continue to have a high burden of subsequent SSTI over time.[101,103,110,147] Thus, novel strategies are needed for the prevention of recurrent staphylococcal infections.

Vaccine

Vaccine development for S aureus has been stymied by multiple factors, including lack of understanding of human immunity to staphylococci, redundancy of virulence determinants within the staphylococcal genome, and failure of previous vaccine candidates. The first of these failures involved a capsular polysaccharide vaccine (StaphVAX) given to hemodialysis patients at high risk for S aureus disease.[199] In this study, the vaccine adequately elicited anticapsular antibodies but failed to protect recipients from clinical disease. This vaccine has been modified significantly to include other targets and is currently in clinical development (PentaStaph). The second clinical failure occurred with a monovalent iron-regulated surface determinant (isd) B-based vaccine (V710)[200] in which vaccine recipients, who were undergoing cardiothoracic surgery, experienced greater mortality than placebo recipients.

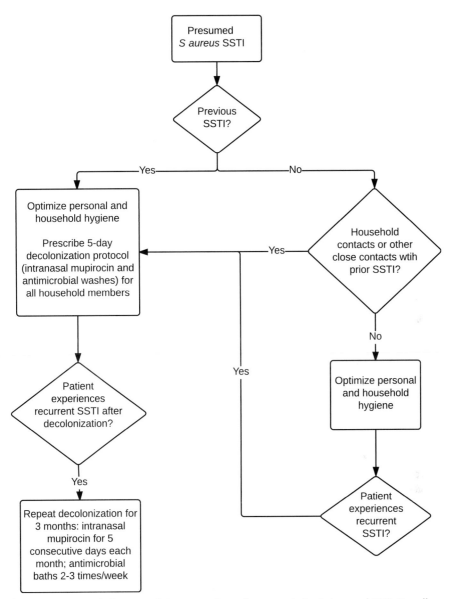

Fig. 1. Recommended approach to prevention of recurrent staphylococcal SSTI. For all patients with *S aureus* SSTI, the authors recommend optimizing hygiene measures. For those experiencing recurrent SSTI, or for households in which multiple members have experienced *S aureus* infection, the authors recommend decolonization with a regimen that includes the application of an intranasal antibiotic (twice daily for 5 days) and daily antimicrobial body washes (performed daily for 5 days; for individuals with sensitive skin, these washes may be performed every other day for 7–10 days). These measures should be performed by all household members and may be considered for other close contacts on a case-by-case basis. Patients and their household contacts should change their bedding at the onset and again at the completion of the decolonization regimen, and towels should be changed daily during the 5-day protocol. For individuals experiencing recurrent SSTI after the optimization of personal and household hygiene measures and the performance of decolonization by all household members, clinicians may consider prescribing a 3-month regimen of periodic decolonization, in which an intranasal antibiotic is applied to the anterior nares twice daily for 5 consecutive days each month and antimicrobial body washes are performed 2 to 3 times each week.

448 Creech et al

Table 5
Staphylococcus aureus mupirocin and chlorhexidine resistance among selected populations

Study Reference	Population; Years Study Performed	Study Design/Intervention	Mupirocin Resistance	Chlorhexidine Resistance	Other Findings/Notes
McNeil et al,[196] 2011	68 Children presenting with recurrent community-onset SSTI (136 *S aureus* isolates) in Houston, TX; 2001–2009	Retrospective study	14.7% of *S aureus* infecting isolates were positive for mupirocin resistance	N/A	• Mupirocin resistance occurred more commonly among *S aureus* isolates recovered from recurrent SSTI cultures than initial SSTI cultures • Mupirocin resistance was more common in MSSA than MRSA isolates • Mupirocin resistance was associated with clindamycin resistance
Fritz et al,[189] 2013	1089 Adults and children presenting with community-onset SSTI (2425 *S aureus* isolates) in St Louis, MO; 483 patients were enrolled in decolonization trials, of which 408 were assigned intranasal mupirocin and/or chlorhexidine body washes; 2007–2009	Cross-sectional study followed by a randomized controlled trial	2.1% of patients were colonized or infected with a mupirocin-resistant *S aureus* strain at baseline	0.9% of patients were colonized or infected with an *S aureus* strain harboring *qacA/B* at baseline	• Colonization with a mupirocin-resistant *S aureus* strain precluded decolonization efforts • A higher proportion of colonizing isolates recovered at longitudinal samplings (following decolonization) were mupirocin-resistant and/or chlorhexidine-resistant compared with those obtained at baseline

Al-Zubeidi et al,[131] 2014	105 Children presenting to the emergency department with community-onset MRSA SSTI (248 isolates) in St Louis, MO; 2005–2011	Retrospective study	6.7% of patients were infected with a mupirocin-resistant MRSA isolate	N/A	—
Johnson et al,[183] 2013	281 MRSA isolates obtained from pediatric emergency department and hospitalized patients in Nashville, TN; 2004–2009	Retrospective study	N/A	18.5% of MRSA-infecting isolates harbored qacA/B or smr (13.9% harbored smr only, 4.3% harbored qacA/B only, and 1 isolate contained both smr and qacA/B)	• USA 300 MRSA isolates were less likely to harbor qacA/B or smr compared with non-USA 300 isolates
McNeil et al,[184] 2013	179 Patients with underlying malignancy with S aureus infection (most commonly bacteremia, yielding 156 S aureus isolates for analysis) in Houston, TX; 2001–2011	Retrospective study	N/A	7.6% of infecting S aureus isolates harbored qacA/B	• The prevalence of qacA/B-positive S aureus isolates increased significantly over the study period (from 4.5% in 2007 to 22.2% in 2011), coinciding with increased chlorhexidine use • Ciprofloxacin-resistance was associated with the presence of qacA/B

(continued on next page)

Table 5
(continued)

Study Reference	Population; Years Study Performed	Study Design/Intervention	Mupirocin Resistance	Chlorhexidine Resistance	Other Findings/Notes
McNeil et al,[185] 2013	216 Patients with congenital heart disease with S aureus infection (most commonly SSTI, surgical site infection, and bacteremia/infective endocarditis, yielding 183 S aureus isolates for analysis) in Houston, TX; 2001–2011	Retrospective study	N/A	16.9% of Infecting S aureus isolates harbored qacA/B	• The prevalence of qacA/B-positive S aureus isolates increased significantly over the study period (from 5.0% in 2006 to 45.5% in 2011) • The presence of qacA/B in S aureus isolates was associated with the presence of central lines, nosocomial acquisition, bacteremia, and prolonged hospitalization
McNeil et al,[182] 2014	400 Children presenting with community-onset S aureus SSTI in Houston, TX (200 isolates from patients with a first-time S aureus SSTI episodes and 200 isolates from patients with ≥3 S aureus SSTI episodes); 2010–2012	Retrospective study	9.8% of patients were infected with a mupirocin-resistant S aureus isolate	14% of patients were infected with an S aureus isolate harboring smr	• 9.5% of patients were infected with a retapamulin-resistant S aureus isolate • Previous mupirocin use was associated with increased mupirocin resistance • Mupirocin resistance was more prevalent in patients with a higher number of recurrent SSTIs • Chlorhexidine resistance was more prevalent in isolates recovered from recurrent SSTI (vs first-time SSTI)

Abbreviation: N/A, not applicable.

Despite these failures, staphylococcal vaccine development as well as strategies for passive immunization[201] continue. Once available, a suitable vaccine will be targeted to individuals at high risk for SSTI and those with recurrent infections.

Bacterial Interference and Probiotics

The endogenous microbiota (ie, normal flora) exist in a delicate balance, vying for nutrients and adhesion sites. In this competition, commensal bacteria may interfere with the adherence and pathogenesis of potential pathogens, thereby protecting the host.[202,203] Additionally, the endogenous microbiota may activate or augment the host defenses against bacterial invaders. The concept of bacterial interference, or the use of a nonpathogenic organism to interfere with colonization and infection of a potentially pathogenic organism, is not novel. Indeed, the practice was implemented in the 1960s in an effort to abate *S aureus* outbreaks among newborns caused by the epidemic strain type 80/81. The concept emerged from an observation that infants colonized with a nonepidemic strain type with apparent low pathogenicity, known as 502A, were at a decreased risk for colonization and infection with strain type 80/81. Newborns intentionally inoculated with 502A in the nares and/or umbilicus were less likely to acquire strain type 80/81 and had a reduced incidence of infection with this epidemic strain.[129,204–209] It is important to note, however, that following dissemination of this practice, reports emerged of infants developing pustulosis, conjunctivitis, and other infections, including one infant who died of meningitis and septicemia, all caused by the 502A strain.[210–212]

The balance of organisms within the host microbiota may play an important role in *S aureus* colonization and development of symptomatic infection. In this contemporary CA-MRSA era, a US military study comparing microbial communities within the anterior nares between soldiers with and without SSTI revealed a significantly higher abundance of *Proteobacteria* in the anterior nares of the non-SSTI group compared with soldiers with active SSTI.[213] Thus, perhaps manipulation of heterologous components of host microbiota may provide resilience against *S aureus* colonization and infection. Uehara and colleagues[214] conducted a trial in Japan in which persistent *S aureus* nasal carriers were inoculated with a strain of *Corynebacterium* sp (Co304) versus sequential inoculation with saline and *S epidermidis*. Of the 17 participants receiving *Corynebacterium* inoculation, *S aureus* was completely eradicated in 71%. In contrast, eradication of *S aureus* carriage was not demonstrated when sodium chloride and *S epidermidis* were applied to the nares. A trial conducted in Switzerland showed that consumption of a probiotic (a fermented milk drink containing *Lactobacillus* GG, *L acidophilus*, *Streptococcus thermophilus*, and *Bifidobacterium* sp) reduced nasal carriage of potentially pathogenic bacteria (*S aureus*, *Streptococcus pyogenes*, β-hemolytic streptococci, and *H influenzae*) compared with eating standard yogurt.[215]

SUMMARY

Ultimately, the optimal regimen for long-term *S aureus* eradication and prevention of recurrent infections remains unclear. Until a more definitive prevention strategy is available, disruption of colonization, targeting multiple anatomic sites with topical antimicrobials, and effective hygiene are the cornerstones of SSTI prevention. At present, the low rate of staphylococcal resistance to commonly prescribed topical agents makes these agents highly effective in temporarily decolonizing the anterior nares and skin. Given the transmission dynamics of *S aureus* within households, decolonization of all household members optimizes this approach.

REFERENCES

1. Holt LE, Howland J, Holt LE, et al. Holt's diseases of infancy and childhood; a textbook for the use of students and practitioners. 11th edition. New York; London: D. Appleton-Century Company; 1940.
2. Hersh AL, Chambers HF, Maselli JH, et al. National trends in ambulatory visits and antibiotic prescribing for skin and soft-tissue infections. Arch Intern Med 2008;168(14):1585–91.
3. Wertheim HF, Melles DC, Vos MC, et al. The role of nasal carriage in *Staphylococcus aureus* infections. Lancet Infect Dis 2005;5(12):751–62.
4. Faden H, Lesse AJ, Trask J, et al. Importance of colonization site in the current epidemic of staphylococcal skin abscesses. Pediatrics 2010;125(3):e618–24.
5. Fritz SA, Hogan PG, Hayek G, et al. *Staphylococcus aureus* colonization in children with community-associated *Staphylococcus aureus* skin infections and their household contacts. Arch Pediatr Adolesc Med 2012;166(6):551–7.
6. Kluytmans J, van Belkum A, Verbrugh H. Nasal carriage of *Staphylococcus aureus*: epidemiology, underlying mechanisms, and associated risks. Clin Microbiol Rev 1997;10(3):505–20.
7. Mertz D, Frei R, Jaussi B, et al. Throat swabs are necessary to reliably detect carriers of *Staphylococcus aureus*. Clin Infect Dis 2007;45(4):475–7.
8. Weems JJ Jr. The many faces of *Staphylococcus aureus* infection. Recognizing and managing its life-threatening manifestations. Postgrad Med 2001;110(4): 24–6, 29–31, 35–6.
9. Lindsay JA, Holden MT. *Staphylococcus aureus*: superbug, super genome? Trends Microbiol 2004;12(8):378–85.
10. Klevens RM, Morrison MA, Nadle J, et al. Invasive methicillin-resistant *Staphylococcus aureus* infections in the United States. JAMA 2007;298(15):1763–71.
11. Barrett FF, McGehee RF Jr, Finland M. Methicillin-resistant *Staphylococcus aureus* at Boston city hospital. Bacteriologic and epidemiologic observations. N Engl J Med 1968;279(9):441–8.
12. Lowy FD. *Staphylococcus aureus* infections. N Engl J Med 1998;339(8):520–32.
13. Boyce JM, Causey WA. Increasing occurrence of methicillin-resistant *Staphylococcus aureus* in the United States. Infect Control 1982;3(5):377–83.
14. Kline MW, Mason EO Jr. Methicillin-resistant *Staphylococcus aureus*: pediatric perspective. Pediatr Clin North Am 1988;35(3):613–24.
15. Mulligan ME, Murray-Leisure KA, Ribner BS, et al. Methicillin-resistant *Staphylococcus aureus*: a consensus review of the microbiology, pathogenesis, and epidemiology with implications for prevention and management. Am J Med 1993;94(3):313–28.
16. National Nosocomial Infections Surveillance System. National Nosocomial Infections Surveillance (NNIS) system report, data summary from January 1992 through June 2004, issued October 2004. Am J Infect Control 2004;32(8):470–85.
17. Kuehnert MJ, Hill HA, Kupronis BA, et al. Methicillin-resistant-*Staphylococcus aureus* hospitalizations, United States. Emerg Infect Dis 2005;11(6):868–72.
18. Centers for Disease Control and Prevention. Four pediatric deaths from community-acquired methicillin-resistant *Staphylococcus aureus* – Minnesota and North Dakota, 1997–1999. MMWR Morb Mortal Wkly Rep 1999;48(32): 707–10.
19. Gopal Rao G, Wong J. Interaction between methicillin-resistant *Staphylococcus aureus* (MRSA) and methicillin-sensitive *Staphylococcus aureus* (MSSA). J Hosp Infect 2003;55(2):116–8.

20. Hulten KG, Kaplan SL, Gonzalez BE, et al. Three-year surveillance of community onset health care-associated *Staphylococcus aureus* infections in children. Pediatr Infect Dis J 2006;25(4):349–53.
21. Kluytmans-Vandenbergh MF, Kluytmans JA. Community-acquired methicillin-resistant *Staphylococcus aureus*: current perspectives. Clin Microbiol Infect 2006;12(Suppl 1):9–15.
22. Hanssen AM, Ericson Sollid JU. SCC*mec* in staphylococci: genes on the move. FEMS Immunol Med Microbiol 2006;46(1):8–20.
23. Tenover FC, McDougal LK, Goering RV, et al. Characterization of a strain of community-associated methicillin-resistant *Staphylococcus aureus* widely disseminated in the United States. J Clin Microbiol 2006;44(1):108–18.
24. Boyle-Vavra S, Ereshefsky B, Wang CC, et al. Successful multiresistant community-associated methicillin-resistant *Staphylococcus aureus* lineage from Taipei, Taiwan, that carries either the novel staphylococcal chromosome cassette mec (SCCmec) type VT or sccmec type IV. J Clin Microbiol 2005; 43(9):4719–30.
25. Katayama Y, Robinson DA, Enright MC, et al. Genetic background affects stability of *mecA* in *Staphylococcus aureus*. J Clin Microbiol 2005;43(5):2380–3.
26. Ito T, Ma XX, Takeuchi F, et al. Novel type V staphylococcal cassette chromosome *mec* driven by a novel cassette chromosome recombinase, ccrC. Antimicrob Agents Chemother 2004;48(7):2637–51.
27. Katayama Y, Zhang HZ, Hong D, et al. Jumping the barrier to beta-lactam resistance in *Staphylococcus aureus*. J Bacteriol 2003;185(18):5465–72.
28. Daum RS, Ito T, Hiramatsu K, et al. A novel methicillin-resistance cassette in community-acquired methicillin-resistant *Staphylococcus aureus* isolates of diverse genetic backgrounds. J Infect Dis 2002;186(9):1344–7.
29. Hiramatsu K, Katayama Y, Yuzawa H, et al. Molecular genetics of methicillin-resistant *Staphylococcus aureus*. Int J Med Microbiol 2002;292(2):67–74.
30. Diep BA, Chambers HF, Graber CJ, et al. Emergence of multidrug-resistant, community-associated, methicillin-resistant *Staphylococcus aureus* clone USA300 in men who have sex with men. Ann Intern Med 2008;148(4):249–57.
31. Han LL, McDougal LK, Gorwitz RJ, et al. High frequencies of clindamycin and tetracycline resistance in methicillin-resistant *Staphylococcus aureus* pulsed-field type USA300 isolates collected at a Boston ambulatory health center. J Clin Microbiol 2007;45(4):1350–2.
32. Otter JA, French GL. Nosocomial transmission of community-associated methicillin-resistant *Staphylococcus aureus*: an emerging threat. Lancet Infect Dis 2006;6(12):753–5.
33. Gonzalez BE, Rueda AM, Shelburne SA 3rd, et al. Community-associated strains of methicillin-resistant *Staphylococcus aureus* as the cause of healthcare-associated infection. Infect Control Hosp Epidemiol 2006;27(10): 1051–6.
34. Hulten KG, Kaplan SL, Lamberth LB, et al. Hospital-acquired *Staphylococcus aureus* infections at Texas Children's Hospital, 2001–2007. Infect Control Hosp Epidemiol 2010;31(2):183–90.
35. Diekema DJ, Richter SS, Heilmann KP, et al. Continued emergence of USA300 methicillin-resistant *Staphylococcus aureus* in the United States: results from a nationwide surveillance study. Infect Control Hosp Epidemiol 2014;35(3): 285–92.
36. McDougal LK, Fosheim GE, Nicholson A, et al. Emergence of resistance among USA300 methicillin-resistant *Staphylococcus aureus* isolates causing invasive

disease in the United States. Antimicrob Agents Chemother 2010;54(9): 3804–11.

37. Lina G, Piemont Y, Godail-Gamot F, et al. Involvement of Panton-Valentine leukocidin-producing *Staphylococcus aureus* in primary skin infections and pneumonia. Clin Infect Dis 1999;29(5):1128–32.

38. Diep BA, Gill SR, Chang RF, et al. Complete genome sequence of USA300, an epidemic clone of community-acquired methicillin-resistant *Staphylococcus aureus*. Lancet 2006;367(9512):731–9.

39. Goering RV, McDougal LK, Fosheim GE, et al. Epidemiologic distribution of the arginine catabolic mobile element among selected methicillin-resistant and methicillin-susceptible *Staphylococcus aureus* isolates. J Clin Microbiol 2007; 45(6):1981–4.

40. DeLeo FR, Diep BA, Otto M. Host defense and pathogenesis in *Staphylococcus aureus* infections. Infect Dis Clin North Am 2009;23(1):17–34.

41. Loughman JA, Fritz SA, Storch GA, et al. Virulence gene expression in human community-acquired *Staphylococcus aureus* infection. J Infect Dis 2009; 199(3):294–301.

42. Naimi TS, LeDell KH, Como-Sabetti K, et al. Comparison of community- and health care-associated methicillin-resistant *Staphylococcus aureus* infection. JAMA 2003;290(22):2976–84.

43. Kaplan SL, Hulten KG, Gonzalez BE, et al. Three-year surveillance of community-acquired *Staphylococcus aureus* infections in children. Clin Infect Dis 2005;40(12):1785–91.

44. Gonzalez BE, Martinez-Aguilar G, Hulten KG, et al. Severe staphylococcal sepsis in adolescents in the era of community-acquired methicillin-resistant *Staphylococcus aureus*. Pediatrics 2005;115(3):642–8.

45. Fritz SA, Garbutt J, Elward A, et al. Prevalence of and risk factors for community-acquired methicillin-resistant and methicillin-sensitive *Staphylococcus aureus* colonization in children seen in a practice-based research network. Pediatrics 2008;121(6):1090–8.

46. Creech CB 2nd, Kernodle DS, Alsentzer A, et al. Increasing rates of nasal carriage of methicillin-resistant *Staphylococcus aureus* in healthy children. Pediatr Infect Dis J 2005;24(7):617–21.

47. Gorwitz RJ, Kruszon-Moran D, McAllister SK, et al. Changes in the prevalence of nasal colonization with *Staphylococcus aureus* in the United States, 2001–2004. J Infect Dis 2008;197(9):1226–34.

48. McCaskill ML, Mason EO Jr, Kaplan SL, et al. Increase of the USA300 clone among community-acquired methicillin-susceptible *Staphylococcus aureus* causing invasive infections. Pediatr Infect Dis J 2007;26(12):1122–7.

49. Orscheln RC, Hunstad DA, Fritz SA, et al. Contribution of genetically restricted, methicillin-susceptible strains to the ongoing epidemic of community-acquired *Staphylococcus aureus* infections. Clin Infect Dis 2009;49(4):536–42.

50. Witt WP, Weiss AJ, Elixhauser A. Overview of hospital stays for children in the United States. 2012. Available at: http://www.hcup-us.ahrq.gov/reports/statbriefs/sb187-Hospital-Stays-Children-2012.jsp. Accessed January 29, 2015.

51. Purcell K, Fergie J. Epidemic of community-acquired methicillin-resistant *Staphylococcus aureus* infections: a 14-year study at Driscoll Children's Hospital. Arch Pediatr Adolesc Med 2005;159(10):980–5.

52. Levison ME, Fung S. Community-associated methicillin-resistant *Staphylococcus aureus*: reconsideration of therapeutic options. Curr Infect Dis Rep 2006;8(1):23–30.

53. Stankovic C, Mahajan PV. Healthy children with invasive community-acquired methicillin-resistant *Staphylococcus aureus* infections. Pediatr Emerg Care 2006;22(5):361–3.

54. Creech CB, Johnson BG, Bartilson RE, et al. Increasing use of extracorporeal life support in methicillin-resistant *Staphylococcus aureus* sepsis in children. Pediatr Crit Care Med 2007;8(3):231–5 [quiz: 47].

55. Gerber JS, Coffin SE, Smathers SA, et al. Trends in the incidence of methicillin-resistant *Staphylococcus aureus* infection in children's hospitals in the United States. Clin Infect Dis 2009;49(1):65–71.

56. Eveillard M, de Lassence A, Lancien E, et al. Evaluation of a strategy of screening multiple anatomical sites for methicillin-resistant *Staphylococcus aureus* at admission to a teaching hospital. Infect Control Hosp Epidemiol 2006;27(2):181–4.

57. Nilsson P, Ripa T. *Staphylococcus aureus* throat colonization is more frequent than colonization in the anterior nares. J Clin Microbiol 2006;44(9):3334–9.

58. Peters PJ, Brooks JT, Limbago B, et al. Methicillin-resistant *Staphylococcus aureus* colonization in HIV-infected outpatients is common and detection is enhanced by groin culture. Epidemiol Infect 2011;139(7):998–1008.

59. Kaplan SL, Forbes A, Hammerman WA, et al. Randomized trial of "bleach baths" plus routine hygienic measures vs. routine hygienic measures alone for prevention of recurrent infections. Clin Infect Dis 2014;58(5):679–82.

60. von Eiff C, Becker K, Machka K, et al. Nasal carriage as a source of *Staphylococcus aureus* bacteremia. N Engl J Med 2001;344(1):11–6.

61. Toshkova K, Annemuller C, Akineden O, et al. The significance of nasal carriage of *Staphylococcus aureus* as risk factor for human skin infections. FEMS Microbiol Lett 2001;202(1):17–24.

62. Davis KA, Stewart JJ, Crouch HK, et al. Methicillin-resistant *Staphylococcus aureus* (MRSA) nares colonization at hospital admission and its effect on subsequent MRSA infection. Clin Infect Dis 2004;39(6):776–82.

63. Ellis MW, Hospenthal DR, Dooley DP, et al. Natural history of community-acquired methicillin-resistant *Staphylococcus aureus* colonization and infection in soldiers. Clin Infect Dis 2004;39(7):971–9.

64. Fritz SA, Epplin EK, Garbutt J, et al. Skin infection in children colonized with community-associated methicillin-resistant *Staphylococcus aureus*. J Infect 2009;59(6):394–401.

65. Macal CM, North MJ, Collier N, et al. Modeling the transmission of community-associated methicillin-resistant *Staphylococcus aureus*: a dynamic agent-based simulation. J Transl Med 2014;12:124.

66. Ray GT, Suaya JA, Baxter R. Incidence, microbiology, and patient characteristics of skin and soft-tissue infections in a U.S. population: a retrospective population-based study. BMC Infect Dis 2013;13:252.

67. Ray GT, Suaya JA, Baxter R. Microbiology of skin and soft tissue infections in the age of community-acquired methicillin-resistant *Staphylococcus aureus*. Diagn Microbiol Infect Dis 2013;76(1):24–30.

68. David MZ, Mennella C, Mansour M, et al. Predominance of methicillin-resistant *Staphylococcus aureus* among pathogens causing skin and soft tissue infections in a large urban jail: risk factors and recurrence rates. J Clin Microbiol 2008;46(10):3222–7.

69. Wright MO, Furuno JP, Venezia RA, et al. Methicillin-resistant *Staphylococcus aureus* infection and colonization among hospitalized prisoners. Infect Control Hosp Epidemiol 2007;28(7):877–9.

70. Centers for Disease Control and Prevention. Methicillin-resistant *Staphylococcus aureus* infections in correctional facilities – Georgia, California, and Texas, 2001–2003. MMWR Morb Mortal Wkly Rep 2003;52(41):992–6.
71. Creech CB, Saye E, McKenna BD, et al. One-year surveillance of methicillin-resistant *Staphylococcus aureus* nasal colonization and skin and soft tissue infections in collegiate athletes. Arch Pediatr Adolesc Med 2010;164(7): 615–20.
72. Centers for Disease Control and Prevention. Methicillin-resistant *Staphylococcus aureus* infections among competitive sports participants – Colorado, Indiana, Pennsylvania, and Los Angeles county, 2000–2003. MMWR Morb Mortal Wkly Rep 2003;52(33):793–5.
73. Kazakova SV, Hageman JC, Matava M, et al. A clone of methicillin-resistant *Staphylococcus aureus* among professional football players. N Engl J Med 2005;352(5):468–75.
74. Jimenez-Truque N, Saye EJ, Soper N, et al. Longitudinal assessment of colonization with *Staphylococcus aureus* in healthy collegiate athletes. J Pediatric Infect Dis Soc, in press.
75. Nouwen J, Schouten J, Schneebergen P, et al. *Staphylococcus aureus* carriage patterns and the risk of infections associated with continuous peritoneal dialysis. J Clin Microbiol 2006;44(6):2233–6.
76. Nouwen JL, van Belkum A, Verbrugh HA. Determinants of *Staphylococcus aureus* nasal carriage. Neth J Med 2001;59(3):126–33.
77. Wertheim HF, Walsh E, Choudhurry R, et al. Key role for clumping factor b in *Staphylococcus aureus* nasal colonization of humans. PLoS Med 2008;5(1):e17.
78. Bubeck Wardenburg J, Schneewind O. Vaccine protection against *Staphylococcus aureus* pneumonia. J Exp Med 2008;205(2):287–94.
79. Maresso AW, Schneewind O. Iron acquisition and transport in *Staphylococcus aureus*. Biometals 2006;19(2):193–203.
80. de Haas CJ, Veldkamp KE, Peschel A, et al. Chemotaxis inhibitory protein of *Staphylococcus aureus*, a bacterial antiinflammatory agent. J Exp Med 2004; 199(5):687–95.
81. Chavakis T, Hussain M, Kanse SM, et al. *Staphylococcus aureus* extracellular adherence protein serves as anti-inflammatory factor by inhibiting the recruitment of host leukocytes. Nat Med 2002;8(7):687–93.
82. Dumont AL, Nygaard TK, Watkins RL, et al. Characterization of a new cytotoxin that contributes to *Staphylococcus aureus* pathogenesis. Mol Microbiol 2011; 79(3):814–25.
83. Tomita T, Kamio Y. Molecular biology of the pore-forming cytolysins from *Staphylococcus aureus*, alpha- and gamma-hemolysins and leukocidin. Biosci Biotechnol Biochem 1997;61(4):565–72.
84. Wang R, Braughton KR, Kretschmer D, et al. Identification of novel cytolytic peptides as key virulence determinants for community-associated MRSA. Nat Med 2007;13(12):1510–4.
85. Foster TJ. Immune evasion by staphylococci. Nat Rev Microbiol 2005;3(12): 948–58.
86. Liu GY, Essex A, Buchanan JT, et al. *Staphylococcus aureus* golden pigment impairs neutrophil killing and promotes virulence through its antioxidant activity. J Exp Med 2005;202(2):209–15.
87. Clauditz A, Resch A, Wieland KP, et al. Staphyloxanthin plays a role in the fitness of *Staphylococcus aureus* and its ability to cope with oxidative stress. Infect Immun 2006;74(8):4950–3.

88. Cosgrove K, Coutts G, Jonsson IM, et al. Catalase (KatA) and alkyl hydroperoxide reductase (AhpC) have compensatory roles in peroxide stress resistance and are required for survival, persistence, and nasal colonization in *Staphylococcus aureus*. J Bacteriol 2007;189(3):1025–35.

89. Mandell GL. Catalase, superoxide dismutase, and virulence of *Staphylococcus aureus*. In vitro and in vivo studies with emphasis on staphylococcal–leukocyte interaction. J Clin Invest 1975;55(3):561–6.

90. Karavolos MH, Horsburgh MJ, Ingham E, et al. Role and regulation of the superoxide dismutases of *Staphylococcus aureus*. Microbiology 2003;149(Pt 10): 2749–58.

91. Liu C, Bayer A, Cosgrove SE, et al. Clinical practice guidelines by the Infectious Diseases Society of America for the treatment of methicillin-resistant *Staphylococcus aureus* infections in adults and children. Clin Infect Dis 2011;52(3):e18–55.

92. Mistry RD. Skin and soft tissue infections. Pediatr Clin North Am 2013;60(5): 1063–82.

93. Llera JL, Levy RC. Treatment of cutaneous abscess: a double-blind clinical study. Ann Emerg Med 1985;14(1):15–9.

94. Lee MC, Rios AM, Aten MF, et al. Management and outcome of children with skin and soft tissue abscesses caused by community-acquired methicillin-resistant *Staphylococcus aureus*. Pediatr Infect Dis J 2004;23(2):123–7.

95. Chen AE, Carroll KC, Diener-West M, et al. Randomized controlled trial of cephalexin versus clindamycin for uncomplicated pediatric skin infections. Pediatrics 2011;127(3):e573–80.

96. Schmitz GR, Bruner D, Pitotti R, et al. Randomized controlled trial of trimethoprim-sulfamethoxazole for uncomplicated skin abscesses in patients at risk for community-associated methicillin-resistant *Staphylococcus aureus* infection. Ann Emerg Med 2010;56(3):283–7.

97. Duong M, Markwell S, Peter J, et al. Randomized, controlled trial of antibiotics in the management of community-acquired skin abscesses in the pediatric patient. Ann Emerg Med 2010;55(5):401–7.

98. National Institute of Allergy and Infectious Diseases. Uncomplicated skin and soft tissue infections caused by community-associated methicillin-resistant *Staphylococcus aureus* (NCT00730028). Available at: https://clinicaltrials.gov/ct2/show/NCT00730028. Accessed January 2, 2015.

99. Williams DJ, Cooper WO, Kaltenbach LA, et al. Comparative effectiveness of antibiotic treatment strategies for pediatric skin and soft-tissue infections. Pediatrics 2011;128(3):e479–87.

100. Chen AE, Cantey JB, Carroll KC, et al. Discordance between *Staphylococcus aureus* nasal colonization and skin infections in children. Pediatr Infect Dis J 2009;28(3):244–6.

101. Fritz SA, Camins BC, Eisenstein KA, et al. Effectiveness of measures to eradicate *Staphylococcus aureus* carriage in patients with community-associated skin and soft-tissue infections: a randomized trial. Infect Control Hosp Epidemiol 2011;32(9):872–80.

102. Miller LG, Quan C, Shay A, et al. A prospective investigation of outcomes after hospital discharge for endemic, community-acquired methicillin-resistant and -susceptible *Staphylococcus aureus* skin infection. Clin Infect Dis 2007; 44(4):483–92.

103. Fritz SA, Hogan PG, Hayek G, et al. Household versus individual approaches to eradication of community-associated *Staphylococcus aureus* in children: a randomized trial. Clin Infect Dis 2012;54(6):743–51.

104. Bocchini CE, Mason EO, Hulten KG, et al. Recurrent community-associated *Staphylococcus aureus* infections in children presenting to Texas Children's Hospital in Houston, Texas. Pediatr Infect Dis J 2013;32(11):1189–93.

105. Miller LG, Eells SJ, David MZ, et al. *Staphylococcus aureus* skin infection recurrences among household members: an examination of host, behavioral, and pathogen-level predictors. Clin Infect Dis 2015;60(5):753–63.

106. Uhlemann AC, Dordel J, Knox JR, et al. Molecular tracing of the emergence, diversification, and transmission of *S. aureus* sequence type 8 in a New York community. Proc Natl Acad Sci U S A 2014;111(18):6738–43.

107. Tacconelli E. Antimicrobial use: risk driver of multidrug resistant microorganisms in healthcare settings. Curr Opin Infect Dis 2009;22(4):352–8.

108. Frazee BW, Lynn J, Charlebois ED, et al. High prevalence of methicillin-resistant *Staphylococcus aureus* in emergency department skin and soft tissue infections. Ann Emerg Med 2005;45(3):311–20.

109. Miller LG, Diep BA. Clinical practice: colonization, fomites, and virulence: rethinking the pathogenesis of community-associated methicillin-resistant *Staphylococcus aureus* infection. Clin Infect Dis 2008;46(5):752–60.

110. Whitman TJ, Herlihy RK, Schlett CD, et al. Chlorhexidine-impregnated cloths to prevent skin and soft-tissue infection in Marine recruits: a cluster-randomized, double-blind, controlled effectiveness trial. Infect Control Hosp Epidemiol 2010;31(12):1207–15.

111. Cluzet VC, Gerber JS, Nachamkin I, et al. Duration of colonization and determinants of earlier clearance of colonization with methicillin-resistant *Staphylococcus aureus*. Clin Infect Dis 2015;60(10):1489–96.

112. Hogan PG, Rodriguez M, Hunstad DA, et al. Effect of antibiotics on community-associated methicillin-resistant *Staphylococcus aureus* (MRSA) colonization in patients with uncomplicated MRSA skin abscesses. Annual Meeting of the Infectious Diseases Society of America. Boston (MA), October 20-23, 2011.

113. Osterlund A, Kahlmeter G, Bieber L, et al. Intrafamilial spread of highly virulent *Staphylococcus aureus* strains carrying the gene for Panton-Valentine leukocidin. Scand J Infect Dis 2002;34(10):763–4.

114. Jones TF, Creech CB, Erwin P, et al. Family outbreaks of invasive community-associated methicillin-resistant *Staphylococcus aureus* infection. Clin Infect Dis 2006;42(9):e76–8.

115. L'Heriteau F, Lucet JC, Scanvic A, et al. Community-acquired methicillin-resistant *Staphylococcus aureus* and familial transmission. JAMA 1999;282(11):1038–9.

116. Dietrich DW, Auld DB, Mermel LA. Community-acquired methicillin-resistant *Staphylococcus aureus* in southern New England children. Pediatrics 2004; 113(4):e347–52.

117. Hollis RJ, Barr JL, Doebbeling BN, et al. Familial carriage of methicillin-resistant *Staphylococcus aureus* and subsequent infection in a premature neonate. Clin Infect Dis 1995;21(2):328–32.

118. Huijsdens XW, van Santen-Verheuvel MG, Spalburg E, et al. Multiple cases of familial transmission of community-acquired methicillin-resistant *Staphylococcus aureus*. J Clin Microbiol 2006;44(8):2994–6.

119. Nerby JM, Gorwitz R, Lesher L, et al. Risk factors for household transmission of community-associated methicillin-resistant *Staphylococcus aureus*. Pediatr Infect Dis J 2011;30(11):927–32.

120. Mollema FP, Richardus JH, Behrendt M, et al. Transmission of methicillin-resistant *Staphylococcus aureus* to household contacts. J Clin Microbiol 2010; 48(1):202–7.

121. Fritz SA, Hogan PG, Singh LN, et al. Contamination of environmental surfaces with *Staphylococcus aureus* in households with children infected with methicillin-resistant *S. aureus*. JAMA Pediatr 2014;168(11):1030–8.

122. Uhlemann AC, Knox J, Miller M, et al. The environment as an unrecognized reservoir for community-associated methicillin resistant *Staphylococcus aureus* USA300: a case-control study. PLoS One 2011;6(7):e22407.

123. Knox J, Uhlemann AC, Miller M, et al. Environmental contamination as a risk factor for intra-household *Staphylococcus aureus* transmission. PLoS One 2012; 7(11):e49900.

124. Davis MF, Iverson SA, Baron P, et al. Household transmission of methicillin-resistant *Staphylococcus aureus* and other staphylococci. Lancet Infect Dis 2012;12(9):703–16.

125. Rodriguez M, Hogan PG, Burnham CA, et al. Molecular epidemiology of *Staphylococcus aureus* in households of children with community-associated *S. aureus* skin and soft tissue infections. J Pediatr 2014;164(1):105–11.

126. Johansson PJ, Gustafsson EB, Ringberg H. High prevalence of MRSA in household contacts. Scand J Infect Dis 2007;39(9):764–8.

127. Huang YC, Ho CF, Chen CJ, et al. Nasal carriage of methicillin-resistant *Staphylococcus aureus* in household contacts of children with community-acquired diseases in Taiwan. Pediatr Infect Dis J 2007;26(11):1066–8.

128. Eells SJ, David MZ, Taylor A, et al. Persistent environmental contamination with USA300 methicillin-resistant *Staphylococcus aureus* and other pathogenic strain types in households with *S. aureus* skin infections. Infect Control Hosp Epidemiol 2014;35(11):1373–82.

129. Shinefield HR, Ruff NL. Staphylococcal infections: a historical perspective. Infect Dis Clin North Am 2009;23(1):1–15.

130. Fridkin SK. Methicillin-resistant *Staphylococcus aureus* in the community setting: the new reality. 2004 Annual Conference on Antimicrobial Resistance. Bethesda (MD), June 28–30, 2004.

131. Al-Zubeidi D, Burnham CD, Hogan PG, et al. Molecular epidemiology of recurrent cutaneous methicillin-resistant *Staphylococcus aureus* infections in children. J Pediatric Infect Dis Soc 2014;3(3):261–4.

132. Chen CJ, Su LH, Lin TY, et al. Molecular analysis of repeated methicillin-resistant *Staphylococcus aureus* infections in children. PLoS One 2010;5(12):e14431.

133. Laupland KB, Conly JM. Treatment of *Staphylococcus aureus* colonization and prophylaxis for infection with topical intranasal mupirocin: an evidence-based review. Clin Infect Dis 2003;37(7):933–8.

134. Perl TM, Cullen JJ, Wenzel RP, et al. Intranasal mupirocin to prevent postoperative *Staphylococcus aureus* infections. N Engl J Med 2002;346(24):1871–7.

135. Sandri AM, Dalarosa MG, Ruschel de Alcantara L, et al. Reduction in incidence of nosocomial methicillin-resistant *Staphylococcus aureus* (MRSA) infection in an intensive care unit: role of treatment with mupirocin ointment and chlorhexidine baths for nasal carriers of MRSA. Infect Control Hosp Epidemiol 2006;27(2):185–7.

136. Tacconelli E, Carmeli Y, Aizer A, et al. Mupirocin prophylaxis to prevent *Staphylococcus aureus* infection in patients undergoing dialysis: a meta-analysis. Clin Infect Dis 2003;37(12):1629–38.

137. Climo MW, Sepkowitz KA, Zuccotti G, et al. The effect of daily bathing with chlorhexidine on the acquisition of methicillin-resistant *Staphylococcus aureus*, vancomycin-resistant enterococcus, and healthcare-associated bloodstream infections: results of a quasi-experimental multicenter trial. Crit Care Med 2009; 37(6):1858–65.

138. Milstone AM, Elward A, Song X, et al. Daily chlorhexidine bathing to reduce bacteraemia in critically ill children: a multicentre, cluster-randomised, crossover trial. Lancet 2013;381(9872):1099–106.

139. Calfee DP, Salgado CD, Milstone AM, et al. Strategies to prevent methicillin-resistant *Staphylococcus aureus* transmission and infection in acute care hospitals: 2014 update. Infect Control Hosp Epidemiol 2014;35(Suppl 2):S108–32.

140. Huang SS, Septimus E, Kleinman K, et al. Targeted versus universal decolonization to prevent ICU infection. N Engl J Med 2013;368(24):2255–65.

141. Noto MJ, Domenico HJ, Byrne DW, et al. Chlorhexidine bathing and health care-associated infections: a randomized clinical trial. JAMA 2015;313(4):369–78.

142. van Rijen M, Bonten M, Wenzel R, et al. Mupirocin ointment for preventing *Staphylococcus aureus* infections in nasal carriers. Cochrane Database Syst Rev 2008;(4):CD006216.

143. Loeb M, Main C, Walker-Dilks C, et al. Antimicrobial drugs for treating methicillin-resistant *Staphylococcus aureus* colonization. Cochrane Database Syst Rev 2003;(4):CD003340.

144. Wendt C, Schinke S, Wurttemberger M, et al. Value of whole-body washing with chlorhexidine for the eradication of methicillin-resistant *Staphylococcus aureus*: a randomized, placebo-controlled, double-blind clinical trial. Infect Control Hosp Epidemiol 2007;28(9):1036–43.

145. Creech CB, Beekmann SE, Chen Y, et al. Variability among pediatric infectious diseases specialists in the treatment and prevention of methicillin-resistant *Staphylococcus aureus* skin and soft tissue infections. Pediatr Infect Dis J 2008;27(3):270–2.

146. Kaplan SL. Community-acquired methicillin-resistant *Staphylococcus aureus* infections in children. Semin Pediatr Infect Dis 2006;17(3):113–9.

147. Ellis MW, Griffith ME, Dooley DP, et al. Targeted intranasal mupirocin to prevent colonization and infection by community-associated methicillin-resistant *Staphylococcus aureus* strains in soldiers: a cluster randomized controlled trial. Antimicrob Agents Chemother 2007;51(10):3591–8.

148. Climo MW, Yokoe DS, Warren DK, et al. Effect of daily chlorhexidine bathing on hospital-acquired infection. N Engl J Med 2013;368(6):533–42.

149. Doebbeling BN, Reagan DR, Pfaller MA, et al. Long-term efficacy of intranasal mupirocin ointment. A prospective cohort study of *Staphylococcus aureus* carriage. Arch Intern Med 1994;154(13):1505–8.

150. Mascitti KB, Gerber JS, Zaoutis TE, et al. Preferred treatment and prevention strategies for recurrent community-associated methicillin-resistant *Staphylococcus aureus* skin and soft-tissue infections: a survey of adult and pediatric providers. Am J Infect Control 2010;38(4):324–8.

151. Centers for Disease Control and Prevention. Methicillin-resistant Staphylococcus aureus (MRSA) infections. Available at: http://www.cdc.gov/mrsa/community/index.html. Accessed January 2, 2015.

152. Hardy KJ, Oppenheim BA, Gossain S, et al. A study of the relationship between environmental contamination with methicillin-resistant *Staphylococcus aureus* (MRSA) and patients' acquisition of MRSA. Infect Control Hosp Epidemiol 2006;27(2):127–32.

153. Milstone AM. Uncovering reservoirs of methicillin-resistant *Staphylococcus aureus*: children contaminating households or households contaminating children? JAMA Pediatr 2014;168(11):994–5.

154. Weber DJ, Rutala WA. Understanding and preventing transmission of healthcare-associated pathogens due to the contaminated hospital environment. Infect Control Hosp Epidemiol 2013;34(5):449–52.

155. Boyce JM. Environmental contamination makes an important contribution to hospital infection. J Hosp Infect 2007;65(Suppl 2):50–4.
156. McConeghy KW, Mikolich DJ, LaPlante KL. Agents for the decolonization of methicillin-resistant *Staphylococcus aureus*. Pharmacotherapy 2009;29(3): 263–80.
157. Thomas CM, Hothersall J, Willis CL, et al. Resistance to and synthesis of the antibiotic mupirocin. Nat Rev Microbiol 2010;8(4):281–9.
158. Patel JB, Gorwitz RJ, Jernigan JA. Mupirocin resistance. Clin Infect Dis 2009; 49(6):935–41.
159. Hetem DJ, Bonten MJ. Clinical relevance of mupirocin resistance in *Staphylococcus aureus*. J Hosp Infect 2013;85(4):249–56.
160. Morton TM, Johnston JL, Patterson J, et al. Characterization of a conjugative staphylococcal mupirocin resistance plasmid. Antimicrob Agents Chemother 1995;39(6):1272–80.
161. Jones RN, Fritsche TR, Sader HS, et al. Activity of retapamulin (sb-275833), a novel pleuromutilin, against selected resistant gram-positive cocci. Antimicrob Agents Chemother 2006;50(7):2583–6.
162. Rittenhouse S, Biswas S, Broskey J, et al. Selection of retapamulin, a novel pleuromutilin for topical use. Antimicrob Agents Chemother 2006;50(11):3882–5.
163. Champney WS, Rodgers WK. Retapamulin inhibition of translation and 50S ribosomal subunit formation in *Staphylococcus aureus* cells. Antimicrob Agents Chemother 2007;51(9):3385–7.
164. Yan K, Madden L, Choudhry AE, et al. Biochemical characterization of the interactions of the novel pleuromutilin derivative retapamulin with bacterial ribosomes. Antimicrob Agents Chemother 2006;50(11):3875–81.
165. Saravolatz LD, Pawlak J, Saravolatz SN, et al. In vitro activity of retapamulin against *Staphylococcus aureus* resistant to various antimicrobial agents. Antimicrob Agents Chemother 2013;57(9):4547–50.
166. Naderer OJ, Anderson M, Roberts K, et al. Nasal decolonization of persistent Staphylococcus aureus (SA) carriers with twice daily application of retapamulin ointment, 1%, (Ret) for 3 or 5 days. 48th Annual Interscience Conference on Antimicrobial Agents and Chemotherapy and the Infectious Disease Society of America 46th Annual Meeting Washington, DC, October 25–28, 2008.
167. University of California, Irvine. Retapamulin for reducing MRSA nasal carriage (NCT01461668). Available at: https://clinicaltrials.gov/ct2/show/NCT01461668. Accessed February 2, 2015.
168. McDonnell G, Russell AD. Antiseptics and disinfectants: activity, action, and resistance. Clin Microbiol Rev 1999;12(1):147–79.
169. Longtin J, Seah C, Siebert K, et al. Distribution of antiseptic resistance genes *qacA, qacB,* and *smr* in methicillin-resistant *Staphylococcus aureus* isolated in Toronto, Canada, from 2005 to 2009. Antimicrob Agents Chemother 2011; 55(6):2999–3001.
170. Edmiston CE Jr, Seabrook GR, Johnson CP, et al. Comparative of a new and innovative 2% chlorhexidine gluconate-impregnated cloth with 4% chlorhexidine gluconate as topical antiseptic for preparation of the skin prior to surgery. Am J Infect Control 2007;35(2):89–96.
171. Milstone AM, Passaretti CL, Perl TM. Chlorhexidine: expanding the armamentarium for infection control and prevention. Clin Infect Dis 2008;46(2):274–81.
172. Huang JT, Abrams M, Tlougan B, et al. Treatment of *Staphylococcus aureus* colonization in atopic dermatitis decreases disease severity. Pediatrics 2009; 123(5):e808–14.

173. Heggers JP, Sazy JA, Stenberg BD, et al. Bactericidal and wound-healing properties of sodium hypochlorite solutions: the 1991 Lindberg Award. J Burn Care Rehabil 1991;12(5):420–4.

174. Fisher RG, Chain RL, Hair PS, et al. Hypochlorite killing of community-associated methicillin-resistant *Staphylococcus aureus*. Pediatr Infect Dis J 2008;27(10):934–5.

175. Paller AS, Mancini AJ. Hurwitz clinical pediatric dermatology. 3rd edition. Philadelphia: Elsevier; 2006.

176. Ryan C, Shaw RE, Cockerell CJ, et al. Novel sodium hypochlorite cleanser shows clinical response and excellent acceptability in the treatment of atopic dermatitis. Pediatr Dermatol 2013;30(3):308–15.

177. Falagas ME, Bliziotis IA, Fragoulis KN. Oral rifampin for eradication of *Staphylococcus aureus* carriage from healthy and sick populations: a systematic review of the evidence from comparative trials. Am J Infect Control 2007;35(2):106–14.

178. Buehlmann M, Frei R, Fenner L, et al. Highly effective regimen for decolonization of methicillin-resistant *Staphylococcus aureus* carriers. Infect Control Hosp Epidemiol 2008;29(6):510–6.

179. Ellis MW, Schlett CD, Millar EV, et al. Hygiene strategies to prevent methicillin-resistant *Staphylococcus aureus* skin and soft tissue infections: a cluster-randomized controlled trial among high-risk military trainees. Clin Infect Dis 2014;58(11):1540–8.

180. Miller LG, Tan J, Eells SJ, et al. Prospective investigation of nasal mupirocin, hexachlorophene body wash, and systemic antibiotics for prevention of recurrent community-associated methicillin-resistant *Staphylococcus aureus* infections. Antimicrob Agents Chemother 2012;56(2):1084–6.

181. Raz R, Miron D, Colodner R, et al. 1-year trial of nasal mupirocin in the prevention of recurrent staphylococcal nasal colonization and skin infection. Arch Intern Med 1996;156(10):1109–12.

182. McNeil JC, Hulten KG, Kaplan SL, et al. Decreased susceptibilities to retapamulin, mupirocin, and chlorhexidine among *Staphylococcus aureus* isolates causing skin and soft tissue infections in otherwise healthy children. Antimicrob Agents Chemother 2014;58(5):2878–83.

183. Johnson JG, Saye EJ, Jimenez-Truque N, et al. Frequency of disinfectant resistance genes in pediatric strains of methicillin-resistant *Staphylococcus aureus*. Infect Control Hosp Epidemiol 2013;34(12):1326–7.

184. McNeil JC, Hulten KG, Kaplan SL, et al. *Staphylococcus aureus* infections in pediatric oncology patients: high rates of antimicrobial resistance, antiseptic tolerance and complications. Pediatr Infect Dis J 2013;32(2):124–8.

185. McNeil JC, Ligon JA, Hulten KG, et al. *Staphylococcus aureus* infections in children with congenital heart disease. J Pediatric Infect Dis Soc 2013;2(4):337–44.

186. Robicsek A, Beaumont JL, Thomson RB Jr, et al. Topical therapy for methicillin-resistant *Staphylococcus aureus* colonization: impact on infection risk. Infect Control Hosp Epidemiol 2009;30(7):623–32.

187. Lee AS, Macedo-Vinas M, Francois P, et al. Impact of combined low-level mupirocin and genotypic chlorhexidine resistance on persistent methicillin-resistant *Staphylococcus aureus* carriage after decolonization therapy: a case-control study. Clin Infect Dis 2011;52(12):1422–30.

188. Simor AE, Phillips E, McGeer A, et al. Randomized controlled trial of chlorhexidine gluconate for washing, intranasal mupirocin, and rifampin and doxycycline versus no treatment for the eradication of methicillin-resistant *Staphylococcus aureus* colonization. Clin Infect Dis 2007;44(2):178–85.

189. Fritz SA, Hogan PG, Camins BC, et al. Mupirocin and chlorhexidine resistance in *Staphylococcus aureus* in patients with community-onset skin and soft tissue infections. Antimicrob Agents Chemother 2013;57(1):559–68.

190. Upton A, Lang S, Heffernan H. Mupirocin and *Staphylococcus aureus*: a recent paradigm of emerging antibiotic resistance. J Antimicrob Chemother 2003; 51(3):613–7.

191. Conly JM, Johnston BL. Mupirocin - are we in danger of losing it? Can J Infect Dis 2002;13(3):157–9.

192. Miller MA, Dascal A, Portnoy J, et al. Development of mupirocin resistance among methicillin-resistant *Staphylococcus aureus* after widespread use of nasal mupirocin ointment. Infect Control Hosp Epidemiol 1996;17(12):811–3.

193. Vasquez JE, Walker ES, Franzus BW, et al. The epidemiology of mupirocin resistance among methicillin-resistant *Staphylococcus aureus* at a veterans' affairs hospital. Infect Control Hosp Epidemiol 2000;21(7):459–64.

194. Batra R, Cooper BS, Whiteley C, et al. Efficacy and limitation of a chlorhexidine-based decolonization strategy in preventing transmission of methicillin-resistant *Staphylococcus aureus* in an intensive care unit. Clin Infect Dis 2010;50(2): 210–7.

195. Mayer S, Boos M, Beyer A, et al. Distribution of the antiseptic resistance genes qacA, qacB and qacC in 497 methicillin-resistant and -susceptible European isolates of *Staphylococcus aureus*. J Antimicrob Chemother 2001;47(6):896–7.

196. McNeil JC, Hulten KG, Kaplan SL, et al. Mupirocin resistance in *Staphylococcus aureus* causing recurrent skin and soft tissue infections in children. Antimicrob Agents Chemother 2011;55(5):2431–3.

197. Cadilla A, David MZ, Daum RS, et al. Association of high-level mupirocin resistance and multidrug-resistant methicillin-resistant *Staphylococcus aureus* at an academic center in the Midwestern United States. J Clin Microbiol 2011;49(1): 95–100.

198. Sheng WH, Wang JT, Lauderdale TL, et al. Epidemiology and susceptibilities of methicillin-resistant *Staphylococcus aureus* in Taiwan: emphasis on chlorhexidine susceptibility. Diagn Microbiol Infect Dis 2009;63(3):309–13.

199. Nabi Biopharmaceuticals announces results of staphvax(r) confirmatory phase III clinical trial. Available at: http://www.prnewswire.com/news-releases/nabi-biopharmaceuticals-announces-results-of-staphvaxr-confirmatory-phase-iii-clinical-trial-55039197.html. Accessed February 20, 2015.

200. Fowler VG, Allen KB, Moreira ED, et al. Effect of an investigational vaccine for preventing *Staphylococcus aureus* infections after cardiothoracic surgery: a randomized trial. JAMA 2013;309(13):1368–78.

201. Sampedro GR, DeDent AC, Becker RE, et al. Targeting *Staphylococcus aureus* alpha-toxin as a novel approach to reduce severity of recurrent skin and soft-tissue infections. J Infect Dis 2014;210(7):1012–8.

202. Cogen AL, Nizet V, Gallo RL. Skin microbiota: a source of disease or defence? Br J Dermatol 2008;158(3):442–55.

203. Reid G, Howard J, Gan BS. Can bacterial interference prevent infection? Trends Microbiol 2001;9(9):424–8.

204. Shinefield HR, Ribble JC, Boris M, et al. Bacterial interference: its effect on nursery-acquired infection with *Staphylococcus aureus*. I. Preliminary observations on artificial colonization of newborns. Am J Dis Child 1963;105:646–54.

205. Shinefield HR, Boris M, Ribble JC, et al. Bacterial interference: its effect on nursery-acquired infection with *Staphylococcus aureus*. III. The Georgia epidemic. Am J Dis Child 1963;105:663–73.

206. Shinefield HR, Sutherland JM, Ribble JC, et al. Bacterial interference: its effect on nursery-acquired infection with *Staphylococcus aureus*. II. The Ohio epidemic. Am J Dis Child 1963;105:655–62.
207. Shinefield HR, Ribble JC, Eichenwald HF, et al. Bacterial interference: its effect on nursery-acquired infection with *Staphylococcus aureus*. V. An analysis and interpretation. Am J Dis Child 1963;105:683–8.
208. Boris M, Shinefield HR, Ribble JC, et al. Bacterial interference: it's effect on nursery-acquired infection with *Staphylococcus aureus*: IV. The Louisiana epidemic. Am J Dis Child 1963;105:174–82.
209. Light IJ, Sutherland JM, Schott JE. Control of a staphylococcal outbreak in a nursery, use of bacterial interference. JAMA 1965;193:699–704.
210. Drutz DJ, Van Way MH, Schaffner W, et al. Bacterial interference in the therapy of recurrent staphylococcal infections. Multiple abscesses due to the implantation of the 502A strain of *Staphylococcus*. N Engl J Med 1966;275(21):1161–5.
211. Blair EB, Tull AH. Multiple infections among newborns resulting from colonization with *Staphylococcus aureus* 502A. Am J Clin Pathol 1969;52(1):42–9.
212. Houck PW, Nelson JD, Kay JL. Fatal septicemia due to *Staphylococcus aureus* 502A. Report of a case and review of the infectious complications of bacterial interference programs. Am J Dis Child 1972;123(1):45–8.
213. Johnson RC, Ellis MW, Lanier JB, et al. Correlation between nasal microbiome composition and remote purulent skin and soft tissue infections. Infect Immun 2015;83(2):802–11.
214. Uehara Y, Nakama H, Agematsu K, et al. Bacterial interference among nasal inhabitants: eradication of *Staphylococcus aureus* from nasal cavities by artificial implantation of *Corynebacterium* sp. J Hosp Infect 2000;44(2):127–33.
215. Gluck U, Gebbers JO. Ingested probiotics reduce nasal colonization with pathogenic bacteria (*Staphylococcus aureus*, *Streptococcus pneumoniae*, and beta-hemolytic streptococci). Am J Clin Nutr 2003;77(2):517–20.

Pitfalls in Diagnosis of Pediatric *Clostridium difficile* Infection

Julia S. Sammons, MD, MSCE[a],*, Philip Toltzis, MD[b]

KEYWORDS

- *Clostridium difficile* • Diagnosis • Diarrhea • Pediatrics

KEY POINTS

- *Clostridium difficile* testing should only be performed in children with diarrhea and prioritized to those with known risk factors for *C difficile* infection (CDI).
- *C difficile* testing is most appropriate in children older than 2 years; for children younger than 2, *C difficile* testing should be pursued only if symptoms persist in the absence of alternative diagnoses or if the clinical presentation is severe or CDI-consistent.
- For otherwise healthy children with diarrhea in the community and no known exposures or risk factors for CDI, *C difficile* testing is likely rarely indicated, particularly if diarrhea is mild.
  - Efforts should be made to remove the inciting agent or identify alternative diagnoses before pursuing testing or treatment.
  - *C diffiicle* testing should be sought only in the child with persistent symptoms despite these interventions and when no alternative pathogens have been identified.

Clostridium difficile is the most common identifiable cause of health care–associated diarrhea in North America and Europe[1,2] and is now the most common health care–associated infection in the United States.[3,4] The pathogenicity of *C difficile* results from expression of 2 homologous enterotoxins labeled toxins A and B, which undermine the integrity of the cytoskeleton of colonic epithelial cells[5]; this in turn produces intense inflammation and often profound and prolonged diarrhea. Strains of *C difficile* that do not encode these toxins do not produce disease. Outside the body, the organisms sporulate, rendering them resistant to many disinfectants and enabling them to survive on inanimate surfaces for prolonged periods of time.[6,7] Inadvertent ingestion of even small numbers of spores, especially in patients with a disturbed colonic microbiome as occurs after antibiotic exposure,[8,9] can result in symptomatic infection.

[a] Division of Infectious Diseases, Department of Infection Prevention and Control, The Children's Hospital of Philadelphia, Perelman School of Medicine at the University of Pennsylvania, Philadelphia, PA 19104, USA; [b] Division of Pediatric Critical Care, Rainbow Babies and Children's Hospital, Case Western Reserve University School of Medicine, Cleveland, OH 44106, USA
* Corresponding author.
E-mail address: sammonsj@email.chop.edu

Infect Dis Clin N Am 29 (2015) 465–476
http://dx.doi.org/10.1016/j.idc.2015.05.010
id.theclinics.com
0891-5520/15/$ – see front matter © 2015 Elsevier Inc. All rights reserved.

Given the prominence of this pathogen and its propensity to spread within closed environments, accurate and expeditious diagnosis is important. However, the diagnosis of CDI in adults is beset with dilemmas, and these are compounded in children. The tests that are available for the diagnosis of *C difficile* infection (CDI) in children are the same as in adults, with similar sensitivities and specificities. However, the diagnosis of CDI in children has a number of pitfalls. Of particular importance is the issue of specificity and the resultant low positive predictive value (PPV; the ratio of true positives to the sum of true positives and false positives) in populations with low CDI prevalence, as is common in many groups of tested children. Furthermore, many persons (particularly young infants) become colonized asymptomatically after exposure to *C difficile* spores, but may excrete detectable quantities of toxigenic *C difficile*, making the interpretation of test results and diagnosis of clinical disease challenging. This leads to the possibility of identifying "biological false positives," where false positivity is not related to the intrinsic characteristics of the test, but to identification of organisms in circumstances in which they are irrelevant clinically. Thus, when used indiscriminately in children, the PPV of *C difficile* tests can be unacceptably low. As a consequence, a falsely positive test may prompt the ordering of isolation precautions and antimicrobial treatment, which are unnecessary and costly and may distract caregivers away from more important alternative diagnoses. This article discusses these issues in detail.

CHANGING EPIDEMIOLOGY OF *C DIFFICILE* INFECTION
Increased Incidence of C difficile Infection

The epidemiology of CDI has changed dramatically in recent years. Between 2000 and 2010, the incidence of CDI more than doubled in adults and CDI-related hospitalizations increased by nearly 300%.[10] The changing epidemiology of CDI is likely multifactorial, owing in part to the emergence of an epidemic strain of *C difficile*, the North American pulsed-field gel electrophoresis type 1 (NAP1) strain, which has been associated with increased morbidity and mortality[11,12] and linked with outbreaks in North America, Europe, and Asia.[1] Increased antibiotic use, growing awareness of CDI among clinicians, and the emergence of highly sensitive detection methods for *C difficile* likely also have contributed to the changing landscape.[13] CDI is now the most common cause of health care–associated infection in the United States, with excess health care costs approaching $5 billion.[3,4,14] Recent data from active population- and laboratory-based surveillance by the Emerging Infections Program in 2011 estimated the number of incident cases of CDI in the United States at 453,000 with 29,300 deaths.[13] These estimates may include some patients with asymptomatic colonization owing to use of a case definition based solely on positive results from *C difficile* stool testing, but signal a significant national burden of disease.

Similar to the findings in adults, several pediatric studies have shown that the incidence of CDI has risen among children[15–21] and CDI is increasingly recognized as an important pathogen among pediatric patients.[17,22] The majority of studies have used administrative data to evaluate the incidence of CDI-related hospitalizations among multicenter cohorts of hospitalized children.[15,17,19] One of the first and largest of these studies evaluated incidence of CDI among 4895 hospitalized children at 22 US children's hospitals using a combination of discharge diagnosis codes and charges for *C difficile* tests and treatment; in this study, Kim and colleagues[15] found an increase from 2.6 to 4 cases per 1000 admissions from 2001 to 2006, whereas the rates of *C difficile* testing remained stable. More recently, data from population-based surveillance of CDI among children in the United States have revealed similar findings.[21,23] Khanna and colleagues[21] performed a population-based cohort study of CDI among children residing in Olmsted County, Minnesota, from 1991 to 2009 and identified an increased incidence of CDI from 2.6 (1991–1997) to 32.6 per 100,000 (2004–2009; $P<.001$) using standard surveillance definitions, although the authors note that the method for *C difficile* testing in stool changed from toxin immunoassay to more sensitive nucleic acid amplification testing methods (NAAT) in 2007.

Increase in Community-Associated Cases

In addition to the increase in the incidence of CDI in general, there has been a concurrent increase in identification of CDI among populations previously believed to be at low risk for disease, namely those in the community or outpatient settings.[24–26] According to recent surveillance by the Emerging Infections Program, more than 300,000 cases of CDI occurred outside of hospitals in 2011, 46% of which were deemed to be community-associated CDI (CA-CDI).[13] Studies in pediatric patients have identified a similar increase in CA-CDI.[18,20,21,23] Using surveillance from the Emerging Infections Program, Wendt and colleagues[20] found that 71% of pediatric CDI identified by positive *C difficile* stool testing arose from the community. As noted, these estimates are limited by reliance on laboratory surveillance, particularly in the era of more sensitive NAAT methods. Still, these findings indicate an important shift in epidemiology and a need for further studies to understand the implications of positive *C difficile* testing in a pediatric ambulatory setting. A study using the same surveillance program in adults suggests that health care exposure may still play a role in CA-CDI; in this study, Chitnis and colleagues[27] found that, although patients with CA-CDI had no documented overnight health care exposures within the prior 12 weeks, 82% reported recent outpatient health care contact during telephone interviews. Given the frequent outpatient health care contact in children, particularly in the first year of life, this finding warrants further investigation in the pediatric population.

AVAILABLE *C DIFFICILE* DIAGNOSTIC TESTS AND THEIR CHARACTERISTICS IN ADULTS AND CHILDREN

For both children and adults, several laboratory tests are available to diagnose CDI. The 2 tests frequently used as "gold standards" are not readily available outside of research settings because they are technically complicated; however, it is against these standards that the performance of the other tests usually is compared. Still, even the gold standard tests are imperfect, because neither unequivocally identifies the patient whose symptoms are owing to *C difficile*; indeed, these 2 tests may yield discordant results in the same stool sample. The first of the standards is cytotoxigenic culture (CC), through which toxin-producing *C difficile* are cultivated from the stool. This technique requires plating and growth in a strictly anaerobic environment on pre-reduced specialized medium. Toxigenicity then is determined by testing the supernatant of subcultured colonies for toxin using one of the assays described elsewhere in this article. CC requires several days to complete, and although it is able to detect the presence of toxigenic organisms even in small quantities of stool or from rectal swabs, it does not identify them categorically as the cause for the diarrhea, because the toxin may be produced in subclinical quantities in vivo. The second gold standard test is the cell cytotoxicity assay (CCTA). Filtrates of the stool specimen are added to cell cultures, one of which is incubated in the presence of antitoxins and the other not. Cytopathic effect detected after 24 to 48 hours in the sample without antitoxin putatively identifies free *C difficile* toxin in the stool. CCTA establishes the association of symptoms to *C difficile* more reliably than CC, because it identifies a surrogate for the biological effect of the toxins, but it may be negative if the concentrations of those toxins are low.

Three additional assays have been introduced that are easier to perform technically and have rapid turnaround time, and thus have supplanted the gold standard tests in many clinical microbiology laboratories. Two of these detect the presence of organism rather than toxin and thus are surrogates for CC. The first of these identifies glutamate dehydrogenase (GDH) by enzyme immunoassay in stool specimens, using monoclonal antibodies specific to *C difficile* GDH. This enzyme is expressed uniformly in high quantities by *C* difficile, but is positive in both toxigenic and nontoxigenic strains. The second assay that identifies the presence of organism is the NAAT noted, which uses the polymerase chain reaction or loop-mediated isothermal amplification to detect genes encoding *C difficile* toxins. The third assay detects free toxin in stool samples by immunoassay ("toxin EIA") and thus is equivalent biologically to CCTA. The toxin immunoassays are easy to perform and until recently they have been the mainstay of *C difficile* diagnosis.

Because diagnostic tests for CDI measure 2 different but related phenomena— the presence of organism (CC, GDH, NAAT) and the presence of toxin (CCTA, toxin EIA)— it is not surprising that they may yield discordant results. Tests measuring the presence of organisms characteristically are more sensitive than those measuring toxin,[28–30] but detection of *C difficile* without detection of toxin frequently reflects *C difficile* colonization rather than disease. Planche and colleagues[31] recently prospectively performed a battery of *C difficile* diagnostic tests, including both gold standard tests, on thousands of mostly adult samples submitted to 4 academic hospitals in the UK, and tested their association with outcome. The 30-day all-cause mortality was significantly higher in patients whose samples were CCTA (and thus toxin) positive (16.6%), than in those who were CC positive but CCTA negative (9.7%, indicating the presence of toxigenic *C difficile* but undetectable toxin) and those in whom neither test was positive (8.6%). Similar results have been derived by other investigators[32,33] (although not by all authors[28,34]). Thus, the 2 classes of tests may have different implications: detection of toxin is likely one of several markers of risk of severe disease, whereas detection of organisms in the absence of toxin may be associated with mild disease or asymptomatic excretion, but nevertheless identifies patients who pose a risk of transmission.[34,35]

In adult samples, the sensitivity of GDH is greater than 90% when compared with culture of *C difficile*, and the sensitivity of NAAT usually is in the 85% to 90% range when compared with CC or CCAT.[36] Sensitivity of toxin EIA generally is much lower,[37] frequently 50% to 80%, and hence has been abandoned recently by many clinical microbiology laboratories as a stand-alone test. The specificities of virtually all of these tests exceed 95%. Published sensitivities and specificities within each class of test are quite variable, however, particularly when 1 commercial test is compared with another. This variability is owing to several factors: (a) the small numbers of specimens that have been used to determine test characteristics, precluding precise measurements, (b) the use of varying gold standards, and the inaccuracies intrinsic in the gold standards themselves,[38] and (c) possible strain–strain variation in test performance.[39–42] In practice, there are additional reasons that may account for variable and sometimes poor performance characteristics. The accuracy of *C difficile* diagnostic tests depends on whether the assay is restricted to liquid stools to reduce the likelihood of detection of colonization,[1] and on the manner of sample handling before testing. Moreover, in the quest to treat a patient with suspected CDI expeditiously, some clinicians may prescribe specific anti–*C difficile* therapy before the specimen being collected for a diagnostic assay. Recently published data in adult patients indicate that metronidazole or oral vancomycin may decrease the diagnostic yield in stool specimens by approximately 15% per day of exposure.[43]

Some authorities have suggested enhancing the performance of *C difficile* diagnostic tests by using a 2-step or even 3-step algorithm.[30] The first step in these algorithms frequently is the GDH immunoassay, because it is inexpensive, has a rapid turnaround, its presence defines a population of samples with a high prevalence of *C difficile*, and its absence has a high negative predictive value across population prevalences ranging between 5% and 50%.[44] This last characteristic allows specimens that are negative for GDH to be reported as negative without further testing. Specimens positive for GDH then are subjected to a second test, namely, toxin EIA or CCTA, to confirm the presence of toxin. The GDH followed by CCTA combination has both biological and logistic appeal, because the second test is the more sensitive assay for toxin and the strategy reserves the complex and expensive CCTA to a relatively small subset of submitted samples.[45] Alternatively, some laboratories unable to maintain the cell culture lines required for CCTA follow a positive GDH assay with NAAT, although positivity of both tests does not guarantee pathologic concentrations of enterotoxin. There is no consensus regarding the ideal testing strategy, however, and a survey of diagnostic laboratories in the UK revealed the use of multiple different *C difficile* diagnostic algorithms.[31]

These tests have not been evaluated extensively in exclusively pediatric samples.[46–48] When they have, the sensitivity and specificity values are similar to those documented for adults, although 1 survey conducted in a large pediatric tertiary care center found an unusually low sensitivity for GDH compared with CCTA (81%).[48] Similar to adult specimens, pediatric stool subjected to different CDI diagnostic tests may yield discordant results; specimens that are positive by NAAT but negative by other tests likewise usually do not reflect CDI-consistent disease[46] and probably represent colonization. Hart and colleagues[47] assessed *C difficile* diagnostic test performances in 150 consecutive pediatric stool specimens and compared these values with those derived in 3 other studies in children. As in adults, toxin EIA had a measured sensitivity of only 35% to 56%. The sensitivity of NAAT was approximately 89%. The specificity of both tests in pediatric specimens exceeded 97%. The addition of the GDH assay as a first test in a multitest algorithm, however, added little to diagnostic accuracy. The combination GDH plus toxin EIA yielded sensitivity of 28% to 71%, similar to that of toxin EIA alone, and GDH plus toxin EIA plus NAAT had a sensitivity of 81% to 89%, similar to NAAT alone; specificity values also were essentially unchanged.

In addition, variation in testing strategies to establish the diagnosis of CDI in children and exclude alternative diagnoses can make longitudinal and interinstitutional comparisons challenging.[49] A survey of pediatric hospital epidemiologists revealed that 13% of respondents reported no restrictions at their institution requiring that *C difficile* testing only be performed on diarrheal stool samples.[49] Similarly, a survey of pediatric infectious diseases physicians showed that although the majority of respondents reported use of NAAT testing at their institution, nearly 10% reported using toxin EIA alone.[50]

CHALLENGES TO ACCURATE DIAGNOSIS OF PEDIATRIC *C DIFFICILE* INFECTION

Although the application of different *C difficile* testing methods can lead to diagnostic difficulties by yielding discordant results, there are additional challenges to the evaluation of CDI in pediatric populations. These issues can be classified into 2 major categories: the issue of low PPV resulting from true false positives in low-prevalence populations, and the concern for "biological false positives," in which the test accurately identifies the presence of *C difficile* or its toxins in children in whom the organism is incidental. Two overlapping populations of children, namely infants and young toddlers and those with community-acquired diarrhea, may have large numbers with biologically false-positive CDI tests.

Low C difficile Infection Prevalence in Many Populations of Children

Regardless of the test, PPV values decrease as the prevalence decreases. As detailed, no CDI test is 100% specific, and a given test's PPV is diminished in populations with low CDI prevalence relative to the test's performance in high prevalence groups. For example, in a group of 100 children with a CDI prevalence of 5% assessed with a test with 97% specificity, the test will be truly positive in 5 children and falsely positive in 3, and thus the PPV = 5/8, or only 62.5%.

In a survey of published articles reporting the performance of C difficile NAAT in adults, the PPV in a population with CDI prevalence less than 10%, 10% to 20%, and greater than 20% was estimated at 71%, 79%, and 93%, respectively.[51] Although prevalence data regarding CDI among pediatric inpatients doubtlessly varies from hospital to hospital and the studied population, common experience and indirect evidence would suggest it is substantially lower than in adults.[52] This is likely the result of the absence of many risk factors for CDI in the general pediatric population, such as significant comorbidities or requirement for prolonged hospitalization or long-term care.[53] That said, this is not apparent in published studies measuring the test characteristics of C difficile diagnostic tests in children. In the review of pediatric CDI test performances by Hart and colleagues[47] the prevalence of CDI that is reported in the tested population ranged from 15% to 30%, similar to that reported in publications assessing C difficile test performance in adults.[36] By contrast, in the assessment of a C difficile toxin EIA test in 2 referral pediatric hospitals, the prevalence (as judged by CC) was only 7%, and the resulting PPV for toxin EIA was accordingly low (64%).[54]

Biologic False Positives Owing to Toxigenic C difficile in Infants

Infants pose a unique challenge in the diagnosis of CDI. Clostridium species are normal commensals in the developing microbiome of the infant colon. Multiple studies performed in the early 1980s showed that toxigenic C difficile colonizes the infant gut at high prevalence.[55–57] Babies hospitalized in neonatal intensive care units are colonized more frequently than healthy infants,[55] but studies performed longitudinally over the first year of life in healthy term infants demonstrate that asymptomatic excretion occurs intermittently throughout.[58] Although the prevalence of C difficile colonization is decreased by nearly one-half in the first year (from 35%–40% during the first month of life to approximately 15% by the 12th month), nearly 10% of infants continue to asymptomatically excrete toxigenic organisms beyond 1 year,[59] and the asymptomatic excretion rates among healthy adults of 1% to 3% are not established until at least age 2 years. Moreover, although standard surveillance definitions for CDI include the documentation of at least 3 unformed stools over a 24-hour period,[1] poorly formed stool is common and intermittent in infants and, thus, the presence of diarrhea is more difficult to use as a discriminating factor.

Despite these issues, CDI testing among infants is common. Some clinical microbiology laboratories refuse to process stool from any infant less than 1 to 2 years of age for C difficile, but many others do. In a recent survey of pediatric infectious diseases physicians, nearly two-thirds of respondents reported no restrictions on C difficile testing by age at their institutions.[50] Likewise, several recent epidemiologic studies show that many infants are diagnosed and treated for CDI.[15,18,60] Analysis of administrative data using a multicenter cohort of hospitalized children showed that CDI-related hospitalizations nearly doubled among infants between 2000 and 2005.[19] More recently, a large population- and laboratory-based surveillance performed by

Wendt and colleagues[20] showed that the greatest incidence of CDI was identified among children in the 1-year-old age group. These data however, cannot distinguish between true disease and asymptomatic carriage.

Still, there are data to suggest that *C difficile* may be pathologic in infants in select circumstances.[61] Although rare, fulminant cases of CDI, including findings of pseudomembranous colitis on autopsy, have been reported among infants.[62–64] In addition, although the study by Wendt and colleagues[20] showed that most CDI cases were clinically mild and severe disease was uncommon, the clinical presentation, disease severity, and outcomes were similar across age groups (including 1-year-olds), suggesting a causative role for *C difficile* in these infants. Furthermore, in the survey of pediatric infectious diseases specialists referenced, respondents differed in their approach to positive *C difficile* test results in infants. When asked to react to a positive *C difficile* test in a preterm infant with frequent diarrhea, multiple antibiotic exposures, and no alternative source identified, 43% reported that they would recommend CDI-directed therapy, indicating that some practitioners consider CDI a viable diagnosis in infants depending on the circumstances.[50] This finding suggests that the diagnosis of CDI in infants remains a controversial topic, even among pediatric infectious diseases specialists.[20] Taken together, the available information suggests that, in most instances, isolation of *C difficile* in an infant represents colonization, that in unusual cases the organism is a true pathogen producing disease similar to adults, but that routine testing in infants should be discouraged.

Biologic False Positives in Community-Associated *C difficile* Infection

The second population in which the presence of *C difficile* may be difficult to interpret is in CA-CDI.[65] *C difficile* has been shown to be particularly problematic for special populations of children, namely those with oncologic disease, transplantation, or inflammatory bowel disease,[66–70] which could manifest in community settings remote from hospitalization owing to the presence of several CDI risk factors. However, the role of CDI in otherwise healthy children in the community is more difficult to define. As described, 2 recent population-based studies of CDI in children[20,21] showed that nearly three-quarters were classified as community associated. Khanna and colleagues[21] utilized standard surveillance definitions and defined CDI based on the presence of diarrhea (3 or more loose stools per day), a positive *C difficile* test, and no other identified cause of diarrhea. However, because there was a disproportionate representation of young infants in these studies, as would be expected given that otherwise healthy children presenting for medical care for diarrhea tend to be young, the population is biased to one known to frequently and asymptomatically excrete toxigenic *C difficile*.

Prior studies evaluating the role of *C difficile* in community-associated diarrhea among otherwise healthy children showed no association between *C difficile* and ambulatory diarrhea.[71–73] In these studies, the organism was more frequently isolated in children without diarrhea than in children with gastrointestinal symptoms. Similar findings were observed in more recent studies. In a study conducted in the emergency department at Seattle Children's Hospital,[74] the odds ratio for isolation of *C difficile* in children younger than 36 months of age who were experiencing diarrhea compared with control children without gastrointestinal illness was 0.6 (95% CI, 0.3–1.3). Although there was a positive association between *C difficile* and diarrhea among children older than 3 years (odds ratio, 4.6; 95% CI, 0.8–27), this difference was not significant.

The association between *C difficile* and diarrhea in otherwise healthy children is confounded further by the common isolation of viruses or other gastrointestinal copathogens in the same stool sample.[75,76] However, the frequency of coinfection in CDI in children has varied from study to study. In the study by Wendt and colleagues,[20] only 3% of those with *C difficile* had other pathogens identified from their stool specimens, although alternatives were not sought systematically. By contrast, a recent study prospectively documenting the etiology of children hospitalized for diarrheal disease in Italy noted that 83% of children found to be *C difficile* positive were coinfected with at least 1 other gastrointestinal pathogen, most commonly rotavirus.[77] Indeed, the degree to which alternative sources for diarrhea are sought are variable, as are the methods used to detect them. In a recent study comparing the yield of standard microbiologic testing to a rapid multiplex PCR platform, an additional pathogen was identified in 65% of samples using the FimArray gastrointestinal panel versus 46% with standard laboratory methods.[78] In studies prospectively evaluating the etiology of community-associated diarrhea in children in general, the frequency in which no pathogen is identified can exceed 50%,[79] raising the possibility that even children in whom *C difficile* has been identified as the sole pathogen may be coinfected with another, albeit undetected, organism.

SUMMARY

The epidemiology of CDI has changed dramatically over the past decade and *C difficile* remains a growing public health concern across North America and Europe. Likewise, the incidence of CDI has increased among children and *C difficile* is increasingly recognized as an important cause of health care–associated diarrhea among pediatric patients. Still, the increased identification of CDI in healthy children in the community and increased testing among infants requires cautious interpretation, given the high prevalence of asymptomatic colonization in young infants and the frequent detection of viruses and other copathogens in stool specimens in these age groups. The significance of CDI among infants as well as the epidemiology of CA-CDI in pediatric patients and the implications of positive *C difficile* testing among healthy children in the community are areas in need of further study.

REFERENCES

1. Cohen SH, Gerding DN, Johnson S, et al. Clinical practice guidelines for *Clostridium difficile* infection in adults: 2010 update by the society for healthcare epidemiology of America (SHEA) and the infectious diseases society of America (IDSA). Infect Control Hosp Epidemiol 2010;31:431–55.
2. Dubberke ER, Wertheimer AI. Review of current literature on the economic burden of *Clostridium difficile* infection. Infect Control Hosp Epidemiol 2009;30:57–66.
3. Miller BA, Chen LF, Sexton DJ, et al. Comparison of the burdens of hospital-onset, healthcare facility-associated *Clostridium difficile* infection and of healthcare-associated infection due to methicillin-resistant *Staphylococcus aureus* in community hospitals. Infect Control Hosp Epidemiol 2011;32:387–90.
4. Magill SS, Edwards JR, Bamberg W, et al. Multistate point-prevalence survey of health care-associated infections. N Engl J Med 2014;370:1198–208.
5. Voth DE, Ballard JD. *Clostridium difficile* toxins: mechanism of action and role in disease. Clin Microbiol Rev 2005;18:247–63.
6. Kaatz GW, Gitlin SD, Schaberg DR, et al. Acquisition of *Clostridium difficile* from the hospital environment. Am J Epidemiol 1988;127:1289–94.
7. Shaughnessy MK, Micielli RL, DePestel DD, et al. Evaluation of hospital room assignment and acquisition of *Clostridium difficile* infection. Infect Control Hosp Epidemiol 2011;32:201–6.

8. Owens RC Jr, Donskey CJ, Gaynes RP, et al. Antimicrobial-associated risk factors for *Clostridium difficile* infection. Clin Infect Dis 2008;46(Suppl 1):S19–31.
9. Seekatz AM, Young VB. *Clostridium difficile* and the microbiota. J Clin Invest 2014;124:4182–9.
10. Steiner C, Barrett M, Terrel L. HCUP projections: *Clostridium difficile* hospitalizations 2011 to 2012. HCUP Projections Report # 2012-01. Rockville (MD): U.S. Agency for Healthcare Research and Quality; 2012.
11. Goorhuis A, Bakker D, Corver J, et al. Emergence of *Clostridium difficile* infection due to a new hypervirulent strain, polymerase chain reaction ribotype 078. Clin Infect Dis 2008;47:1162–70.
12. Loo VG, Poirier L, Miller MA, et al. A predominantly clonal multi-institutional outbreak of *Clostridium difficile*-associated diarrhea with high morbidity and mortality. N Engl J Med 2005;353:2442–9.
13. Lessa FC, Mu Y, Bamberg WM, et al. Burden of *Clostridium difficile* infection in the United States. N Engl J Med 2015;372:825–34.
14. Dubberke ER, Olsen MA. Burden of *Clostridium difficile* on the healthcare system. Clin Infect Dis 2012;55(Suppl 2):S88–92.
15. Kim J, Smathers SA, Prasad P, et al. Epidemiological features of *Clostridium difficile*-associated disease among inpatients at children's hospitals in the United States, 2001–2006. Pediatrics 2008;122:1266–70.
16. Zilberberg MD, Tillotson GS, McDonald C. *Clostridium difficile* infections among hospitalized children, United States, 1997–2006. Emerg Infect Dis 2010;16:604–9.
17. Nylund CM, Goudie A, Garza JM, et al. *Clostridium difficile* infection in hospitalized children in the United States. Arch Pediatr Adolesc Med 2011;165:451–7.
18. Benson L, Song X, Campos J, et al. Changing epidemiology of *Clostridium difficile*-associated disease in children. Infect Control Hosp Epidemiol 2007;28:1233–5.
19. Zilberberg MD, Shorr AF, Kollef MH. Increase in *Clostridium difficile*-related hospitalizations among infants in the United States, 2000–2005. Pediatr Infect Dis J 2008;27:1111–3.
20. Wendt JM, Cohen JA, Mu Y, et al. *Clostridium difficile* infection among children across diverse US geographic locations. Pediatrics 2014;133:651–8.
21. Khanna S, Baddour LM, Huskins WC, et al. The epidemiology of *Clostridium difficile* infection in children: a population-based study. Clin Infect Dis 2013;56:1401–6.
22. Sammons JS, Localio R, Xiao R, et al. *Clostridium difficile* infection is associated with increased risk of death and prolonged hospitalization in children. Clin Infect Dis 2013;57:1–8.
23. Rhee SM, Tsay R, Nelson DS, et al. *Clostridium difficile* in the pediatric population of Monroe County, New York. J Pediatric Infect Dis Soc 2014;3:183–8.
24. Centers for Disease Control and Prevention (CDC). Severe *Clostridium difficile*-associated disease in populations previously at low risk–four states, 2005. MMWR Morb Mortal Wkly Rep 2005;54:1201–5.
25. Centers for Disease Control and Prevention (CDC). Surveillance for community-associated *Clostridium difficile*–Connecticut, 2006. MMWR Morb Mortal Wkly Rep 2008;57:340–3.
26. Centers for Disease Control and Prevention (CDC). Vital signs: preventing *Clostridium difficile* infections. MMWR Morb Mortal Wkly Rep 2012;61:157–62.
27. Chitnis AS, Holzbauer SM, Belflower RM, et al. Epidemiology of community-associated *Clostridium difficile* infection, 2009 through 2011. JAMA Intern Med 2013;173:1359–67.

28. Humphries RM, Uslan DZ, Rubin Z. Performance of *Clostridium difficile* toxin enzyme immunoassay and nucleic acid amplification tests stratified by patient disease severity. J Clin Microbiol 2013;51:869–73.
29. Kaltsas A, Simon M, Unruh LH, et al. Clinical and laboratory characteristics of *Clostridium difficile* infection in patients with discordant diagnostic test results. J Clin Microbiol 2012;50:1303–7.
30. Peterson LR, Manson RU, Paule SM, et al. Detection of toxigenic *Clostridium difficile* in stool samples by real-time polymerase chain reaction for the diagnosis of *C. difficile*-associated diarrhea. Clin Infect Dis 2007;45:1152–60.
31. Planche TD, Davies KA, Coen PG, et al. Differences in outcome according to *Clostridium difficile* testing method: a prospective multicentre diagnostic validation study of *C difficile* infection. Lancet Infect Dis 2013;13:936–45.
32. Baker I, Leeming JP, Reynolds R, et al. Clinical relevance of a positive molecular test in the diagnosis of *Clostridium difficile* infection. J Hosp Infect 2013;84:311–5.
33. Longtin Y, Trottier S, Brochu G, et al. Impact of the type of diagnostic assay on *Clostridium difficile* infection and complication rates in a mandatory reporting program. Clin Infect Dis 2013;56:67–73.
34. Guerrero DM, Chou C, Jury LA, et al. Clinical and infection control implications of *Clostridium difficile* infection with negative enzyme immunoassay for toxin. Clin Infect Dis 2011;53:287–90.
35. Guerrero DM, Becker JC, Eckstein EC, et al. Asymptomatic carriage of toxigenic *Clostridium difficile* by hospitalized patients. J Hosp Infect 2013;85:155–8.
36. Crobach MJ, Dekkers OM, Wilcox MH, et al. European Society of Clinical Microbiology and Infectious Diseases (ESCMID): data review and recommendations for diagnosing *Clostridium difficile*-infection (CDI). Clin Microbiol Infect 2009; 15:1053–66.
37. Planche T, Aghaizu A, Holliman R, et al. Diagnosis of *Clostridium difficile* infection by toxin detection kits: a systematic review. Lancet Infect Dis 2008;8:777–84.
38. O'Horo JC, Jones A, Sternke M, et al. Molecular techniques for diagnosis of *Clostridium difficile* infection: systematic review and meta-analysis. Mayo Clin Proc 2012;87:643–51.
39. Leslie JL, Cohen SH, Solnick JV, et al. Role of fecal *Clostridium difficile* load in discrepancies between toxin tests and PCR: is quantitation the next step in *C. difficile* testing? Eur J Clin Microbiol Infect Dis 2012;31:3295–9.
40. Dionne LL, Raymond F, Corbeil J, et al. Correlation between *Clostridium difficile* bacterial load, commercial real-time PCR cycle thresholds, and results of diagnostic tests based on enzyme immunoassay and cell culture cytotoxicity assay. J Clin Microbiol 2013;51:3624–30.
41. Warny M, Pepin J, Fang A, et al. Toxin production by an emerging strain of *Clostridium difficile* associated with outbreaks of severe disease in North America and Europe. Lancet 2005;366:1079–84.
42. Tenover FC, Novak-Weekley S, Woods CW, et al. Impact of strain type on detection of toxigenic *Clostridium difficile*: comparison of molecular diagnostic and enzyme immunoassay approaches. J Clin Microbiol 2010;48:3719–24.
43. Sunkesula VC, Kundrapu S, Muganda C, et al. Does empirical *Clostridium difficile* infection (CDI) therapy result in false-negative CDI diagnostic test results? Clin Infect Dis 2013;57:494–500.
44. Shetty N, Wren MW, Coen PG. The role of glutamate dehydrogenase for the detection of *Clostridium difficile* in faecal samples: a meta-analysis. J Hosp Infect 2011;77:1–6.

45. Ticehurst JR, Aird DZ, Dam LM, et al. Effective detection of toxigenic *Clostridium difficile* by a two-step algorithm including tests for antigen and cytotoxin. J Clin Microbiol 2006;44:1145–9.
46. Selvaraju SB, Gripka M, Estes K, et al. Detection of toxigenic *Clostridium difficile* in pediatric stool samples: an evaluation of Quik Check Complete Antigen assay, BD GeneOhm Cdiff PCR, and ProGastro Cd PCR assays. Diagn Microbiol Infect Dis 2011;71:224–9.
47. Hart J, Putsathit P, Knight DR, et al. *Clostridium difficile* infection diagnosis in a paediatric population: comparison of methodologies. Eur J Clin Microbiol Infect Dis 2014;33:1555–64.
48. Ota KV, McGowan KL. *Clostridium difficile* testing algorithms using glutamate dehydrogenase antigen and *C. difficile* toxin enzyme immunoassays with *C. difficile* nucleic acid amplification testing increase diagnostic yield in a tertiary pediatric population. J Clin Microbiol 2012;50:1185–8.
49. Kociolek LK, Sandora TJ. National variability in surveillance, testing, and infection prevention for *Clostridium difficile* infection in pediatric populations. Am J Infect Control 2013;41:933–5.
50. Sammons JS, Gerber JS, Tamma PD, et al. Diagnosis and management of *Clostridium difficile* infection by pediatric infectious diseases physicians. J Pediatric Infect Dis Soc 2013;3:43–8.
51. Deshpande A, Pasupuleti V, Rolston DD, et al. Diagnostic accuracy of real-time polymerase chain reaction in detection of *Clostridium difficile* in the stool samples of patients with suspected *Clostridium difficile* infection: a meta-analysis. Clin Infect Dis 2011;53:e81–90.
52. Rutledge-Taylor K, Matlow A, Gravel D, et al. A point prevalence survey of health care-associated infections in Canadian pediatric inpatients. Am J Infect Control 2012;40:491–6.
53. Campbell RJ, Giljahn L, Machesky K, et al. *Clostridium difficile* infection in Ohio hospitals and nursing homes during 2006. Infect Control Hosp Epidemiol 2009; 30:526–33.
54. Toltzis P, Nerandzic MM, Saade E, et al. High proportion of false-positive *Clostridium difficile* enzyme immunoassays for toxin A and B in pediatric patients. Infect Control Hosp Epidemiol 2012;33:175–9.
55. Donta ST, Myers MG. *Clostridium difficile* toxin in asymptomatic neonates. J Pediatr 1982;100:431–4.
56. Larson HE, Barclay FE, Honour P, et al. Epidemiology of *Clostridium difficile* in infants. J Infect Dis 1982;146:727–33.
57. Sherertz RJ, Sarubbi FA. The prevalence of *Clostridium difficile* and toxin in a nursery population: a comparison between patients with necrotizing enterocolitis and an asymptomatic group. J Pediatr 1982;100:435–9.
58. Rousseau C, Poilane I, De Pontual L, et al. *Clostridium difficile* carriage in healthy infants in the community: a potential reservoir for pathogenic strains. Clin Infect Dis 2012;55:1209–15.
59. Jangi S, Lamont JT. Asymptomatic colonization by *Clostridium difficile* in infants: implications for disease in later life. J Pediatr Gastroenterol Nutr 2010;51:2–7.
60. Kim J, Shaklee JF, Smathers S, et al. Risk factors and outcomes associated with severe *Clostridium difficile* infection in children. Pediatr Infect Dis J 2012;31: 134–8.
61. Schutze GE, Willoughby RE, Committee on Infectious Disease, American Academy of Pediatrics. *Clostridium difficile* infection in infants and children. Pediatrics 2013;131:196–200.

62. Adler SP, Chandrika T, Berman WF. *Clostridium difficile* associated with pseudo-membranous colitis. Occurrence in a 12-week-old infant without prior antibiotic therapy. Am J Dis Child 1981;135:820–2.

63. Qualman SJ, Petric M, Karmali MA, et al. *Clostridium difficile* invasion and toxin circulation in fatal pediatric pseudomembranous colitis. Am J Clin Pathol 1990; 94:410–6.

64. Singer DB, Cashore WJ, Widness JA, et al. Pseudomembranous colitis in a pre-term neonate. J Pediatr Gastroenterol Nutr 1986;5:318–20.

65. McDonald LC, Coignard B, Dubberke E, et al. Recommendations for surveillance of *Clostridium difficile*-associated disease. Infect Control Hosp Epidemiol 2007; 28:140–5.

66. Pai S, Aliyu SH, Enoch DA, et al. Five years experience of *Clostridium difficile* infection in children at a UK tertiary hospital: proposed criteria for diagnosis and management. PLoS One 2012;7:e51728.

67. de Blank P, Zaoutis T, Fisher B, et al. Trends in *Clostridium difficile* infection and risk factors for hospital acquisition of *Clostridium difficile* among children with cancer. J Pediatr 2013;163:699–705.e1.

68. Tschudin-Sutter S, Tamma PD, Naegeli AN, et al. Distinguishing community-associated from hospital-associated *Clostridium difficile* infections in children: implications for public health surveillance. Clin Infect Dis 2013;57:1665–72.

69. Pascarella F, Martinelli M, Miele E, et al. Impact of *Clostridium difficile* infection on pediatric inflammatory bowel disease. J Pediatr 2009;154:854–8.

70. Sandora TJ, Fung M, Flaherty K, et al. Epidemiology and risk factors for *Clostridium difficile* infection in children. Pediatr Infect Dis J 2011;30:580–4.

71. Boenning DA, Fleisher GR, Campos JM, et al. *Clostridium difficile* in a pediatric outpatient population. Pediatr Infect Dis 1982;1:336–8.

72. Ellis ME, Mandal BK, Dunbar EM, et al. *Clostridium difficile* and its cytotoxin in infants admitted to hospital with infectious gastroenteritis. Br Med J (Clin Res Ed) 1984;288:524–6.

73. Vesikari T, Isolauri E, Maki M, et al. *Clostridium difficile* in young children. Association with antibiotic usage. Acta Paediatr Scand 1984;73:86–91.

74. Denno DM, Shaikh N, Stapp JR, et al. Diarrhea etiology in a pediatric emergency department: a case control study. Clin Infect Dis 2012;55:897–904.

75. Tang P, Roscoe M, Richardson SE. Limited clinical utility of *Clostridium difficile* toxin testing in infants in a pediatric hospital. Diagn Microbiol Infect Dis 2005; 52:91–4.

76. El Feghaly RE, Stauber JL, Tarr PI, et al. Viral co-infections are common and are associated with higher bacterial burden in children with *clostridium difficile* infection. J Pediatr Gastroenterol Nutr 2013;57:813–6.

77. Valentini D, Vittucci AC, Grandin A, et al. Coinfection in acute gastroenteritis predicts a more severe clinical course in children. Eur J Clin Microbiol Infect Dis 2013;32:909–15.

78. Stockmann C, Rogatcheva M, Harrel B, et al. How well does physician selection of microbiologic tests identify *Clostridium difficile* and other pathogens in paediatric diarrhoea? Insights using multiplex PCR-based detection. Clin Microbiol Infect 2015;21:179.e9–15.

79. Vernacchio L, Vezina RM, Mitchell AA, et al. Diarrhea in American infants and young children in the community setting: incidence, clinical presentation and microbiology. Pediatr Infect Dis J 2006;25:2–7.

New Diagnostics for Childhood Tuberculosis

Silvia S. Chiang, MD[a,c], Douglas S. Swanson, MD[b], Jeffrey R. Starke, MD[a,*]

KEYWORDS

- Childhood tuberculosis • Diagnosis • Drug susceptibility testing
- Interferon-γ release assay • Microscopic-observation drug-susceptibility assay
- Xpert MTB/RIF • Nitrate reductase assay • Line probe assays

KEY POINTS

- Mycobacterial culture, the gold standard for diagnosing tuberculosis, provides microbiological confirmation in only 30% to 40% of childhood pulmonary tuberculosis cases and takes up to 6 weeks to result.
- Conventional drug susceptibility testing requires an additional 2 to 4 weeks after culture confirmation.
- New assays, including Xpert MTB/RIF, have shortened time to microbiological confirmation and drug susceptibility testing results.
- No new assay offers greater diagnostic sensitivity than culture for childhood disease.
- The need for further development and evaluation of new TB diagnostics in children remains.

INTRODUCTION

Recent studies estimate that less than two-thirds of tuberculosis (TB) cases occurring in childhood—defined by the World Health Organization (WHO) as 0 to 14 years of age—are detected worldwide.[1,2] Because TB disproportionately strikes poor, marginalized populations, socioeconomic barriers, such as lack of health care access, lead to underdiagnosis among patients of all ages. However, 2 biological factors exacerbate the problem for children. First, the inability of most children to expectorate complicates sputum collection for microbiological examination. Two simple, inexpensive procedures, gastric aspiration and sputum induction, can circumvent this obstacle,

Disclosures: J.R. Starke serves on Otsuka Pharmaceuticals' Data Safety Monitoring Board for pediatric studies of delamanid.
[a] Section of Infectious Diseases, Department of Pediatrics, Baylor College of Medicine, 1102 Bates Street, Suite 1150, Houston, TX 77030, USA; [b] Division of Infectious Diseases, Department of Pediatrics, University of Missouri-Kansas City School of Medicine, 2401 Gillham Road, Kansas City, MO 64108, USA; [c] Department of Global Health and Social Medicine, Harvard Medical School, 641 Huntington Avenue, Boston, MA 02115, USA
* Corresponding author.
E-mail address: jrstarke@texaschildrens.org

but they require supplies and training that not all health establishments have. A newer alternative is the string test, a 4-hour procedure in which the child swallows a dissolvable capsule containing a string, the proximal end of which has been taped to the child's cheek for retrieval purposes. The string unravels as peristalsis propels the capsule into the stomach, where it collects swallowed sputum. Although well tolerated by children, the string test's efficacy for pediatric diagnosis has not been reported, and its use is limited to children who can swallow pills.[3]

Second, the paucibacillary nature of childhood TB decreases the sensitivities of acid-fast smear microscopy and mycobacterial culture, the traditional tests of microbiological confirmation. Even with rigorous specimen collection and laboratory methods, only 10% to 15% of children with pulmonary TB are smear-positive, and only 30% to 40% of children are culture-positive.[4–6] Microbiological confirmation of extrapulmonary TB is also elusive.[7–10] In the absence of smear- and culture-positivity, physicians make a clinical diagnosis using signs and symptoms, a test of infection (tuberculin skin test [TST] or interferon-γ release assay [IGRA]), exposure history, and radiographic findings. However, the imperfections of the tests of infection, unclear exposure history in high-burden areas, and nonspecific clinical and radiographic findings all introduce uncertainty to the clinical diagnosis.

Another disadvantage of conventional TB diagnosis is the wait time of up to 6 weeks for culture confirmation, followed by another 2 to 4 weeks for drug susceptibility testing (DST). During this delay, patients may receive empiric anti-TB treatment. However, without DST results to tailor therapy, patients with drug-resistant disease may receive suboptimal regimens that exacerbate resistance. In addition, adolescents and adults with inadequately treated or untreated TB may continue to spread infection. Diagnostic delay also postpones contact investigation, which identifies other TB-infected individuals.

In response to these challenges, many new tools have entered the TB diagnostic pipeline (**Fig. 1**). Because most of the world's TB burden falls on resource-poor countries, these technologies ideally should be inexpensive, simple to perform, and able to withstand a variety of environmental conditions. With a focus on the needs of children, this article reviews diagnostics for TB infection, disease, and drug resistance that have come into use in the last 15 years as well as promising candidates currently in development.

FROM CONCEPTUALIZATION TO LARGE-SCALE IMPLEMENTATION

The new diagnostics discussed in this article have reached various stages of the development pipeline (see **Fig. 1**).[11,12] The first stage is the identification of diagnostic needs, followed by the conceptualization of a product to meet these needs. The product is then developed and optimized with feedback from prototype performance evaluations. Then, diagnostic accuracy in adults is evaluated against the existing reference standard. Next, the new assay's cost-effectiveness, ease of implementation, and impact on patient outcome and public health are assessed in programmatic settings. These data inform industry and policymakers, who decide whether to scale up delivery and access. Pediatric studies may be conducted at any stage, but most are performed after large-scale implementation. In other words, policy decisions infrequently consider the interests of children.

Although mycobacterial culture serves as the reference standard for diagnosing TB disease, its low sensitivity in paucibacillary disease limits its utility as a yardstick for evaluating new tests in children. In 2012, an expert panel standardized and published clinical case definitions for childhood intrathoracic TB to increase the rigor and

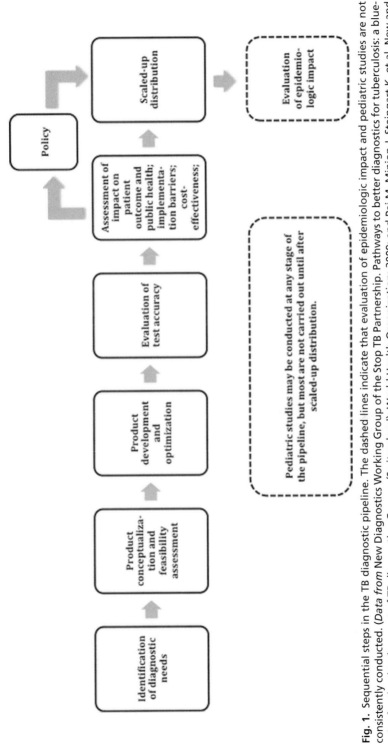

Fig. 1. Sequential steps in the TB diagnostic pipeline. The dashed lines indicate that evaluation of epidemiologic impact and pediatric studies are not consistently conducted. (*Data from* New Diagnostics Working Group of the Stop TB Partnership. Pathways to better diagnostics for tuberculosis: a blueprint for the development of TB diagnostics. Geneva (Switzerland): World Health Organization; 2009; and Pai M, Minion J, Steingart K, et al. New and improved tuberculosis diagnostics: evidence, policy, practice, and impact. Curr Opin Pulm Med 2010;16:271–84.)

comparability of studies with culture-negative cases.[13] Similar research definitions of childhood TB meningitis also were published in 2010.[14] The studies reviewed in this article did not use the standardized definitions because the definitions were published too recently. Instead, the studies used widely varying, ambiguous definitions, leading to difficult-to-interpret results. For this reason, this article discusses only sensitivities and specificities derived from comparison to culture.

APPROACHES TO TESTING

To diagnose an infection, a test can detect either the pathogen or the host response to the pathogen. TB diagnosis is complicated by the need to distinguish between disease—defined by the appearance of signs, symptoms, or radiologic findings (other than calcified Ghon focus) caused by *Mycobacterium tuberculosis*—and latent TB infection (LTBI)—defined by the presence of *M tuberculosis* in the body without these manifestations. Currently available immune-based tests cannot discriminate between LTBI and disease. Conversely, no existing pathogen-based test can diagnose LTBI because the bacterial load in LTBI is small and the organisms are walled off inside lung parenchyma and other tissues.

Pathogen-based diagnostics are divided into genotypic tests, which detect nucleic acid fragments from *M tuberculosis*, and phenotypic tests, which detect whole microbes or their components. The sensitivity of pathogen-based methods depends on bacterial burden and is therefore low in children because of the paucibacillary nature of childhood disease.

DST methods are characterized in 2 ways: first, as indirect or direct, and second, as phenotypic or genotypic. Direct tests are performed on the patient specimen, whereas indirect tests are performed on culture isolates of *M tuberculosis*. Phenotypic DST evaluates the strain's growth or metabolic activity in the drug's presence, whereas genotypic DST detects resistance-conferring mutations. Discrepancies between phenotypic and genotypic DST are incompletely understood but may stem from several factors. First, correlations between certain mutations and treatment outcomes are incompletely understood. Second, because of randomly occurring mutations in drug resistance genes, bacilli sampled from the same patient at different times may have different resistance patterns. Third, in a patient infected with multiple TB strains with distinct resistance patterns, sampling of different strains may account for disparate results.

ASSAYS FOR DETECTING INFECTION
No Reference Standard

The TST, the oldest test of TB infection, has suboptimal sensitivity in immunocompromised individuals and poor specificity in patients with prior Bacille Calmette-Guérin (BCG) vaccination or exposure to nontuberculous mycobacteria (NTM) (**Table 1**). These limitations preclude its use as a reference standard. Therefore, evaluations of new tests of infection use culture-confirmed TB or degree of exposure to a documented source case as surrogate reference standards.

Interferon-γ Release Assays

QuantiFERON-TB Gold (QFT; Cellestis/Qiagen, Carnegie, Australia) and T-SPOT.*TB* (T-SPOT; Oxford Immunotec, Abingdon, UK) are the 2 commercially available IGRAs. In terms of performance, neither test is preferred over the other.[15] QFT uses enzyme-linked immunosorbent assay (ELISA) to measure interferon-γ (IFN-γ) secreted by the patient's T lymphocytes on stimulation with 3 *M tuberculosis*-specific antigens: early secreted antigenic target 6 (ESAT6), culture filtered protein 10 (CFP10), and TB7.7.

T-SPOT use enzyme-linked immunosorbent spot (ELISPOT) to quantify the T lympho-cytes that produce IFN-γ after incubation with ESAT6 and CFP10. Both tests use pos-itive and negative controls; if either control fails, the result is deemed indeterminate (QFT) or invalid (T-SPOT).

Like the TST, IGRAs produce continuous results, and cutoff values are used to inter-pret results as positive or negative (or borderline for T-SPOT). Unlike the TST, each IGRA has only one cutoff value regardless of the patient's exposure history or immune status. Discordance between IGRA and TST results in household contacts of confirmed TB cases have called this lack of risk stratification into question.[16,17] More-over, studies of serially tested individuals at low risk of TB infection have demon-strated conversions and reversions between positive and negative results, particularly when values are near the cutoff.[18–22] These data suggest a need for further refinement of IGRA cutoff values.

Four meta-analyses of pediatric IGRA studies concurred that IGRAs have higher specificity for TB infection than the TST, particularly in settings of low TB burden and among BCG-vaccinated children.[23–26] One meta-analysis estimated pooled specificities of 100%, 90%, and 56% for QFT, T-SPOT, and TST, respectively.[26] This finding is unsurprising because ESAT6, CFP10, and TB7.7 are not found in BCG vaccines or most NTM species.

IGRAs do not offer greater sensitivity than the TST. Sensitivities for both tests range between 62% and 90% for children with culture-confirmed TB disease.[23–26] Further-more, like the TST, IGRAs have poor sensitivity among immunocompromised patients and cannot differentiate LTBI from disease.[27–31]

Of note, a lack of data on IGRA performance in children aged 0 to 4 years has led to hesitancy to use these assays in this age group.[15] In contrast, the TST is routinely used in children as young as 6 months of age (**Box 1**).

Interferon-γ-Inducible Protein 10 Assays

Given the IGRAs' imperfections, other tools have been examined as alternatives for detecting infection. The leading candidate is an assay that uses ELISA to measure IFN-γ-inducible protein 10 (IP-10) levels in whole blood after stimulation with ESAT6, CFP10, and TB7.7. Variable ELISA platforms and cutoff values for a positive result limit the current literature on IP-10 assay performance. However, IP-10 assays appear to be comparable to IGRAs in terms of their accuracy, poor sensitivity in immu-nocompromised patients, and inability to distinguish LTBI from disease.[32–38] Two studies suggested that IP-10 assays outperform IGRAs in children aged 0–4 years,[34,38] but other reports contradicted this finding.[32,36]

Even though IP-10 assays are not more accurate than IGRAs, they may have value. When used in conjunction with IGRAs and the TST, they increase the sensitivity of TB screening.[33,36] In addition, IGRAs require conditions for sample storage, transport, and processing that are difficult to achieve in resource-limited settings. Because IP-10 is secreted in higher quantities than IFN-γ, IP-10 assays lack such stringent re-quirements.[39] Presently, IP-10 assays are not commercially available or recommen-ded for TB diagnosis.

ASSAYS FOR DETECTING THE ORGANISM AND DRUG RESISTANCE
Reference Standards: Mycobacterial Culture and the Proportion Method

Mycobacterial culture, the gold standard for confirming TB disease, has poor sensitivity and a long processing time (**Table 2**). BACTEC (Becton-Dickinson, Franklin Lakes, NJ, USA) and other automated liquid media systems, which capitalize on the capacity of *M*

Table 1
Assays that detect tuberculosis infection

Characteristic	TST	IGRA	IP-10
Current stage in the diagnostic pipeline	Scaled-up distribution globally	Scaled-up distribution in high-income countries	Product development/optimization
Commercially available	Yes	Yes	No
Antigens used	PPD, among many others	ESAT-6, CFP-10, TB7.7[a]	ESAT-6, CFP-10, TB7.7
Sample	Intradermal injection	Blood draw	Blood draw
Patient visits required	2	1	1
Recommended age group	≥6 mo	≥5 y	Unknown
Distinguish between LTBI and TB disease	No	No	No
Cross-reactivity with BCG	Yes	No	No
Cross-reactivity with NTM	Yes	Only 4 species[b]	Only 4 species[b]
Cutoff values for positive result	High risk: 5 mm Medium risk: 10 mm Low risk: 15 mm[c]	QFT: 0.35 IU T-SPOT: 8 spots (5–7 spots is considered borderline)	Not standardized
Causes boosting	Yes	No	No
Subject to boosting by previous TST	Yes	Possible	Unknown
Recommended timing in relation to live virus vaccines	On the same day or postponed for 4–6 wk[d]	On the same day or postponed for 4–6 wk[e]	No recommendation
Difficulties with test reproducibility	Yes	Yes	Unknown

Relative commercial cost	Lower	Higher	Not commercially available
Location of need for trained staff	Clinical	Laboratory	Laboratory
Estimated specificity in BCG-unvaccinated children[f]	95%–100%	90%–95%	Unknown
Estimated specificity in BCG-vaccinated children[f]	49%–65%	89%–100%	Unknown
Estimated sensitivity in immunocompetent hosts[f]	75%–85%	80%–85%	43%–91%[g]
Performance in immunocompromised hosts	Poor	Poor	Poor

Abbreviations: BCG, Bacille Calmette-Guérin; CFP-10, culture-filtered protein 10; ESAT-6, early secreted antigenic target 6; IU, international unit; LTBI, latent tuberculosis infection; NA, not applicable; NTM, nontuberculous mycobacteria; PPD, purified protein derivative; TB, tuberculosis; T-SPOT, T-SPOT.*TB*.

[a] QFT uses all 3 antigens; T-SPOT uses only CFP-10 and ESAT-6.

[b] *M marinum, M kansasii, M szulgai, M flavescens.*

[c] High risk: immunocompromise or household contact with confirmed TB case. Low risk: no TB exposures.

[d] This recommendation from the US Centers for Disease Control and Prevention (CDC) is based on evidence of measles-mumps-rubella vaccine-associated suppression of TST response. Because of theoretic concerns, the CDC has extended this recommendation to varicella zoster vaccine and live-attenuated influenza vaccine.[132]

[e] This recommendation is based on theoretic concerns only. No studies have measured the impact of live virus vaccines on IGRA response.[133]

[f] Using culture-confirmed disease as the reference standard.

[g] The widely variable sensitivities likely result from the lack of a standardized technique and cutoff value.

Data from Starke JR, Committee On Infectious Diseases. Interferon-gamma release assays for diagnosis of tuberculosis infection and disease in children. Pediatrics 2014;134:e1763–73.

Box 1
Recommendations for diagnosing latent tuberculosis infection in children

Low-burden, high-resource settings

IGRAs may be used in lieu of TSTs in children 5 years of age and older who have received BCG vaccine or who are unlikely to return for TST interpretation. In children with previous BCG vaccination, an initial positive TST, and no significant TB risk factors, an IGRA may be used to confirm infection. For children less than age 5, TSTs are preferred, although some experts will use an IGRA in children as young as 2 years old, particularly if they have received BCG and have no significant TB risk factors. Many experts recommend performing all 3 tests (QFT, T-SPOT, and TST) in immunocompromised patients to increase diagnostic sensitivity, especially because these patients have a higher risk of progression from LTBI to disease. Because sensitivities are imperfect, negative results cannot rule out TB and must be interpreted in concert with epidemiologic, clinical, and radiographic data.[15]

High-burden, resource-limited settings

The WHO recommends exclusive use of the TST. There are insufficient data on IGRA performance in resource-limited settings. Second, compared with the TST, IGRAs are more expensive and technically complex to perform. This added strain on LMIC resources is not justified because IGRAs do not increase diagnostic sensitivity.[134]

---

tuberculosis to grow faster in liquid media compared with solid media, have shortened the time to positive culture to 3 weeks but have not increased test sensitivity.

The most commonly used reference standard for DST is the proportion method, a phenotypic, indirect test traditionally performed on Löwenstein-Jensen (LJ) agar (**Table 3**). The use of a liquid media system shortens time to result from 4 weeks to 1 week. The conceptual basis of the proportion method is as follows: because *M tuberculosis* resistance genes have fixed mutations rates, any large population of a single *M tuberculosis* strain will have individual bacilli resistant to a particular antibiotic, even if the strain responds clinically to that drug. Therefore, it is the *proportion* of resistant bacilli that determines whether an antibiotic can be used successfully. To perform the test, a critical concentration of the drug—the amount that inhibits wild-type organisms but not resistant mutants—is placed in the medium. If the proportion of resistant bacilli exceeds 1%, the strain is considered resistant. DST is routinely performed with more than one critical concentration for isoniazid. This practice is clinically significant because higher doses of the drug may overcome low-level resistance.

Of note, the proportion method lacks standardized techniques and interpretations for ethambutol, pyrazinamide, and second-line drugs. Thus, there is uncertainty about the reliability of this—or any other—method for detecting resistance to these drugs.[40]

Microscopic-Observation Drug-Susceptibility Assay

The microscopic-observation drug-susceptibility (MODS) assay is a variation on mycobacterial culture that uses inverted light microscopy to visualize cord formation—an early indication of *M tuberculosis* growth in liquid media. Patient samples are placed in wells with Middlebrook 7H9 broth-based medium and examined daily. Some wells contain antibiotics. The appearance of cords in drug-free wells indicates the presence of *M tuberculosis*, and the concurrent appearance of cords in antibiotic-containing wells indicates resistance.[41]

The MODS assay has performed favorably in large pediatric studies. Among Vietnamese children with a clinical diagnosis of pulmonary TB, the assay was positive in 46%, whereas LJ culture was positive in only 39%.[42] In 2 Peruvian cohorts with microbiologically confirmed TB, 87% to 91% had a positive MODS assay, while only 55% to 59% had a positive LJ culture.[43,44] Moreover, median time to TB detection was only 7 to 10 days for the MODS assay compared with 24 to 32 days for LJ culture.

In the sole pediatric study that evaluated the assay's diagnostic utility for extrapulmonary TB, the MODS assay and LJ culture detected *M tuberculosis* in the same percentage (67%) of cerebrospinal fluid (CSF) samples among children with clinically diagnosed TB meningitis.[42] The MODS assay's accuracy has not been assessed in immunocompromised children, but a meta-analysis of human immunodeficiency virus (HIV)-infected adults showed 88% sensitivity and 98% specificity compared with conventional culture.[45]

Since its inception, the MODS assay has been used for direct detection of isoniazid and rifampin resistance. Most studies have demonstrated 95% to 100% sensitivity and specificity for isoniazid (at the low critical concentration of 0.1 μg/mL) and rifampin.[46] Raising the critical concentration of isoniazid widens the range of sensitivities to 82% to 100%.[46,47] Evaluations of the assay for second-line drugs have yielded sensitivities and specificities of 88% to 100%.[48–51]

Although the MODS assay is appealing because of its high accuracy and low cost, its extensive laboratory requirements have limited its use to reference-level laboratories.[52] The TB MODS Kit (Hardy Diagnostics, Santa Maria, CA, USA), the first commercial MODS assay, addresses this limitation by simplifying the procedure. In an evaluation of more than 2000 sputum samples, the TB MODS Kit performed as well as the conventional assay.[53]

Data from Peru have shown an association between implementation of the MODS assay and reduced rates of treatment failure among adults with multidrug-resistant TB (MDR-TB).[54] No published studies have evaluated the assay's impact on pediatric outcomes.

Xpert MTB/RIF

Xpert MTB/RIF (Xpert; Cepheid, Sunnyvale, CA, USA) uses an automated, cartridge-based polymerase chain reaction (PCR) platform and probes to detect *M tuberculosis* and mutations in *rpoB*, the gene responsible for almost all rifampin resistance. Because Xpert produces results in less than 2 hours and has higher sensitivity than smear microscopy,[55] the WHO committed to a roll-out of 1.4 million cartridges and more than 200 instruments in 21 countries.[56]

A 2013 meta-analysis of 13 studies with greater than 2600 pediatric participants reported 98% or greater specificity for Xpert when evaluated against sputum or gastric lavage culture.[55] However, Xpert's pooled sensitivity was only 66%—higher than smear microscopy but lower than culture—and there was significant heterogeneity.[55] Subgroup analyses revealed the primary source of heterogeneity: Xpert performed better among smear-positive (95%–96% sensitivity) compared with smear-negative (55%–62% sensitivity) samples.[55] This finding again highlights the diagnostic challenge of paucibacillary disease. Further subgroup analyses failed to show a statistically significant difference in the assay's performance in HIV-infected versus HIV-uninfected children (57%).[55] Finally, specimen type—sputum or gastric aspirate—did not affect Xpert's performance.[55]

Few reports have described the diagnostic utility of Xpert for childhood extrapulmonary TB. In a large cohort study that used culture as the reference standard, Xpert

Table 2
Assays that detect *M tuberculosis*

Test	Myco-bacterial Culture	MODS Assay	Xpert MTB/RIF	Phage-Based Assays	TB-LAMP	Urinary LAM	Tr-DNA	Host Gene Expression Signatures	African Pouched Rats	Electronic Noses
Sample type	Any body fluid or tissue	Any body fluid or tissue	Any body fluid or tissue	Sputum[a]	Sputum[a]	Urine	Urine	Blood	Sputum	Sputum and breath
Time to result	≤6 wk[b]	7–14 d	≤2 h	2 d for *FastPlaque* assays	≤1 h	≤30 min for ELISA or lateral flow assay	Estimated ≤1 d; variable[c]	NA[d]	≤1 min	3–15 min, depending on equipment
Phenotypic or genotypic	Phenotypic	Phenotypic	Genotypic	Phenotypic	Genotypic	Phenotypic	Genotypic	Genotypic (host)	Phenotypic	Phenotypic
Simultaneous DST	No	Yes	Yes	Yes	No	No	No	No	No	No
Current stage in diagnostic pipeline	Scaled-up distribution globally	Scaled-up distribution in some countries	Scaled-up distribution in some countries	Evaluation of test accuracy	Evaluation of test accuracy	Evaluation of test accuracy	Product development/optimization	Product development/optimization	Assessment of impact on patient outcome	Product development/optimization
Commercially available	Yes	Yes	Yes	Yes	Yes	Yes	No	No	Yes	Yes

WHO-endorsed	Yes	Yes	Yes	No	No	No	No	No	No	No
Pediatric data	Yes	Yes	Yes	No	No	Yes	Yes[e]	Yes	No	No
Estimated sensitivity for childhood PTB[f]	Reference standard	Reference standard[c]	66%	Unknown	Unknown	2%–48%	Unknown	78%[g]	Unknown	Unknown
Estimated specificity for childhood PTB[f]	Reference standard	Reference standard[c]	≥98%	Unknown	Unknown	61% for lateral flow assay; 96% for ELISA	Unknown	74%[g]	Unknown	Unknown

Abbreviations: AFB, acid-fast bacilli; DST, drug susceptibility testing; ELISA, enzyme-linked immunosorbent assay; LAM, lipoarabinomannan; MODS, microscopic-observation drug-susceptibility; NA, not applicable; PTB, pulmonary tuberculosis; TB-LAMP, tuberculosis-loop-mediated isothermal amplification; Tr-DNA, transrenal deoxyribonucleic acid; WHO, World Health Organization.

[a] Test may be used on other specimen types, but diagnostic utility has been reported only for sputum samples.
[b] Automated liquid culture systems have shortened detection time to 3 weeks or less.
[c] Time to result varies with urine volume, batch size, and processing methods.
[d] Host gene expression signatures have not been adapted for clinical use.
[e] The use of Tr-DNA to diagnose childhood TB has been described in only a single case report.
[f] Compared with mycobacterial culture; MODS is a variation on culture.
[g] Sensitivity and specificity depend on selected RNA expression signature and cutoff value. The values reported here are from one study.[97]

demonstrated sensitivities of 100% and 75% for lymph node tissue and CSF, respectively.[57] In other studies that included children but did not disaggregate pediatric results, sensitivities ranged between 50% and 100% for both CSF and lymph node tissue.[55,58–60]

Compared with reference standards, Xpert's pooled sensitivity and specificity for rifampin resistance are 95% and 98%, respectively.[55] False positive results may stem from the detection of silent *rpoB* mutations that do not affect phenotypic susceptibility.[61,62] Therefore, in countries with low prevalence of rifampin resistance, confirmation of a positive result is recommended (**Box 2**).[63]

The Xpert roll-out has encountered several implementation issues, including inconsistent power supply and high cost.[64,65] Although data have shown Xpert to be cheaper than conventional assays for diagnosing TB in HIV-infected patients and MDR-TB in all patients, the cost of testing all TB suspects is beyond the reach of low-income countries. Randomized trials in Brazil and South Africa have demonstrated an association between Xpert use in community settings and higher rates of microbiological confirmation and faster treatment initiation among adults.[66–68] However, the one study that included children did not show any associations between Xpert use and microbiological confirmation of childhood TB and did not age-stratify data regarding time to treatment initiation.[67] In addition, these trials found no improvements in case notifications, morbidity, and mortality after Xpert implementation.[66–68]

Phage-Based Assays

FASTPlaque TB (Biotec Laboratories, Ipswich, UK) and other phage-based assays use plaque-forming mycobacteria-specific phages to detect the presence of *M tuberculosis*. Phages are added to the sputum specimen, which is then incubated to allow phage infection of and replication within *M tuberculosis* organisms. The subsequent addition of a virucidal solution ensures that no phages remain in specimens that do not contain *M tuberculosis*. The presence of 20 plaques or more after 2 days' incubation indicates a positive result. *FASTPlaque* TB can also detect rifampin resistance,

---

Box 2
Recommendations for diagnosing tuberculosis disease in children

The tools used to diagnose TB in children will vary depending on the patient's clinical situation and the availability of technology. However, some general guiding principles should be followed:

1. All children suspected of having TB should undergo a careful history, including review of possible source cases, physical examination (including growth assessment), test of infection (TST or IGRA), and relevant radiologic examinations if available (eg, chest radiography for pulmonary disease, neuroimaging for TB meningitis). Each of these elements may provide important diagnostic clues.

2. Bacteriologic confirmation should be pursued with culture, which remains the most sensitive diagnostic tool. Nonetheless, molecular methods play an important role in shortening the time to diagnosis, which is particularly important for suspected drug-resistant TB or severe, life-threatening disease. In the case of limited sample volumes, the WHO has strongly recommended prioritizing Xpert MTB/RIF over conventional microscopy and culture in children suspected of having MDR-TB, HIV-associated TB, or TB meningitis. However, there are few data to support this recommendation. When sample volumes are adequate, both culture and molecular testing should be obtained to increase diagnostic yield.[135]

3. In the United States and other countries with low prevalence of rifampin resistance, the detection of rifampin resistance by Xpert should be confirmed with DNA sequencing or phenotypic DST.[63]

indicated by the presence of 20 plaques or more after incubation with the drug.[69] With the original *FASTPlaque* TB, DST could only be performed indirectly from culture isolates, but the newer *FASTPlaque*-Response allows direct DST from patient specimens. As an alternative to plaque visualization, phage-based assays may use genetically engineered luciferase reporter phages, which emit quantifiable light, to signal the presence of *M tuberculosis*.[70]

With greater than 97% specificity, *FASTPlaque* TB detects 75% to 88% of culture-confirmed adult pulmonary TB cases but only 54% to 67% of smear-negative cases.[71–73] For rifampin resistance, *FASTPlaque* TB and other phage-based assays have sensitivities of 81% to 100% and specificities of 73% to 100% compared with traditional DST.[74] No studies have evaluated phage-based assays' accuracy in children or impact on pediatric outcomes.

ADDITIONAL ASSAYS FOR DETECTING THE ORGANISM
Tuberculosis-Loop-Mediated Isothermal Amplification

TB-LAMP (Eiken Chemical, Tokyo, Japan) adapts loop-mediated isothermal amplification (LAMP) technology to detect *M tuberculosis*. TB-LAMP has several features that facilitate its implementation in resource-poor areas: it is fast, isothermal (requiring only a heat block), and immune to inhibitors and reaction conditions that damage other molecular tests. TB-LAMP's few simple steps consist of transferring the patient sample between tubes of pre-prepared reagents and then placing the sample on a warming block for 40 minutes to facilitate amplification. The fluorescent result can be visualized with the naked eye.

The WHO evaluated TB-LAMP's accuracy for diagnosing adult pulmonary TB in 5 countries. Compared with culture, TB-LAMP's overall sensitivity was 78% to 84%. Like Xpert and *FASTPlaque* TB, TB-LAMP has higher sensitivity for smear-positive cases (97%) than for smear-negative cases (62%). In addition, sensitivity was lower in HIV-infected patients. This multisite assessment also uncovered technical issues with TB-LAMP and high rates of operational error in the absence of extensive operator training.[75] The assay was modified in response to these findings, and independent evaluations of TB-LAMP at 14 different sites are currently underway.[76] To date, no pediatric data have been published.

Urinary Lipoarabinomannan

Commercial ELISA kits that detect urinary lipoarabinomannan (LAM), a glycolipid component of the mycobacterial cell wall that is excreted into urine, have become available in the last few years. Urinary LAM showed promise as a diagnostic test for TB in adults with advanced HIV infection.[77–79] However, in a pediatric cohort of more than 500 children, 20% of whom had HIV infection, urinary LAM—detected by ELISA as well as by lateral flow assay—showed poor sensitivity compared with culture (2%–48%), regardless of HIV status. When children with clinically diagnosed TB were added to the analysis, sensitivity did not improve. Specificity of the ELISA and lateral flow assay were 96% and 61%, respectively.[80]

Transrenal Deoxyribonucleic Acid

Transrenal deoxyribonucleic acid (Tr-DNA)—small, cell-free nucleic acid fragments filtered into the urine after release from dying human and microorganism cells—presents another possibility for TB diagnosis. Tr-DNA assays have gained importance in prenatal care and oncology. In preliminary evaluations, the measurement of *M tuberculosis* Tr-DNA has 7% to 79% sensitivity for diagnosing adult disease.

Differences in urine collection, sample storage, and DNA amplification techniques may account for the variable results.[81–88] Efforts are currently underway to refine, standardize, and further evaluate these methods.[89] The only pediatric data on this diagnostic approach come from a case report that described the detection of *M tuberculosis* Tr-DNA in a child with TB otitis media.[90]

Host Gene Expression Signatures

Various studies have used *M tuberculosis*-induced changes in host gene expression to distinguish between patients with TB disease, LTBI, and healthy controls.[91–96] The sole pediatric study compared host gene expression signatures in blood between children with culture-confirmed TB disease, LTBI, and other diseases with similar presentations. For each of the more than 2000 study participants, the investigators generated a risk score that quantified the degree to which the child's expression signature was consistent with TB disease. The investigators then determined a score cutoff that could differentiate between culture-confirmed TB and other diseases with 78% sensitivity and 74% specificity and between TB disease and LTBI with 96% sensitivity and 91% specificity. Accuracy did not differ between HIV-infected and HIV-uninfected children.[97] Although these results are promising, gene expression signatures require further evaluation as a tool for TB diagnosis, particularly among genetically diverse populations. Furthermore, the procedures described in these studies are too costly and time-consuming for routine use; however, identified expression signatures may be adapted to a clinically feasible format.

Volatile Organic Compound Detection

The identification of *M tuberculosis*-specific volatile organic compounds (VOCs) has led to various lines of diagnostic investigation. For more than 5 years, APOPO, a Belgian organization, has been training African giant pouched rats (*Cricetomys gambianus*) to identify *M tuberculosis*-containing sputum samples by smell. The rats, who are resistant to TB, work in specially designed cages with sniffing holes, under which sputum samples are placed. The rats have been trained to indicate a positive sample by keeping their nose in the corresponding sniffing hole for 5 seconds. In contrast, they linger for less than a second in sniffing holes with negative samples.[98] (Videos of the rats at work are available at www.youtube.com/user/apopovideos.) The rats identify *M tuberculosis*-infected sputum with 87% sensitivity and 89% specificity. In a programmatic setting, the evaluation of sputum samples by trained rats increased early case detection by greater than 40%.[99,100] Further work has shown that the rats detect diverse *M tuberculosis* genotypes and differentiate between *M tuberculosis* and NTM with high accuracy (80% sensitivity, 72% specificity).[101,102]

Electronic noses (e-noses), instruments composed of chemical sensors that measure VOCs, are also undergoing development and evaluation as TB breath and sputum tests. Various e-noses are available commercially. Preliminary studies have demonstrated widely variable sensitivities (68%–96%) and specificities (67%–99%); this variability is likely related to differences in instruments and techniques.[103–107] Pediatric-specific data and results from gastric aspirates have not been reported for the rats or e-noses.

ADDITIONAL ASSAYS FOR DETECTING DRUG RESISTANCE
Nitrate Reductase (Griess) Assay

The nitrate reductase colorimetric assay (NRA), also known as the Griess assay, is based on the ability of *M tuberculosis* to reduce nitrate to nitrite; this reaction produces a color change in the presence of the Griess reagent. To perform the assay, the patient

Table 3
Assays that detect drug resistance

Test	Proportion Method	MODS Assay	Xpert MTB/RIF	Phage-Based Assays	LiPA	Griess Assay	PSQ	WGS
Sample type	Any body fluid or tissue	Any body fluid or tissue	Any body fluid or tissue	Sputum[a]	Sputum[a]	Sputum[a]	Sputum[a]	Sputum[a]
Time to result[b]	2–4 wk	7–14 d	<2 h	2 d	1–2 d	<2 wk	Estimated 5–6 h; variable[c]	Estimated 2 d; variable[c]
Phenotypic or genotypic	Phenotypic	Phenotypic	Genotypic	Phenotypic	Genotypic	Phenotypic	Genotypic	Genotypic
Direct or indirect	Indirect	Indirect	Indirect	Both	Both	Both	Both	Indirect
Commercially available	Yes	Yes	Yes	Yes	Yes	No	No	No
Current stage in diagnostic pipeline	Not applicable	Scaled-up distribution in some countries	Scaled-up distribution in some countries	Evaluation of test accuracy	Scaled-up distribution in some countries	Scaled-up distribution in some countries	Product development/ optimization	Product development/ optimization
WHO endorsed	Yes	Yes	Yes	No	Yes	Yes	No	No
Pediatric data	Yes	Yes	Yes	No	No	No	No	No
Sensitivity for isoniazid resistance[d]	Reference standard	82%–100%	NA	NA	57%–100%	96%	89%–94%	Unknown
Specificity for isoniazid resistance[d]	Reference standard	95%–100%	NA	NA	>99%	99%	96%–100%	Unknown
Sensitivity for rifampin resistance[d]	Reference standard	95%–100%	95%	81%–100%	>98%	97%	95%–96%	Unknown
Specificity for rifampin resistance[d]	Reference standard	95%–100%	98%	73%–100%	>98%	100%	100%	Unknown

Abbreviations: LiPA, line probe assay; MODS, microscopic-observation drug-susceptibility; NA, not applicable; PSQ, pyrosequencing; WGS, whole genome sequencing; WHO, World Health Organization.

[a] Test may be used on other specimen types, but diagnostic utility has been reported only for sputum samples.
[b] For indirect tests, time to result does not include time to positive culture.
[c] Time to result varies with assay design and laboratory conditions.
[d] Compared with the proportional method.

sample is placed in culture medium containing potassium nitrate and an antibiotic. If the addition of the Griess reagent produces a color change, the M tuberculosis strain is resistant to the antibiotic present in the medium. The NRA can be used on patient specimens or culture isolates. As a direct test, the assay produces results in less than 2 weeks; as an indirect test, it provides no time reduction compared with conventional techniques.

A recent meta-analysis showed pooled sensitivities and specificities of 96% and 99% for isoniazid resistance and 97% and 100% for rifampin resistance, respectively, compared with traditional DST. There was no significant heterogeneity. Although pooled specificities for ethambutol and streptomycin resistance were also high, pooled sensitivities were lower (90% for ethambutol, 82% for streptomycin), and there was significant heterogeneity.[108] The NRA recently has been evaluated for ofloxacin and kanamycin resistance; early evaluations have shown sensitivities, specificities, and accuracies of 95% to 100% compared with conventional DST.[109,110] No studies have examined the assay's utility in childhood TB.

The impact of the NRA on patient outcomes has been evaluated in Peru, where the test has been standardized at the district level to screen smear-positive samples from patients with no history of MDR-TB. NRA implementation was associated with statistically significant but modest improvements in treatment outcome and survival. This evaluation did not include children.[111]

Line Probe Assays

Line probe assays (LiPAs) use PCR to isolate and amplify genes that confer drug resistance. The PCR products subsequently hybridize to oligonucleotide probes immobilized on a strip. The appearance of colored bands on the strip indicates the capture of the hybrids. LiPAs, which can be performed on patient samples or culture isolates, produce results in one to 2 days. GenoType MTBDR (Hain Lifesciences, Nehren, Germany), the original model in the widely used GenoType series, detects mutations in rpoB and katG, the latter conferring high-level isoniazid resistance. The second-generation assay, GenoType MTBDRplus, detects mutations in rpoB, katG, and inhA; inhA is responsible for low-level isoniazid resistance. The newest version, GenoTypeMTBDRsl, detects mutations in gyrA, rrs, and embB—which confer resistance to fluoroquinolones, second-line injectable drugs (amikacin, kanamycin, and capreomycin), and ethambutol, respectively. Like Xpert, LiPAs may report falsely positive results with silent mutations.

A meta-analysis of GenoType MTBDR and GenoType MTBDRplus showed pooled sensitivity and specificity estimates of greater than 98% with no significant heterogeneity for rifampin resistance. For isoniazid resistance, specificity was also consistently high (pooled estimate >99%), but sensitivity varied between 57% and 100%. When GenoType MTBDRplus performance was isolated and analyzed, the sensitivity for isoniazid DST improved to nearly 90%.[112] For fluoroquinolone resistance, GenoType MTBDRsl had a pooled sensitivity of 83% and a pooled specificity of 98% compared with conventional DST. Pooled sensitivities for amikacin, kanamycin, and capreomycin were 88%, 67%, and 80%, respectively. Specificities ranged between 95% and 100%.[113] In general, genotypic methods, including GenoType MTBDRsl, have low sensitivity for ethambutol resistance.[114]

The high accuracy and speed of LiPAs for first-line DST led the WHO to endorse their use in 2008 and facilitate their implementation and distribution in high TB-burden countries. LiPA implementation has been associated with decreased time to treatment initiation and lower lost-to-follow-up rates among MDR-TB patients.[115,116] However, no changes in time to culture conversion or treatment outcome have been reported.[116] In addition, no pediatric-specific data have been published.

DNA Sequencing

Unlike Xpert and LiPAs, which use probes to detect a set number of resistance-conferring mutations fixed a priori into the product design, sequencing platforms can identify all possible mutations in target genes and be rapidly adapted to add more genes. Sequencing can also distinguish between silent and phenotypically significant mutations.

Pyrosequencing (PSQ), which quantifies the pyrophosphate released during DNA synthesis to identify the type and number of incorporated nucleotides, has been used to sequence resistance-conferring M tuberculosis genes from both culture isolates and patient samples. Compared with conventional DST, PSQ has demonstrated 89% to 94% sensitivity and 96% to 100% specificity for isoniazid; 95% to 96% sensitivity and 100% specificity for rifampin; 61% sensitivity and 85% specificity for ethambutol; 87% to 93% sensitivity and 100% specificity for fluoroquinolones; and 68% to 88% sensitivity and 97% to 100% specificity for second-line injectable agents.[62,117–119] Of note, Sanger sequencing, which uses a different technology, offers comparable sensitivities and specificities, but PSQ, an easier and shorter procedure, is more suitable for high-throughput processing.[117,118]

Whole genome sequencing (WGS) has emerged as another strategy for DST. WGS has been performed successfully on culture isolates but not sputum samples. Although PSQ examines only certain genes associated with resistance, WGS characterizes the entire genome and offers the possibility of discovering new resistance-conferring mutations. To date, the clinical utility of WGS has been described in only a few cases in which WGS allowed faster diagnosis of extensive drug resistance compared with conventional DST.[120,121]

The high cost of sequencing and the advanced expertise required preclude its use in most TB-prevalent settings. Future studies should further characterize the clinical utility of sequencing methods—including in children—and explore ways to make these techniques accessible for resource-limited countries.

SUMMARY

Despite recent advances in TB diagnostics, many pediatric-specific needs remain. First, none of the new assays has improved on the low sensitivity of mycobacterial culture for confirming clinical pediatric TB disease. Although the paucibacillary nature of childhood TB limits the sensitivity of pathogen-based detection methods, work in TB immunology has identified a burgeoning number of biomarkers of host response. Some of these biomarkers—such as multicytokine transcription profiles, microRNA, and the aforementioned RNA expression signatures—may serve to diagnose TB infection and disease more accurately.[91–97,122–126]

Second, given the challenges of sputum collection in children, new diagnostic tools should ideally use easily obtained specimens such as urine, saliva, stool, or blood. Nonetheless, the accuracy of sputum-based tests should be more thoroughly evaluated in children. Assessments of the string test's value for childhood TB diagnosis are also needed.

Third, the WHO has endorsed MODS, Xpert, and LiPAs for use in high TB-burden countries, yet with the exception of one study (which did not show associations between Xpert use and microbiological confirmation of childhood TB), the impact of these tests on pediatric outcomes has never been reported.[67] Future studies should evaluate new diagnostic tools for both accuracy and their effect on the disease course in children. Studies that include both children and adults should report disaggregated pediatric data.

Fourth, the development, validation, and distribution of a sensitive diagnostic test for childhood TB may be years away. In the meantime, many pediatric cases can be diagnosed clinically using history of TB exposure, signs and symptoms, physical examination, tests of infection, and chest radiography. Nevertheless, because of inadequate training, front-line providers often lack basic knowledge about childhood TB signs and symptoms and the ability to interpret pediatric films.[127–130] Operational research, health system improvements, and health care worker training may help optimize existing tools.

Finally, of the $67.8 million US dollars spent globally on TB diagnostic research and development in 2013, only $2.5 million were explicitly allocated to pediatrics despite the greater difficulty of confirming childhood disease.[131] This funding discrepancy reflects the low priority placed on childhood TB and explains why diagnostic advances in children lag behind those in adults. On a brighter note, total spending for childhood TB research and development has increased since 2010, and the amount doubled between 2012 and 2013, suggesting that donors increasingly recognize the importance of this work.[131]

Childhood TB has been trapped in a cycle of invisibility: diagnostic challenges have contributed to the underestimation of its epidemiologic impact, which has led to lower prioritization by funders, researchers, and public health programs. In turn, insufficient research and public health efforts have compromised pediatric case detection. Fortunately, the cycle shows signs of breaking because of recent increases in childhood TB advocacy and research. This momentum must be sustained in order to harness the financial and political commitments necessary for truly revolutionary advances in childhood TB diagnosis.

REFERENCES

1. Dodd PJ, Gardiner E, Coghlan R, et al. Burden of childhood tuberculosis in 22 high-burden countries: a mathematical modelling study. Lancet Glob Health 2014;2:e453–9 (systematic review and meta-analyses).
2. Jenkins HE, Tolman AW, Yuen CM, et al. Incidence of multidrug-resistant tuberculosis disease in children: systematic review and global estimates. Lancet 2014;383:1572–9 (systematic review and meta-analyses).
3. Chow F, Espiritu N, Gilman RH, et al. La cuerda dulce–a tolerability and acceptability study of a novel approach to specimen collection for diagnosis of paediatric pulmonary tuberculosis. BMC Infect Dis 2006;6:67.
4. Starke JR, Taylor-Watts KT. Tuberculosis in the pediatric population of Houston, Texas. Pediatrics 1989;84:28–35.
5. Iriso R, Mudido PM, Karamagi C, et al. The diagnosis of childhood tuberculosis in an HIV-endemic setting and the use of induced sputum. Int J Tuberc Lung Dis 2005;9:716–26.
6. Zar HJ, Hanslo D, Apolles P, et al. Induced sputum versus gastric lavage for microbiological confirmation of pulmonary tuberculosis in infants and young children: a prospective study. Lancet 2005;365:130–4.
7. Chiang SS, Khan FA, Milstein MB, et al. Treatment outcomes of childhood tuberculous meningitis: a systematic review and meta-analysis. Lancet Infect Dis 2014;14:947–57 (systematic review and meta-analyses).
8. Blount RJ, Tran B, Jarlsberg LG, et al. Childhood tuberculosis in northern Viet Nam: a review of 103 cases. PLoS One 2014;9:e97267.
9. Fanny ML, Beyam N, Gody JC, et al. Fine-needle aspiration for diagnosis of tuberculous lymphadenitis in children in Bangui, Central African Republic. BMC Pediatr 2012;12:191.

10. Wu XR, Yin QQ, Jiao AX, et al. Pediatric tuberculosis at Beijing Children's Hospital: 2002-2010. Pediatrics 2012;130:e1433–40.
11. New Diagnostics Working Group of the Stop TB Partnership. Pathways to better diagnostics for tuberculosis: a blueprint for the development of TB diagnostics. Geneva (Switzerland): World Health Organization; 2009.
12. Pai M, Minion J, Steingart K, et al. New and improved tuberculosis diagnostics: evidence, policy, practice, and impact. Curr Opin Pulm Med 2010;16:271–84.
13. Graham SM, Ahmed T, Amanullah F, et al. Evaluation of tuberculosis diagnostics in children: 1. Proposed clinical case definitions for classification of intrathoracic tuberculosis disease. Consensus from an expert panel. J Infect Dis 2012; 205(Suppl 2):S199–208.
14. Marais S, Thwaites G, Schoeman JF, et al. Tuberculous meningitis: a uniform case definition for use in clinical research. Lancet Infect Dis 2010;10:803–12.
15. Starke JR, Committee On Infectious Diseases. Interferon-gamma release assays for diagnosis of tuberculosis infection and disease in children. Pediatrics 2014; 134:e1763–73.
16. Ribeiro-Rodrigues R, Kim S, Coelho da Silva FD, et al. Discordance of tuberculin skin test and interferon gamma release assay in recently exposed household contacts of pulmonary TB cases in Brazil. PLoS One 2014;9:e96564.
17. Machado A Jr, Emodi K, Takenami I, et al. Analysis of discordance between the tuberculin skin test and the interferon-gamma release assay. Int J Tuberc Lung Dis 2009;13:446–53.
18. Mancuso JD, Bernardo J, Mazurek GH. The elusive "gold" standard for detecting Mycobacterium tuberculosis infection. Am J Respir Crit Care Med 2013;187: 122–4.
19. Metcalfe JZ, Cattamanchi A, McCulloch CE, et al. Test variability of the QuantiFERON-TB gold in-tube assay in clinical practice. Am J Respir Crit Care Med 2013;187:206–11.
20. Pai M, Dheda K, Cunningham J, et al. T-cell assays for the diagnosis of latent tuberculosis infection: moving the research agenda forward. Lancet Infect Dis 2007;7:428–38.
21. Zwerling A, Benedetti A, Cojocariu M, et al. Repeat IGRA testing in Canadian health workers: conversions or unexplained variability? PLoS One 2013;8: e54748.
22. Veerapathran A, Joshi R, Goswami K, et al. T-cell assays for tuberculosis infection: deriving cut-offs for conversions using reproducibility data. PLoS One 2008;3:e1850.
23. Chiappini E, Accetta G, Bonsignori F, et al. Interferon-gamma release assays for the diagnosis of Mycobacterium tuberculosis infection in children: a systematic review and meta-analysis. Int J Immunopathol Pharmacol 2012;25:557–64 (systematic review and meta-analyses).
24. Machingaidze S, Wiysonge CS, Gonzalez-Angulo Y, et al. The utility of an interferon gamma release assay for diagnosis of latent tuberculosis infection and disease in children: a systematic review and meta-analysis. Pediatr Infect Dis J 2011;30:694–700 (systematic review and meta-analyses).
25. Mandalakas AM, Detjen AK, Hesseling AC, et al. Interferon-gamma release assays and childhood tuberculosis: systematic review and meta-analysis. Int J Tuberc Lung Dis 2011;15:1018–32 (systematic review and meta-analyses).
26. Sun L, Xiao J, Miao Q, et al. Interferon gamma release assay in diagnosis of pediatric tuberculosis: a meta-analysis. FEMS Immunol Med Microbiol 2011;63: 165–73.

27. Mandalakas AM, Hesseling AC, Chegou NN, et al. High level of discordant IGRA results in HIV-infected adults and children. Int J Tuberc Lung Dis 2008; 12:417–23.
28. Mandalakas AM, van Wyk S, Kirchner HL, et al. Detecting tuberculosis infection in HIV-infected children: a study of diagnostic accuracy, confounding and interaction. Pediatr Infect Dis J 2013;32:e111–8.
29. Stefan DC, Dippenaar A, Detjen AK, et al. Interferon-gamma release assays for the detection of Mycobacterium tuberculosis infection in children with cancer. Int J Tuberc Lung Dis 2010;14:689–94.
30. Cattamanchi A, Smith R, Steingart KR, et al. Interferon-gamma release assays for the diagnosis of latent tuberculosis infection in HIV-infected individuals: a systematic review and meta-analysis. J Acquir Immune Defic Syndr 2011;56: 230–8 (systematic review and meta-analyses).
31. Santin M, Munoz L, Rigau D. Interferon-gamma release assays for the diagnosis of tuberculosis and tuberculosis infection in HIV-infected adults: a systematic review and meta-analysis. PLoS One 2012;7:e32482 (systematic review and meta-analyses).
32. Holm LL, Rose MV, Kimaro G, et al. A comparison of interferon-gamma and IP-10 for the diagnosis of tuberculosis. Pediatrics 2014;134:e1568–75.
33. Latorre I, Diaz J, Mialdea I, et al. IP-10 is an accurate biomarker for the diagnosis of tuberculosis in children. J Infect 2014;69:590–9.
34. Lighter J, Rigaud M, Huie M, et al. Chemokine IP-10: an adjunct marker for latent tuberculosis infection in children. Int J Tuberc Lung Dis 2009;13:731–6.
35. Ruhwald M, Aabye MG, Ravn P. IP-10 release assays in the diagnosis of tuberculosis infection: current status and future directions. Expert Rev Mol Diagn 2012;12:175–87.
36. Ruhwald M, Petersen J, Kofoed K, et al. Improving T-cell assays for the diagnosis of latent TB infection: potential of a diagnostic test based on IP-10. PLoS One 2008;3:e2858.
37. Whittaker E, Gordon A, Kampmann B. Is IP-10 a better biomarker for active and latent tuberculosis in children than IFNgamma? PLoS One 2008;3:e3901.
38. Alsleben N, Ruhwald M, Russmann H, et al. Interferon-gamma inducible protein 10 as a biomarker for active tuberculosis and latent tuberculosis infection in children: a case-control study. Scand J Infect Dis 2012;44:256–62.
39. Aabye MG, Latorre I, Diaz J, et al. Dried plasma spots in the diagnosis of tuberculosis: IP-10 release assay on filter paper. Eur Respir J 2013;42:495–503.
40. World Health Organization. Policy guidance on drug-susceptibility testing (DST) of second-line antituberculosis drugs. Geneva (Switzerland): World Health Organization; 2008.
41. MODS: a user guide. 2008. Available at: http://www.modsperu.org/MODS_user_guide.pdf. Accessed February 14, 2015.
42. Tran ST, Renschler JP, Le HT, et al. Diagnostic accuracy of microscopic Observation Drug Susceptibility (MODS) assay for pediatric tuberculosis in Hanoi, Vietnam. PLoS One 2013;8:e72100.
43. Oberhelman RA, Soto-Castellares G, Caviedes L, et al. Improved recovery of Mycobacterium tuberculosis from children using the microscopic observation drug susceptibility method. Pediatrics 2006;118:e100–6.
44. Oberhelman RA, Soto-Castellares G, Gilman RH, et al. Diagnostic approaches for paediatric tuberculosis by use of different specimen types, culture methods, and PCR: a prospective case-control study. Lancet Infect Dis 2010;10:612–20.

45. Wikman-Jorgensen P, Llenas-Garcia J, Hobbins M, et al. Microscopic observation drug susceptibility assay for the diagnosis of TB and MDR-TB in HIV-infected patients: a systematic review and meta-analysis. Eur Respir J 2014; 44:973–84 (systematic review and meta-analyses).
46. Minion J, Leung E, Menzies D, et al. Microscopic-observation drug susceptibility and thin layer agar assays for the detection of drug resistant tuberculosis: a systematic review and meta-analysis. Lancet Infect Dis 2010;10:688–98 (systematic review and meta-analyses).
47. Makamure B, Mhaka J, Makumbirofa S, et al. Microscopic-observation drug-susceptibility assay for the diagnosis of drug-resistant tuberculosis in Harare, Zimbabwe. PLoS One 2013;8:e55872.
48. Fitzwater SP, Sechler GA, Jave O, et al. Second-line anti-tuberculosis drug concentrations for susceptibility testing in the MODS assay. Eur Respir J 2013;41: 1163–71.
49. Trollip AP, Moore D, Coronel J, et al. Second-line drug susceptibility breakpoints for Mycobacterium tuberculosis using the MODS assay. Int J Tuberc Lung Dis 2014;18:227–32.
50. Huang Z, Li G, Chen J, et al. Evaluation of MODS assay for rapid detection of Mycobacterium tuberculosis resistance to second-line drugs in a tertiary care tuberculosis hospital in China. Tuberculosis (Edinb) 2014;94:506–10.
51. Huang Z, Qin C, Du J, et al. Evaluation of the microscopic observation drug susceptibility assay for the rapid detection of MDR-TB and XDR-TB in China: a prospective multicentre study. J Antimicrob Chemother 2015;70:456–62.
52. World Health Organization. Noncommercial culture and drug-susceptibility testing methods for screening patients at risk for multidrug-resistant tuberculosis: policy statement. Geneva (Switzerland): World Health Organization; 2011.
53. Martin L, Coronel J, Faulx D, et al. A field evaluation of the Hardy TB MODS Kit for the rapid phenotypic diagnosis of tuberculosis and multi-drug resistant tuberculosis. PLoS One 2014;9:e107258.
54. Mendoza-Ticona EA, Alarcón V, Bissell K, et al. Effect of universal MODS access on pulmonary tuberculosis treatment outcomes in new patients in Peru. Public Health Action 2014;2:162–7.
55. World Health Organization. Xpert MTB/RIF assay for the diagnosis of pulmonary and extrapulmonary TB in adults and children. Policy update. Geneva (Switzerland): World Health Organization; 2013 (systematic review and meta-analyses).
56. TBXpert Project. Available at: http://www.who.int/tb/publications/TBXpert_briefing_note.pdf?ua=1. Accessed February 15, 2015.
57. Tortoli E, Russo C, Piersimoni C, et al. Clinical validation of Xpert MTB/RIF for the diagnosis of extrapulmonary tuberculosis. Eur Respir J 2012;40:442–7.
58. Vadwai V, Boehme C, Nabeta P, et al. Xpert MTB/RIF: a new pillar in diagnosis of extrapulmonary tuberculosis? J Clin Microbiol 2011;49:2540–5.
59. Scott LE, Beylis N, Nicol M, et al. Diagnostic accuracy of Xpert MTB/RIF for extrapulmonary tuberculosis specimens: establishing a laboratory testing algorithm for South Africa. J Clin Microbiol 2014;52:1818–23.
60. Ligthelm LJ, Nicol MP, Hoek KG, et al. Xpert MTB/RIF for rapid diagnosis of tuberculous lymphadenitis from fine-needle-aspiration biopsy specimens. J Clin Microbiol 2011;49:3967–70.
61. Mathys V, van de Vyvere M, de Droogh E, et al. False-positive rifampicin resistance on Xpert(R) MTB/RIF caused by a silent mutation in the rpoB gene. Int J Tuberc Lung Dis 2014;18:1255–7.

62. Ajbani K, Lin SY, Rodrigues C, et al. Evaluation of pyrosequencing for detecting extensively drug-resistant Mycobacterium tuberculosis among clinical isolates from four high-burden countries. Antimicrob Agents Chemother 2015;59: 414–20.

63. Centers for Disease Control and Prevention. Availability of an assay for detecting Mycobacterium tuberculosis, including rifampin-resistant strains, and considerations for its use - United States, 2013. MMWR Morb Mortal Wkly Rep 2013;62:821–7.

64. Creswell J, Codlin AJ, Andre E, et al. Results from early programmatic implementation of Xpert MTB/RIF testing in nine countries. BMC Infect Dis 2014;14:2.

65. Pantoja A, Fitzpatrick C, Vassall A, et al. Xpert MTB/RIF for diagnosis of tuberculosis and drug-resistant tuberculosis: a cost and affordability analysis. Eur Respir J 2013;42:708–20.

66. Cox HS, Mbhele S, Mohess N, et al. Impact of Xpert MTB/RIF for TB diagnosis in a primary care clinic with high TB and HIV prevalence in South Africa: a pragmatic randomised trial. PLoS Med 2014;11:e1001760.

67. Durovni B, Saraceni V, van den Hof S, et al. Impact of replacing smear microscopy with Xpert MTB/RIF for diagnosing tuberculosis in Brazil: a stepped-wedge cluster-randomized trial. PLoS Med 2014;11:e1001766.

68. Theron G, Zijenah L, Chanda D, et al. Feasibility, accuracy, and clinical effect of point-of-care Xpert MTB/RIF testing for tuberculosis in primary-care settings in Africa: a multicentre, randomised, controlled trial. Lancet 2014;383:424–35.

69. Albert H, Trollip AP, Mole RJ, et al. Rapid indication of multidrug-resistant tuberculosis from liquid cultures using FASTPlaqueTB-RIF, a manual phage-based test. Int J Tuberc Lung Dis 2002;6:523–8.

70. Banaiee N, Bobadilla-Del-Valle M, Bardarov S Jr, et al. Luciferase reporter mycobacteriophages for detection, identification, and antibiotic susceptibility testing of Mycobacterium tuberculosis in Mexico. J Clin Microbiol 2001;39: 3883–8.

71. Albert H, Heydenrych A, Brookes R, et al. Performance of a rapid phage-based test, FASTPlaqueTB, to diagnose pulmonary tuberculosis from sputum specimens in South Africa. Int J Tuberc Lung Dis 2002;6:529–37.

72. Kiraz N, Et L, Akgun Y, et al. Rapid detection of Mycobacterium tuberculosis from sputum specimens using the FASTPlaqueTB test. Int J Tuberc Lung Dis 2007;11:904–8.

73. Muzaffar R, Batool S, Aziz F, et al. Evaluation of the FASTPlaqueTB assay for direct detection of Mycobacterium tuberculosis in sputum specimens. Int J Tuberc Lung Dis 2002;6:635–40.

74. Minion J, Pai M. Bacteriophage assays for rifampicin resistance detection in Mycobacterium tuberculosis: updated meta-analysis. Int J Tuberc Lung Dis 2010;14:941–51 (systematic review and meta-analyses).

75. World Health Organization. The use of a commercial loop-mediated isothermal amplification assay (TB-LAMP) for the detection of tuberculosis. Geneva (Switzerland): World Health Organization; 2013.

76. Loop mediated isothermal amplification (LAMP) for TB. Available at: http://www.finddiagnostics.org/programs/tb/find_activities/lamp_assay.html. Accessed February 21, 2015.

77. Boehme C, Molokova E, Minja F, et al. Detection of mycobacterial lipoarabinomannan with an antigen-capture ELISA in unprocessed urine of Tanzanian patients with suspected tuberculosis. Trans R Soc Trop Med Hyg 2005;99: 893–900.

78. Peter JG, Theron G, van Zyl-Smit R, et al. Diagnostic accuracy of a urine lipoar-abinomannan strip-test for TB detection in HIV-infected hospitalised patients. Eur Respir J 2012;40:1211–20.
79. Shah M, Variava E, Holmes CB, et al. Diagnostic accuracy of a urine lipoarabi-nomannan test for tuberculosis in hospitalized patients in a high HIV prevalence setting. J Acquir Immune Defic Syndr 2009;52:145–51.
80. Nicol MP, Allen V, Workman L, et al. Urine lipoarabinomannan testing for diag-nosis of pulmonary tuberculosis in children: a prospective study. Lancet Glob Health 2014;2:e278–84.
81. Aceti A, Zanetti S, Mura MS, et al. Identification of HIV patients with active pul-monary tuberculosis using urine based polymerase chain reaction assay. Tho-rax 1999;54:145–6.
82. Cannas A, Goletti D, Girardi E, et al. Mycobacterium tuberculosis DNA detection in soluble fraction of urine from pulmonary tuberculosis patients. Int J Tuberc Lung Dis 2008;12:146–51.
83. Gopinath K, Singh S. Urine as an adjunct specimen for the diagnosis of active pulmonary tuberculosis. Int J Infect Dis 2009;13:374–9.
84. Green C, Huggett JF, Talbot E, et al. Rapid diagnosis of tuberculosis through the detection of mycobacterial DNA in urine by nucleic acid amplification methods. Lancet Infect Dis 2009;9:505–11.
85. Kafwabulula M, Ahmed K, Nagatake T, et al. Evaluation of PCR-based methods for the diagnosis of tuberculosis by identification of mycobacterial DNA in urine samples. Int J Tuberc Lung Dis 2002;6:732–7.
86. Rebollo MJ, San Juan Garrido R, Folgueira D, et al. Blood and urine samples as useful sources for the direct detection of tuberculosis by polymerase chain re-action. Diagn Microbiol Infect Dis 2006;56:141–6.
87. Sechi LA, Pinna MP, Sanna A, et al. Detection of Mycobacterium tuberculosis by PCR analysis of urine and other clinical samples from AIDS and non-HIV-infected patients. Mol Cell Probes 1997;11:281–5.
88. Torrea G, Van de Perre P, Ouedraogo M, et al. PCR-based detection of the Mycobacterium tuberculosis complex in urine of HIV-infected and uninfected pulmonary and extrapulmonary tuberculosis patients in Burkina Faso. J Med Mi-crobiol 2005;54:39–44.
89. Devonshire AS, Whale AS, Gutteridge A, et al. Towards standardisation of cell-free DNA measurement in plasma: controls for extraction efficiency, fragment size bias and quantification. Anal Bioanal Chem 2014;406:6499–512.
90. Petrucci R, Lombardi G, Corsini I, et al. Use of transrenal DNA for the diagnosis of extrapulmonary tuberculosis in children: a case of tubercular otitis media. J Clin Microbiol 2015;53:336–8.
91. Lesho E, Forestiero FJ, Hirata MH, et al. Transcriptional responses of host pe-ripheral blood cells to tuberculosis infection. Tuberculosis (Edinb) 2011;91: 390–9.
92. Berry MP, Graham CM, McNab FW, et al. An interferon-inducible neutrophil-driven blood transcriptional signature in human tuberculosis. Nature 2010; 466:973–7.
93. Lu C, Wu J, Wang H, et al. Novel biomarkers distinguishing active tuberculosis from latent infection identified by gene expression profile of peripheral blood mononuclear cells. PLoS One 2011;6:e24290.
94. Dawany N, Showe LC, Kossenkov AV, et al. Identification of a 251 gene expres-sion signature that can accurately detect M. tuberculosis in patients with and without HIV co-infection. PLoS One 2014;9:e89925.

95. Jacobsen M, Repsilber D, Kleinsteuber K, et al. Suppressor of cytokine signaling-3 is affected in T-cells from tuberculosisTB patients. Clin Microbiol Infect 2011;17:1323–31.

96. Wang C, Yang S, Sun G, et al. Comparative miRNA expression profiles in individuals with latent and active tuberculosis. PLoS One 2011;6:e25832.

97. Anderson ST, Kaforou M, Brent AJ, et al. Diagnosis of childhood tuberculosis and host RNA expression in Africa. N Engl J Med 2014;370:1712–23.

98. Weetjens BJ, Mgode GF, Machang'u RS, et al. African pouched rats for the detection of pulmonary tuberculosis in sputum samples. Int J Tuberc Lung Dis 2009;13:737–43.

99. Mahoney AM, Weetjens BJ, Cox C, et al. Using giant African pouched rats to detect tuberculosis in human sputum samples: 2010 findings. Pan Afr Med J 2011;9:28.

100. Poling A, Weetjens BJ, Cox C, et al. Using giant African pouched rats to detect tuberculosis in human sputum samples: 2009 findings. Am J Trop Med Hyg 2010;83:1308–10.

101. Mgode GF, Cohen-Bacrie S, Bedotto M, et al. Mycobacterium genotypes in pulmonary tuberculosis infections and their detection by trained african giant pouched rats. Curr Microbiol 2015;70:212–8.

102. Mgode GF, Weetjens BJ, Nawrath T, et al. Diagnosis of tuberculosis by trained African giant pouched rats and confounding impact of pathogens and microflora of the respiratory tract. J Clin Microbiol 2012;50:274–80.

103. Bruins M, Rahim Z, Bos A, et al. Diagnosis of active tuberculosis by e-nose analysis of exhaled air. Tuberculosis (Edinb) 2013;93:232–8.

104. Fend R, Kolk AH, Bessant C, et al. Prospects for clinical application of electronic-nose technology to early detection of Mycobacterium tuberculosis in culture and sputum. J Clin Microbiol 2006;44:2039–45.

105. Kolk A, Hoelscher M, Maboko L, et al. Electronic-nose technology using sputum samples in diagnosis of patients with tuberculosis. J Clin Microbiol 2010;48:4235–8.

106. Phillips M, Basa-Dalay V, Blais J, et al. Point-of-care breath test for biomarkers of active pulmonary tuberculosis. Tuberculosis (Edinb) 2012;92:314–20.

107. Phillips M, Cataneo RN, Condos R, et al. Volatile biomarkers of pulmonary tuberculosis in the breath. Tuberculosis (Edinb) 2007;87:44–52.

108. Coban AY, Deveci A, Sunter AT, et al. Nitrate reductase assay for rapid detection of isoniazid, rifampin, ethambutol, and streptomycin resistance in Mycobacterium tuberculosis: a systematic review and meta-analysis. J Clin Microbiol 2014;52:15–9 (systematic review and meta-analyses).

109. Martin A, Imperiale B, Ravolonandriana P, et al. Prospective multicentre evaluation of the direct nitrate reductase assay for the rapid detection of extensively drug-resistant tuberculosis. J Antimicrob Chemother 2014;69:441–4.

110. Ramos E, Fissette K, de Rijk P, et al. Integrated detection of multi- and extensively drug-resistant tuberculosis using the nitrate reductase assay. Int J Tuberc Lung Dis 2012;16:110–3.

111. Shin SS, Asencios L, Yagui M, et al. Impact of rapid drug susceptibility testing for tuberculosis: program experience in Lima, Peru. Int J Tuberc Lung Dis 2012;16:1538–43.

112. Ling DI, Zwerling AA, Pai M. GenoType MTBDR assays for the diagnosis of multidrug-resistant tuberculosis: a meta-analysis. Eur Respir J 2008;32:1165–74 (systematic review and meta-analyses).

113. Theron G, Peter J, Richardson M, et al. The diagnostic accuracy of the Geno-Type((R)) MTBDRsl assay for the detection of resistance to second-line anti-tuberculosis drugs. Cochrane Database Syst Rev 2014;(10):CD010705.
114. Cheng S, Cui Z, Li Y, et al. Diagnostic accuracy of a molecular drug suscepti-bility testing method for the antituberculosis drug ethambutol: a systematic re-view and meta-analysis. J Clin Microbiol 2014;52:2913–24 (systematic review and meta-analyses).
115. Singla N, Satyanarayana S, Sachdeva KS, et al. Impact of introducing the line probe assay on time to treatment initiation of MDR-TB in Delhi, India. PLoS One 2014;9:e102989.
116. Skenders GK, Holtz TH, Riekstina V, et al. Implementation of the INNO-LiPA Rif. TB(R) line-probe assay in rapid detection of multidrug-resistant tuberculosis in Latvia. Int J Tuberc Lung Dis 2011;15:1546–52, i.
117. Engstrom A, Morcillo N, Imperiale B, et al. Detection of first- and second-line drug resistance in Mycobacterium tuberculosis clinical isolates by pyrose-quencing. J Clin Microbiol 2012;50:2026–33.
118. Lin SY, Rodwell TC, Victor TC, et al. Pyrosequencing for rapid detection of exten-sively drug-resistant Mycobacterium tuberculosis in clinical isolates and clinical specimens. J Clin Microbiol 2014;52:475–82.
119. Zheng R, Zhu C, Guo Q, et al. Pyrosequencing for rapid detection of tubercu-losis resistance in clinical isolates and sputum samples from re-treatment pul-monary tuberculosis patients. BMC Infect Dis 2014;14:200.
120. Koser CU, Bryant JM, Becq J, et al. Whole-genome sequencing for rapid sus-ceptibility testing of M. tuberculosis. N Engl J Med 2013;369:290–2.
121. Witney AA, Gould KA, Arnold A, et al. Clinical application of whole genome sequencing to inform treatment for multi-drug resistant tuberculosis cases. J Clin Microbiol 2015;53:1473–83.
122. Chegou NN, Black GF, Kidd M, et al. Host markers in QuantiFERON superna-tants differentiate active TB from latent TB infection: preliminary report. BMC Pulm Med 2009;9:21.
123. Djoba Siawaya JF, Chegou NN, van den Heuvel MM, et al. Differential cytokine/chemokines and KL-6 profiles in patients with different forms of tuberculosis. Cytokine 2009;47:132–6.
124. Kaforou M, Wright VJ, Oni T, et al. Detection of tuberculosis in HIV-infected and -uninfected African adults using whole blood RNA expression signatures: a case-control study. PLoS Med 2013;10:e1001538.
125. Wu B, Huang C, Kato-Maeda M, et al. Messenger RNA expression of IL-8, FOXP3, and IL-12beta differentiates latent tuberculosis infection from disease. J Immunol 2007;178:3688–94.
126. Walzl G, Ronacher K, Hanekom W, et al. Immunological biomarkers of tubercu-losis. Nat Rev Immunol 2011;11:343–54.
127. Bjerrum S, Rose MV, Bygbjerg IC, et al. Primary health care staff's perceptions of childhood tuberculosis: a qualitative study from Tanzania. BMC Health Serv Res 2012;12:6.
128. Chiang SS, Cruz AT, Del Castillo H, et al. Evaluation of health-care providers' knowledge of childhood tuberculosis in Lima, Peru. Paediatr Int Child Health 2015;35:29–35.
129. Vellema SC, Durrheim DN, Smith JE. Diagnosing childhood tuberculosis in rural clinics in Mpumalanga Province, South Africa. Curationis 2008;31:52–8.
130. Seddon JA, Padayachee T, Du Plessis AM, et al. Teaching chest X-ray reading for child tuberculosis suspects. Int J Tuberc Lung Dis 2014;18:763–9.

131. Frick M. Tuberculosis research and development: 2014 report on tuberculosis research funding trends, 2005–2013. New York: Treatment Action Group; 2014.
132. United States Centers for Disease Control and Prevention. The pink book. 12th edition. Atlanta (GA): United States Centers for Disease Control and Prevention; 2012.
133. Department of TB Elimination, United States Centers for Disease Control and Prevention. TB elimination: interferon-gamma release assays (IGRAs) - blood tests for TB infection. Atlanta (GA): United States Centers for Disease Control and Prevention; 2011.
134. World Health Organization. Use of tuberculosis interferon-gamma release assays (IGRAs) in low- and middle-income countries: policy statement. Geneva (Switzerland): World Health Organization; 2011.
135. World Health Organization. Guidance for national tuberculosis programmes on the management of tuberculosis in children. 2nd edition. Geneva (Switzerland): World Health Organization; 2014.

New Horizons for Pediatric Antibiotic Stewardship

Jennifer L. Goldman, MD, MS[a,b,]*, Jason G. Newland, MD, MEd[c]

KEYWORDS

- Pediatrics • Antimicrobial stewardship • Antimicrobial resistance

KEY POINTS

- Inappropriate antimicrobial prescribing in pediatrics is common and the number of pediatric antimicrobial stewardship programs (ASPs) continues to grow.
- Many targets for pediatric ASP interventions differ compared with targets for adults due to differences in common diseases and prescribed antibiotics unique to children.
- Combating antimicrobial resistance is gaining recognition by government and policy makers, which reinforces the importance of stewardship.
- Collaborative efforts among ASPs nationally will continue to strengthen the approach to pediatric stewardship initiatives.

INTRODUCTION

Antimicrobial resistance is a major health threat resulting in at least 2 million illnesses and 23,000 deaths in the United States annually. The cause of antimicrobial resistance is multifactorial with the overuse and inappropriate use of antimicrobials contributing to the development of resistance. Unfortunately, the threat of bacterial resistance is

---

Conflicts of interest: The authors have no commercial or financial conflicts of interest.
Financial support: J.L. Goldman is supported by a CTSA grant from NCATS awarded to the University of Kansas Medical Center for Frontiers: The Heartland Institute for Clinical and Translational Research # KL2TR000119. The contents are solely the responsibility of the authors and do not necessarily represent the official views of the NIH or NCATS.
J.L. Goldman and J.G. Newland are supported by Pfizer/The Joint Commission. Implementation of Antimicrobial Stewardship Interventions in Children's Hospitals Using Benchmarking.
[a] Division of Pediatric Infectious Diseases, Department of Pediatrics, Children's Mercy Hospitals & Clinics, University of Missouri-Kansas City School of Medicine, 2401 Gillham Road, Kansas City, MO 64108, USA; [b] Division of Clinical Pharmacology, Department of Pediatrics, Children's Mercy Hospitals & Clinics, University of Missouri-Kansas City School of Medicine, 2401 Gillham Road, Kansas City, MO 64108, USA; [c] Department of Pediatrics, Children's Mercy Hospitals & Clinics, University of Missouri-Kansas City School of Medicine, 2401 Gillham Road, Kansas City, MO 64108, USA
* Corresponding author. Division of Pediatric Infectious Diseases, Department of Pediatrics, Children's Mercy Hospital, 2401 Gillham Road, Kansas City, MO 64108.
E-mail address: jlgoldman@cmh.edu

Infect Dis Clin N Am 29 (2015) 503–511
http://dx.doi.org/10.1016/j.idc.2015.05.003
0891-5520/15/$ – see front matter © 2015 Elsevier Inc. All rights reserved.

widespread because these pathogens can be acquired in hospitals, nursing homes, and in the community. The dearth of new antimicrobial development over recent decades to treat highly resistant pathogens has forced clinicians to rely on older antimicrobials. These can be associated with more severe adverse effects. Preservation of available antimicrobials to assure appropriate and optimal use has become a necessity.

Incorporation of antimicrobial stewardship programs (ASPs) into medical care has become a popular strategy to optimize antimicrobial use with the ultimate goal of reducing antimicrobial resistance. Because a high rate of antimicrobial prescribing occurs in children, pediatric ASPs have continued to develop and increase in number. Although many of the overarching principles of stewardship apply to children and adults alike, many factors related to pediatric stewardship are unique to children.

In this article, new developments in pediatric antimicrobial stewardship are reviewed. Current practices and approaches to expand pediatric stewardship are described. Finally, policies and collaborative efforts directed to augment stewardship strategies on a national scale are outlined.

ANTIMICROBIAL STEWARDSHIP GUIDELINES AND STRATEGIES

For more than 25 years, the need to improve the use of antimicrobials has been well-recognized. Guidelines addressing antimicrobial resistance in the hospital setting were originally published in 1988, followed by a joint statement in 1997 from the Society for Healthcare Epidemiology of America and the Infectious Diseases Society of America (IDSA) recognizing the importance of integrating ASPs in health care settings.[1,2] Revised guidelines published in 2007 specifically outlined strategic approaches for implementing stewardship programs.[3] Although, the recommendations are not specific to the pediatric population, the current guidelines provide valuable information concerning ASP implementation in any hospital setting, including pediatric institutions.

The overarching goal of an ASP is to optimize and control the use of antimicrobials to prevent and decrease the emerging resistance of bacterial pathogens. Cost savings and a decrease in the undesired side effects associated with antimicrobials (eg, *Clostridium difficile*, gastrointestinal distress, adverse drug reactions) are additional benefits of stewardship (**Box 1**).

Box 1
Goals of an antimicrobial stewardship program

- Decrease unnecessary use of antimicrobials
- Decrease antimicrobial resistance
- Optimize antimicrobial selection
- Decrease cost
- Avoid unnecessary use of prolonged intravenous antimicrobials if transition to peroral medication can be tolerated
- Decrease side effects of antimicrobials (*C difficile*, allergic reactions) by eliminating unnecessary antimicrobial use
- Improve patient outcomes and safety

In the hospital setting, implementation of antimicrobial monitoring and optimization is frequently performed by implementing one or both of the core stewardship strategies: (1) formulary restriction and preauthorization and (2) prospective audit with feedback intervention and feedback (**Table 1**). As outlined in **Table 1**, both strategies have strengths and limitations and both approaches can be used and are not mutually exclusive. Additional supplemental strategies of ASPs that have been shown to improve antimicrobial use are clinical pathways or clinical practice guidelines,[4,5] conversion from parenteral to oral therapy,[6,7] and integration of computer surveillance and decision support to facilitate stewardship.

The core ASP team should consist of a clinical pharmacist and/or an infectious diseases physician. Additionally, microbiologists, infection preventionists, epidemiologists, and data analysts are essential in improving the use of antimicrobials and monitoring antimicrobial resistance trends (**Fig. 1**). Finally, hospital administration is critical in providing the financial and political support for the implementation and ongoing efforts of an ASP.

TRENDS IN EMERGENCE OF PEDIATRIC ANTIMICROBIAL STEWARDSHIP PROGRAMS

The American Academy of Pediatrics and the Pediatric Infectious Diseases Society endorse the IDSA and the Society for Healthcare Epidemiology of America guidelines for developing an institutional program to enhance antimicrobial stewardship because it recognizes that the pediatric population must be included in stewardship efforts. Several pediatric hospitals have successfully implemented ASPs and the prevalence of pediatric ASPs has increased during the past decade.[8–11] In 2008, just 1 year following publication of the IDSA stewardship guidelines, a national survey was conducted to inquire about pediatric ASP development.[12] Approximately 50% of the institutions surveyed (70:138; 51%) reported either having or planning implementation of an ASP. However, a dedicated full-time equivalent (FTE) to support the programs was limited, with 40% of institutions polled reporting no FTE for the program. Lack of funding and time represented the most commonly perceived challenges for those programs without an active ASP.

A follow-up survey of freestanding children's hospitals was conducted in 2011.[13] Of the 38 hospitals, 16 (42%) reported having a formal ASP, which meant 1 or more

Table 1		
Antimicrobial stewardship program strategies		
Strategy Type	**Strengths**	**Limitations**
Formulary restriction and preauthorization • Prescribing physician must receive approval before or immediately following antimicrobial initiation • Recommendation is provided at antimicrobial initiation	• Influence empirical antimicrobials at initial prescribing	• Potential barrier or delay in initial antimicrobial initiation
Prospective audit with feedback • Antimicrobial indication is evaluated following the initial prescribing • Recommendation is provided after antimicrobial initiation	• Greater clinical information available to guide recommendations • Does not interfere with initial prescribing	• More labor intensive and time consuming

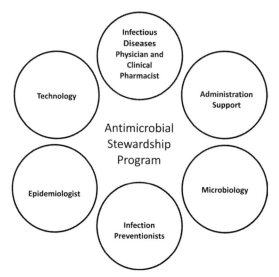

Fig. 1. Key elements of an ASP.

dedicated FTEs were committed to the program. The median number of total FTEs was 0.63 with pharmacists having 0.1 to 1.5 FTEs and physicians having 0.1 to 0.5 FTEs. Among these 16 hospitals, 13 (81%) implemented an ASP after the 2007 stewardship guidelines. Furthermore, another 14 hospitals reported they were developing an ASP. These data demonstrate an emerging trend toward uptake of formal ASPs in children's hospitals across the United States.

These hospitals with dedicated FTEs for stewardship or formal ASPs have been shown to perform better than hospitals with stewardship activity but without FTEs dedicated to supporting the program. Hersh and colleagues[14] demonstrated that a greater decline in use of a select group of broad-spectrum antibiotics was present in hospitals with a formal ASP. Furthermore, a study showed that when support is withdrawn and an ASP is discontinued, the gains made in improving antimicrobial use vanish rapidly.[15]

TARGETS FOR PEDIATRIC STEWARDSHIP

Special considerations specific to children must be recognized when considering implementation of a pediatric ASP. Children are not little adults and, therefore, the disease processes, antimicrobial resistance patterns, dosing strategies, and commonly prescribed antimicrobials differ for children compared with adults. Identifying specific targets for stewardship is critical and priority areas vary by hospitals, communities, and country regions.

Common diagnoses, such as pneumonia, appendicitis, infections in patients with cystic fibrosis, and skin and soft tissue infections, are frequently associated with immense variability in antimicrobial prescribing in children.[16,17] These diagnoses are, therefore, frequent targets for stewardship and interventions because antimicrobial recommendations can be centered on available national guidelines in addition to local resistance patterns.[4,18,19]

In addition to specific diagnoses, ASPs often direct efforts toward broad-spectrum antimicrobial agents in efforts to minimize unnecessary use. Linezolid, carbapenems, vancomycin, and fluoroquinolones are commonly targeted antimicrobials among pediatric stewardship programs, similar to many adult stewardship programs.[12] However, prescribing in children is quite different than adults and the frequency of encountering these broad agents is less frequent in the pediatric population. Targeting antimicrobials that are commonly used and potentially fraught with either selection or dosing errors, such as third-generation cephalosporins, should be considered targets in pediatric ASPs.

The types of recommendations frequently provided by ASPs vary (**Box 2**) and depend on the encountered clinical scenarios. The recommendation to stop antimicrobial therapy due to no indication is not uncommon; however, stewardship programs also provide guidance to optimizing therapy and provide recommendations on when an infectious diseases consultation should be considered.[11] The implementation of local clinical practice guidelines for prescribing clinicians can also be an effective method to enhance best prescribing practices.[5]

EXPANSION OF PEDIATRIC ANTIMICROBIAL STEWARDSHIP PROGRAMS OUTSIDE THE HOSPITAL SETTING

Antimicrobial stewardship needs to extend beyond the hospital setting because most inappropriate prescribing occurs in the ambulatory setting. Antibiotics are prescribed in nearly 1 in 5 pediatric outpatient visits. Nearly 25% of those antimicrobials are unnecessary because they are prescribed for diagnoses such as asthma and viral pneumonia and result in millions of unnecessary antimicrobials prescribed each year.[20] Rapid patient turnover and the filling of prescriptions in the outpatient pharmacy setting makes the traditional prospective-audit with feedback or restriction stewardship strategies used in the hospital setting less pragmatic in the outpatient or emergency department setting.

Nevertheless, antimicrobial stewardship has been effective in the pediatric clinic setting. Clinician education coupled with personalized provider audit and feedback has resulted in a decrease of unnecessary broad-spectrum antimicrobial use for pneumonia and sinusitis in outpatient pediatric practices.[21] However, when these stewardship interventions were removed, previous rates of broad-spectrum antimicrobial

---

Box 2
Types of recommendations provided by an antimicrobial stewardship program

Stop Therapy

- No indication

- Redundant coverage unnecessary

Modify Therapy

- Shorten duration

- Extend duration

- Broaden or narrow empirically

Optimize Therapy

- Intravenous to peroral conversion

- Adjust dose or frequency

- Modify based on culture results

Consult Infectious Diseases

prescribing resumed.[22] Therefore, expansion of ASPs into the outpatient setting requires innovative approaches that are sustainable and adaptable. These will likely depend on the type of outpatient setting (eg, urgent care or pediatrician office).

The transition period during which a hospitalized patient is preparing for discharge is yet another area for which stewardship is needed. Outpatient parental antimicrobial therapy (OPAT) is commonly prescribed at the point of hospital discharge for the continued treatment of infections in the outpatient setting. Although OPAT has proven cost-effective compared with hospitalization, outpatient administration of intravenous antimicrobials is associated with complications, including central line–associated bloodstream infections, thrombosis, and mechanical difficulties resulting in unintended medical care visits.[23,24] When prescribed to children, OPAT is often either not indicated or requires modification in dose or duration.[25] Instead of prolonged parenteral antibiotic administration, the transition to oral antibiotics after an initial course of intravenous antibiotics has proven effective when treating pediatric conditions, such as acute osteomyelitis and intraabdominal infections. This reduces the need for OPAT in some clinical scenarios.[26,27]

Because OPAT is associated with a relatively high risk of complications, standardized approaches involving infectious diseases specialists and a checklist of processes to minimize risk has been recommended.[28] Stewardship programs have the potential to improve safety and efficacy by assuring the appropriate use of OPAT, optimizing drug selection and dosing, and reducing unnecessary OPAT when oral conversion is a therapeutic option. However, involvement of ASPs with OPAT prescribing is rare in children, highlighting the importance of expanding pediatric stewardship beyond the hospital setting.

THE FUTURE OF PEDIATRIC ANTIMICROBIAL STEWARDSHIP PROGRAMS

In September 2014, the President of the United States released an executive order on combating antibiotic-resistant bacteria.[29] Additionally, the White House released a National Strategy on combating antibiotic-resistant bacteria and the President's Council of Advisors on Science and Technology published their report on antibiotic resistance.[30] In total, the executive order and these documents recognized both the health and economic threat of antimicrobial resistance. Several key efforts were highlighted as critical in the fight against antimicrobial resistance, including the development of new, effective antibacterials; the expansion of rapid diagnostic technologies to detect resistance; the preservation of efficacious antimicrobial use; and the enhancement antimicrobial stewardship. The executive order proposed that by the end of the year in 2016, the Department of Health and Human Services will require the implementation of ASPs in hospitals and inpatient health care systems and recommend stewardship programs in outpatient settings.

These national efforts emphasize the critical importance of ASPs and strongly suggest that stewardship will be an expected part of health care in the near future. Therefore, the opportunities to enhance pediatric stewardship are anticipated as more programs develop, mature, and succeed. The ability for pediatric stewardships across the country to gain knowledge about effective stewardship strategies and develop sustainable collaborative efforts to determine best practices is critical to move pediatric stewardship forward. Despite the uniqueness of individual hospitals, many, if not all, centers that provide medical care to children have some overlapping commonality for joined stewardship approaches.

A pediatric ASP collaborative was initiated in the fall of 2013. The SHARPS (Sharing Antimicrobial Reports for Pediatric Stewardship) collaborative is composed of 32 pediatric ASPs across the United States working together to improve antimicrobial use. The collaborative uses benchmarked antimicrobial data to drive stewardship interventions. Individual stewardship programs develop effective interventions based on the needs and data of the respective hospital. The information is then disseminated to all ASPs. This approach is widely beneficial because programs with similar challenges or needs can apply already proven techniques or avoid those that failed. Collaborative efforts such as SHARPS will play a critical role as ASPs strive to develop the best practices to optimize antimicrobial use in children.[31]

SUMMARY

ASPs have proven successful in decreasing inappropriate antimicrobial prescribing. As pediatric ASPs continue to advance and become an expected part of medical care, standardization of best practices directly linked with outcome measures is critical. Collaboration among government, hospital and outpatient health care facilities, and communities is needed to advance stewardship and fully augment effective strategies to battle the threat of bacterial resistance.

REFERENCES

1. Marr JJ, Moffet HL, Kunin CM. Guidelines for improving the use of antimicrobial agents in hospitals: a statement by the Infectious Diseases Society of America. J Infect Dis 1988;157(5):869–76.
2. Shlaes DM, Gerding DN, John JF Jr, et al. Society for Healthcare Epidemiology of America and Infectious Diseases Society of America Joint Committee on the Prevention of Antimicrobial Resistance: guidelines for the prevention of antimicrobial resistance in hospitals. Infect Control Hosp Epidemiol 1997;18(4):275–91.
3. Dellit TH, Owens RC, McGowan JE Jr, et al, Infectious Diseases Society of America, Society for Healthcare Epidemiology of America. Infectious Diseases Society of America and the Society for Healthcare Epidemiology of America guidelines for developing an institutional program to enhance antimicrobial stewardship. Clin Infect Dis 2007;44(2):159–77.
4. Bradley JS, Byington CL, Shah SS, et al, Pediatric Infectious Diseases Society and the Infectious Diseases Society of America. The management of community-acquired pneumonia in infants and children older than 3 months of age: clinical practice guidelines by the Pediatric Infectious Diseases Society and the Infectious Diseases Society of America. Clin Infect Dis 2011;53(7):e25–76.
5. Newman RE, Hedican EB, Herigon JC, et al. Impact of a guideline on management of children hospitalized with community-acquired pneumonia. Pediatrics 2012;129(3):e597–604.
6. Jones M, Huttner B, Madaras-Kelly K, et al. Parenteral to oral conversion of fluoroquinolones: low-hanging fruit for antimicrobial stewardship programs? Infect Control Hosp Epidemiol 2012;33(4):362–7.
7. Kuti JL, Le TN, Nightingale CH, et al. Pharmacoeconomics of a pharmacist-managed program for automatically converting levofloxacin route from i.v. to oral. Am J Health Syst Pharm 2002;59(22):2209–15.
8. Agwu AL, Lee CK, Jain SK, et al. A World Wide Web-based antimicrobial stewardship program improves efficiency, communication, and user satisfaction and reduces cost in a tertiary care pediatric medical center. Clin Infect Dis 2008;47(6):747–53.
9. Di Pentima MC, Chan S, Hossain J. Benefits of a pediatric antimicrobial stewardship program at a children's hospital. Pediatrics 2011;128(6):1062–70.

10. Metjian TA, Prasad PA, Kogon A, et al. Evaluation of an antimicrobial stewardship program at a pediatric teaching hospital. Pediatr Infect Dis J 2008;27(2):106–11.

11. Newland JG, Stach LM, De Lurgio SA, et al. Impact of a prospective-audit-with-feedback antimicrobial stewardship program at a children's hospital. J Pediatric Infect Dis Soc 2012;1(3):179–86.

12. Hersh AL, Beekmann SE, Polgreen PM, et al. Antimicrobial stewardship programs in pediatrics. Infect Control Hosp Epidemiol 2009;30(12):1211–7.

13. Newland JG, Gerber JS, Weissman SJ, et al. Prevalence and characteristics of antimicrobial stewardship programs at freestanding children's hospitals in the United States. Infect Control Hosp Epidemiol 2014;35(3):265–71.

14. Hersh AL, De Lurgio SA, Thurm C, et al. Antimicrobial stewardship programs in freestanding children's hospitals. Pediatrics 2015;135(1):33–9.

15. Standiford HC, Chan S, Tripoli M, et al. Antimicrobial stewardship at a large tertiary care academic medical center: cost analysis before, during, and after a 7-year program. Infect Control Hosp Epidemiol 2012;33(4):338–45.

16. Gerber JS, Kronman MP, Ross RK, et al. Identifying targets for antimicrobial stewardship in children's hospitals. Infect Control Hosp Epidemiol 2013;34(12):1252–8.

17. Gerber JS, Newland JG, Coffin SE, et al. Variability in antibiotic use at children's hospitals. Pediatrics 2010;126(6):1067–73.

18. Liu C, Bayer A, Cosgrove SE, et al. Clinical practice guidelines by the Infectious Diseases Society of America for the treatment of methicillin-resistant *Staphylococcus aureus* infections in adults and children: executive summary. Clin Infect Dis 2011;52(3):285–92.

19. Solomkin JS, Mazuski JE, Bradley JS, et al. Diagnosis and management of complicated intra-abdominal infection in adults and children: guidelines by the Surgical Infection Society and the Infectious Diseases Society of America. Clin Infect Dis 2010;50(2):133–64.

20. Hersh AL, Shapiro DJ, Pavia AT, et al. Antibiotic prescribing in ambulatory pediatrics in the United States. Pediatrics 2011;128(6):1053–61.

21. Gerber JS, Prasad PA, Fiks AG, et al. Effect of an outpatient antimicrobial stewardship intervention on broad-spectrum antibiotic prescribing by primary care pediatricians: a randomized trial. JAMA 2013;309(22):2345–52.

22. Gerber JS, Prasad PA, Fiks AG, et al. Durability of benefits of an outpatient antimicrobial stewardship intervention after discontinuation of audit and feedback. JAMA 2014;312(23):2569–70.

23. Gomez M, Maraqa N, Alvarez A, et al. Complications of outpatient parenteral antibiotic therapy in childhood. Pediatr Infect Dis J 2001;20(5):541–3.

24. Maraqa NF, Gomez MM, Rathore MH. Outpatient parenteral antimicrobial therapy in osteoarticular infections in children. J Pediatr Orthop 2002;22(4):506–10.

25. Knackstedt ED, Stockmann C, Davis CR, et al. Outpatient parenteral antimicrobial therapy in pediatrics: an opportunity to expand antimicrobial stewardship. Infect Control Hosp Epidemiol 2015;36(2):222–4.

26. Fraser JD, Aguayo P, Leys CM, et al. A complete course of intravenous antibiotics vs a combination of intravenous and oral antibiotics for perforated appendicitis in children: a prospective, randomized trial. J Pediatr Surg 2010;45(6):1198–202.

27. Keren R, Shah SS, Srivastava R, et al. Comparative effectiveness of intravenous vs oral antibiotics for postdischarge treatment of acute osteomyelitis in children. JAMA Pediatr 2015;169(2):120–8.

28. Muldoon EG, Snydman DR, Penland EC, et al. Are we ready for an outpatient parenteral antimicrobial therapy bundle? A critical appraisal of the evidence. Clin Infect Dis 2013;57(3):419–24.

29. Available at: http://www.whitehouse.gov/the-press-office/2014/09/18/executive-order-combating-antibiotic-resistant-bacteria. Accessed February 19, 2015.
30. Available at: https://www.whitehouse.gov/blog/2014/09/18/pcast-releases-new-report-combating-antibiotic-resistance. Accessed March 14, 2015.
31. Newland JG, Hersh A, Gerber JS, et al, SHARPS Collaborative. Sharing Antimicrobial Reports for Pediatric Stewardship (SHARPS): a quality improvement collaborative. Philadelphia: Infectious Diseases Society of America (IDSA)-ID Week; 2014. Oral Presentation.

The Changing Epidemiology of Pediatric Endocarditis

Robert W. Elder, MD[a], Robert S. Baltimore, MD[b],*

KEYWORDS

- Endocarditis • Congenital heart disease • Cyanotic • Acyanotic • Streptococci
- Staphylococci • Incidence • Mortality

KEY POINTS

- The mortality from infective endocarditis (IE) has decreased progressively in the past 80 years. Introduction of antibiotics, early detection, surgical management, and advances in postoperative care seem to be responsible.
- Over the past 80 years the predominant bacterial species causing IE have changed from viridans streptococci to staphylococci.
- The underlying conditions in children with IE have changed from unoperated CHD and rheumatic heart disease to postoperative congenital heart disease, and no heart disease (but intravascular cannulae).
- As more children with CHD are treated nonoperatively with transcatheter approaches, the association of IE and CHD remains a concern due to lack of long-term follow-up data.

INTRODUCTION

The epidemiology of pediatric infective endocarditis (IE) is closely intertwined with the evolution of care for the sick child, and in particular infants and children who were born with congenital heart disease (CHD). With data spanning nearly a century of changing surgical and transcatheter interventions, IE in children has substantially evolved.

This article discusses the epidemiology of IE in 3 eras related to the evolution of CHD care and management:

1. The presurgical era, dominated by underlying conditions including principally rheumatic heart disease and unrepaired CHD.

Disclosure: Neither of the authors has any commercial or financial conflicts of interest. There was no funding source used in the production of this article.
ª Section of Pediatric Cardiology, Yale School of Medicine, 333 Cedar Street, New Haven, CT 06520-8064, USA; ᵇ Section of Pediatric Infectious Disease, Department of Pediatrics, School of Public Health, Yale School of Medicine, 333 Cedar Street, New Haven, CT 06520-8064, USA
* Corresponding author.
E-mail address: robert.baltimore@yale.edu

Infect Dis Clin N Am 29 (2015) 513–524
http://dx.doi.org/10.1016/j.idc.2015.05.004
0891-5520/15/$ – see front matter © 2015 Elsevier Inc. All rights reserved.

2. The early years of surgical intervention for CHD, which correlated with the more widespread ability to treat IE with penicillin.
3. The modern era of pediatrics, which includes advances in surgical and catheter therapies for CHD; technologies that benefit many patients but do not eliminate the risk of IE.

This last era also includes critically ill children with normal hearts who depend on advanced technology (eg, premature children dependent on chronic indwelling catheters) who remain at high risk for IE in spite of normal cardiac structure as well as children who have recently undergone surgical correction for congenital cardiac lesions.

INCIDENCE

Only limited data exist about the incidence of pediatric endocarditis in a population-wide analysis. Most estimates of IE incidence in the general population are based on inpatient admission data, which may not be representative of the general population. In one report, between 1943 and 1952, the incidence was 0.22 cases per 1000 pediatric hospital admissions.[1] Blumenthal[2] stated that the incidence was 0.5 per 1000 admissions between 1930 and 1959 and that this did not change between the first and second halves of the time interval. Between 1972 and 1982, the estimated incidence of pediatric IE was 1 in 1280 (0.78 per 1000) pediatric admissions.[3] Three decades later, Pasquali and colleagues[4] in a multicenter report published that the incidence was slightly decreased: between 0.05 and 0.12 cases per 1000 pediatric admissions. These estimates have been fairly consistently over 8 decades of data, with IE cases representing less than 1 per 1000 pediatric admissions.

In 2013, Rushani and colleagues[5] used the Quebec CHD database to conduct a population-based analysis of the incidence of IE among children. Although the study does not account for all cases of IE, CHD has remained the dominant underlying condition associated with IE in children in developed countries throughout the various surgical eras. Following more than 47,000 children with CHD for nearly 500,000 patient years, they identified 185 cases of IE between1988 and 2010. For those children followed since birth, the cumulative incidence of IE was 6.1 per 1000 children, corresponding with an incidence rate of 4.1 per 10,000 patient years.[5] Assuming that CHD substantially increases the risk for IE compared with children with normally formed hearts, the population-based incidence for all children is likely to be considerably less, although data are lacking.

In contrast with reports in adults, among whom men have a higher rate of IE than women, IE seems to be evenly distributed between boys and girls.[5,6] It has been speculated that certain at-risk behaviors may be less common in the pediatric population to account for the difference.

REPORTS ON MICROBIOLOGY OF INFECTIVE ENDOCARDITIS

Spanning more than 8 decades of microbiologic data in pediatric IE, 2 groups of organisms remain dominant: the viridans group of streptococci and *Staphylococcus aureus* (**Table 1**). The trend between these organisms has been a gradual increase in cases related to *S aureus* with a decline in cases caused by streptococcal species. This trend likely reflects the changing risk factors of those children who acquire IE, with more children having a hospitalization with medical issues predisposing to IE.

Table 1
Principal pathogenic bacterial agents in pediatric IE series over 8 decades

Series (First Author)	Blumenthal[2]	Johnson[1]	Stanton[15]	Van Hare[3]	Martin[37]	Saiman[18]	Stockheim[29]	Coward[38]	Day[6]
Number of Subjects	59	149	26	42	76	62	111	57	632
Years Reviewed	1930–1959	1933–1972	1970–1979	1972–1982	1958–1992	1977–1992	1978–1996	1990–2002	2000–2003
Organism (%)									
Viridans group streptococci	68	51	50	31	38	23	32	30	20
S aureus	17	28	12	33	32	39	27	21	57
Coagulase-negative staphylococci	—	1	8	14	4	11	12	7	14
Streptococcus pneumoniae	—	2	—	7	4	—	7	—	1
Enterococcus species	—	—	8	2	7	2	4	16	—
HACEK	—	—	4	5	4	—	5	—	1
Other gram-negative rods	—	3	12	—	4	6	11	12	2
Other	3	—	4	2	1	10	13	5	5
Culture negative	14	13	4	2	7	6	5	9	NA
Survival (%)	47[a]	65[b]	81	86	82	89	NA	88	95

For organisms, not all percentages equal 100 because in some cases infections were polymicrobial.

Abbreviations: HACEK, *Haemophilus aphrophilus, Haemophilus paraphrophilus, Haemophilus influenzae, Haemophilus parainfluenzae, Actinobacillus actinomycetemcomitans, Cardiobacterium hominis, Eikenella corrodens,* and *Kingella* species; NA, information not available.

[a] Era-specific survival 14% (1930–1943) and 68% (1944–1959).
[b] Era-specific survival 0% (1933–1942), 72% (1943–1952), 73% (1953–1962), 81% (1963–1972).

Enterococcus, often associated with nosocomial infections, now occupies a small but important portion of most pediatric IE series; this is also true for hospital-acquired gram-negative rods. Fungal endocarditis remains unusual in the pediatric age group, but can be seen especially in neonates with chronic indwelling central catheters. Throughout these years, a small minority of cases remain culture negative. This percentage has decreased over time with improvements in diagnostic microbiology techniques.

Presurgical Era

As early as 1844, Paget[7] recognized that a "defective development" of the heart predisposed to inflammatory disease. In this era, IE was almost uniformly fatal. For example, in a review series of 149 episodes between the 1930s and 1970s, none of the patients diagnosed with IE between 1933 and 1942 survived. That mortality changed substantially with each passing decade and by the period from 1963 to 1972 more than 80% of patients with IE survived (see **Table 1**).[1]

IE on a normally formed heart was uncommon in this era. Significant prematurity was mostly lethal, and contemporary medicine did not have many of the advanced tools that lead to increased susceptibility in the normally formed heart, such as indwelling central intravascular catheters.

CHD in the presurgical era underlay between two-thirds and three-quarters of all cases.[2,8] The remaining cases tended to be those with rheumatic heart disease following acute rheumatic fever. Occasionally, both CHD and rheumatic heart disease were reported in the same patient with IE.[2]

Viridans streptococci were the dominant species, accounting for between 45% and 65% of pediatric IE cases.[1,2] S aureus was the second most common organism isolated during this era, representing ~20% of cases.[1]

Acyanotic heart disease

One early series published in 1942 focused on 453 cases with "significant congenital cardiac defects." IE was present (and presumably the proximate cause of death) in 6.5% of the cases. However, when some of the lethal CHD lesions associated with infant death were eliminated and the analysis restricted to children who died after 2 years of age, IE accounted for 30 of the 181 such patients, or 16.5%.[9]

Similar to modern data, there were no cases of IE associated with atrial septal defects (ASDs). However, IE was present in 57% of children with uncomplicated ventricular septal defect (VSD) who died after the age of 2 years, suggesting that it comprised a significant proportion of the deaths in this presurgical era.[9] Of the 40 children with CHD who developed IE in the New York series between 1930 and 1959, two-thirds were acyanotic and included, in decreasing order of frequency, VSD, patent ductus arteriosus (PDA), other undiagnosed left-to-right shunt, coarctation of the aorta, and pulmonic stenosis.[2]

Cyanotic heart disease

Most cyanotic lesions in children were ultimately fatal in this era. Between 1933 and 1942, cyanotic CHD was rare as the underlying cause of IE. However, that changed as surgical amelioration became available, enabling the survival of patients with cyanotic lesions, such as tetralogy of Fallot (ToF) and transposition of the great vessels.[1]

Before 1963, various reports estimated that cyanotic CHD accounted for only 6% to 20% of IE cases.[2,10,11] By the time of the establishment of open and closed heart surgery in the 1960s, underlying cyanotic CHD accounted for up to 45% of cases.[1]

ToF was by far the most common cardiac lesion seen in IE cases in the presurgical era,[2] which may reflect that it is the most common cyanotic congenital heart lesion and it may be more survivable without surgical interventions compared with other cyanotic lesions. In that era, before echocardiography, IE often presented late. In some cases, unrepaired patients with ToF who developed IE presented with cyanosis worsening from baseline.[2] This condition was most likely caused by vegetations resulting in further obstruction to pulmonary blood flow.

Rheumatic heart disease

Although acute rheumatic fever is rare in contemporary practice in developed countries, it persists in economically poor and preindustrial countries. In the presurgical era, children with rheumatic heart disease comprised a significant proportion of pediatric patients with IE. It has been estimated that before 1970, 30% to 50% of pediatric cases of IE in the United States had underlying rheumatic heart disease.[12] In a single-center experience that examined IE cases over 7 decades, Rosenthal and colleagues[8] found that rheumatic heart disease accounted for 31% of all cases in the presurgical era (1930–1959), contrasted with 1992 to 2004 when rheumatic heart disease was only present in 1% of new IE cases.

Early Surgical Era

The era including the Second World War was a revolutionary time in developing new technologies for medical care of patients with CHD (**Fig. 1**). In 1938, Robert Gross performed the first successful surgical ligation of a PDA. Shortly thereafter, Blalock and colleagues at Johns Hopkins Hospital dramatically altered the natural history of the so-called blue baby syndrome with the Blalock-Taussig shunt in 1944 (see Vricella and colleagues).[13] Within a decade, C. Walton Lillehei and others developed cross

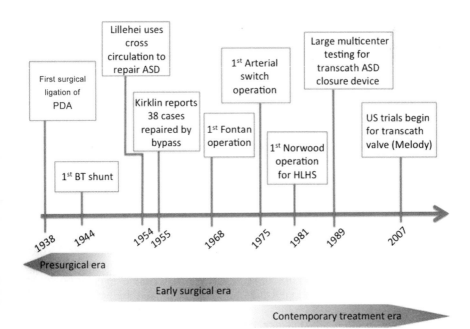

Fig. 1. Selected timeline for advances in surgical and transcatheter treatment of CHD. BT, Blalock-Taussig; HLHS, hypoplastic left heart syndrome; Transcath, transcatheter.

circulation and ultimately bypass to enable open heart procedures to be performed and drastically changed the landscape for patients with simple to complex heart disease. For the first time for many patients with CHD, survival was a distinct possibility.

These surgical CHD treatments had a dramatic impact on the epidemiology of IE. Although many patients were palliated, they often had abnormal vascular flow patterns with turbulence that placed them at risk for the development of endocardial/endothelial infections.

Presurgery and palliation

Morris and colleagues[14] reviewed the experience in Oregon from 1958 onward for patients who had CHD surgery as children. Before surgical repair, IE occurred most frequently in conditions with a large degree of shunting and turbulence: most notably, VSD and ToF with systemic-to-pulmonary shunt. For example, among patients with ToF and a palliative shunt, the risk of IE was 8.2 cases per 1000 patient years. In unoperated VSD, the risk was 3.8 cases per 1000 patient years. No children with ASD, coarctation, complete atrioventricular canal, or pulmonary valve stenosis had IE in this study.

Van Hare and colleagues[3] examined the experience with pediatric IE between 1972 and 1982 in Cleveland. There were a total of 42 IE cases in 41 patients, which were divided fairly evenly between those with no history of previous surgical intervention and those who had undergone CHD surgery. In the preoperative group, the lesion at highest risk was again VSD, accounting for 7 of 24 cases in that category. After repair, the rate decreased to 2 of 18 cases.

Endocarditis after surgical intervention

In a study that examined 3 eras of IE at a single institution, demographic and epidemiologic changes relating to surgical intervention were evident.[8] In the years between 1977 and 1992, the proportion of patients with IE who had CHD was 40 out of 62 patients (65%), similar to those of an earlier era from 1930 to 1959. However, more than half of the group had surgically treated CHD compared with about one-quarter in the earlier era (closed heart procedures).[8] Similarly, between 1970 and 1979 at Yale, among 26 pediatric IE cases, 54% occurred in postoperative patients with CHD, 35% occurred in unoperated patients with CHD, and only 11% had no underlying cardiac disorder.[15]

For patients with ToF, surgery dramatically reduced the risk of IE. Patients with complete repair of ToF had a risk that was less than one-tenth of those with palliative systemic-to-pulmonary shunts (0.7 cases vs 8.2 cases per 1000 patient years, respectively).[14] This reduction in risk is particularly important given the trend to perform complete repair of this cardiac lesion at an earlier age, in many cases obviating an interval systemic to pulmonary shunt.[16]

Following cardiac surgery, the highest risk group for IE was those with aortic valve stenosis. Over 30 years of follow-up, the cumulative risk of IE in this patient population was 7.2 cases per 1000 patient years.[14] Those with a prosthetic valve had the highest risk. Ten years following aortic valve surgery the incidence of IE was 26% in the group with a prosthetic valve replacement versus 5% in the native valvuloplasty group.[14] Similarly, another study found that the risk of aortic valve IE was greater postoperatively: 8% of cases in the nonoperative group versus 28% in the postsurgical repair group.[3]

In a study by Van Hare and colleagues,[3] from 1972 to 1982, following cardiac repair the main pathogens were divided into roughly thirds with one-third S aureus, one-third Staphylococcus epidermidis, and one-third alpha-hemolytic streptococci with small numbers of other organisms. Among the 6 deaths in this series, 3 cases of IE were caused by *S aureus*, which accounted for 21% of mortality compared with 14% for other species.

Contemporary Treatment Era

In the ensuing decades, advances in interventions for CHD have focused on complete repair of common lesions, palliation of more complex lesions, and earlier surgical intervention to normalize hemodynamics. As the era of neonatal surgical intervention began in the 1970s and 1980s, many of the prior palliative procedures, such as systemic-to-pulmonary shunts, were used less frequently.

In this era, IE is less often community acquired and more often health care associated. For example, in one study, for the period between 1992 and 2004, more than half of all IE cases were hospital acquired, and most (68 of 85; 80%) had underlying CHD.[8]

Because IE complicates care of CHD, it is important to recognize the risks of the two together. In a large multi-institutional study of IE cases based on International Classification of Diseases, 9th Revision (ICD-9) codes, children with IE who had preexisting CHD had significantly longer and more costly hospital stays as well as a tendency toward higher in-hospital mortality.[6]

Unrepaired and palliated lesions in the contemporary era

Cyanosis has long been thought to be a risk for IE. Among the most recent antibiotic prophylaxis guidelines from the American Heart Association, cyanotic patients occupy a distinct group for whom dental prophylaxis continues to be recommended.[17] In a population-wide analysis of cases of IE among patients with CHD, cyanotic patients had more than 6 times the rate of endocarditis compared with acyanotic controls with CHD.[5]

The risk of IE related to cyanosis is particularly relevant to the population of patients with a functionally single ventricle. These patients often undergo multiple surgical interventions. Most have varying degrees of cyanosis though the first stage (eg, Norwood operation for hypoplastic left heart syndrome, or systemic-to-pulmonary shunt for others) and second stage of palliation (Glenn shunt). Ultimately, the Fontan operation is typically performed between 2 and 4 years of age. The risk of IE in this group is high. In a population-based study, patients with single ventricles had a relative risk of 5.9 compared with other controls with biventricular CHD.[5]

Postoperative

Approximately half of all cases of pediatric IE complicating CHD have had previous cardiac surgery, particularly palliative shunts or complex intracardiac repair.[18] Discharge records from 2000 and 2003 show that 33.8% (224 of 662) of patients with preexisting heart disease had some form of cardiac surgery performed during the same admission. Among those, 55.4% had CHD surgery, with others related to acquired heart disease (eg, rheumatic heart disease, previous IE).[6]

Risk of IE postoperatively depends greatly on the type of surgery. For example, following complete repair of ToF, the risk of IE was low in the first postoperative month and less than that of preoperative patients with palliative shunts.[14] However, the same does not hold true for placement of a prosthetic valve. The cumulative risk at 25 years following surgery for aortic valve stenosis was 13.3% in one study.[14] In another study that examined 153 IE cases in patients with CHD diagnosed between 1966 and 2001, individuals diagnosed in the second half of the interval had higher rates of infection related to prosthetic material, including conduits related to Rastelli-type repair and prosthetic valves.[19]

In a large population-based study of IE risk in CHD, the investigators compared 185 IE cases with 3700 calendar time-matched controls with CHD without IE. In the final multivariate analysis, pediatric patients who had undergone cardiac surgery in the prior 6 months were greater than 5 times more likely to develop IE than those who had not. Shunt surgery in particular was more common, and had occurred in 7% of IE cases but 0% of the CHD population who did not develop IE.[5]

Catheter-based interventions

Since the 1990s, catheter-based interventions to treat CHD have become more common. For some cardiac lesions, such as a simple secundum ASD, catheter-based treatment is often the default choice. Interventional cardiac procedures are frequently used to intervene in complex postsurgical repair, such as stenting of narrowed pulmonary arteries after ToF repair, or ballooning or stenting of recurrent stenosis after coarctation repair.

As these catheter-based interventions have become more widely available, IE has remained a concern. The risk of IE is likely greatest in the early postinterventional period. Following placement of foreign material (eg, a vascular plug, ASD device, PDA device), IE prophylaxis is typically recommended for 6 months to allow for endothelialization.[17]

In a long-term study following ASD repair, at 10-year follow-up among the 168 transcatheter-treated patients with ASD, no patient developed IE.[20] In the literature, there are sporadic case reports of IE among patients with ASD devices, although in some cases they seem to be caused by poor endothelialization.[21,22] Similarly, several case reports of endocarditis related to transcatheter device treatment of VSD and PDA with residual shunting suggest that continued turbulence around a device may be a long-term risk for IE.[23–25]

In 2007, the first US trials of a nonsurgical, catheter-based valve known as the Melody valve to treat right ventricular outflow tract lesions began.[26] As more experience has been gained with this technique, reports of IE have emerged.[27] In a recent study examining trial data from 3 large trials, there were 6 cases of transcatheter pulmonary valve–related IE. The 4-year survival free from Melody valve–related IE was 97%, with a linearized rate of Melody-related IE of 0.88% per patient year.[28] Long-term data in this group are lacking, but this will become an important issue to follow as more such valves are implanted.

Children with anatomically normal hearts

In the contemporary era, IE in the anatomically normal heart comprises a smaller but growing proportion of pediatric IE. Estimates as to the size of this group are still unclear. Conservatively, 8% to 10% of IE cases have been estimated to occur in structurally normal hearts.[29] In a multi-institutional study based on ICD-9 codes, 58% of cases had no codes for preexisting heart disease. This finding may simply indicate a limitation in terms of the methodology relying on coding accuracy to reflect underlying cardiac status.[6]

One of the major risk factors among patients with structurally normal hearts is a central indwelling intravascular catheter. In a large national sample of the Kids Inpatient Database examining health care cost and use, Day and colleagues[6] examined hospital discharge records using ICD-9 codes for IE cases in patients less than 21 years of age, from 2000 and 2003. They identified 1588 admissions for IE, with a bimodal distribution with peaks of infants (31 days to 11 months) and late adolescents (17–20 years of age). Outside of traditional risk factors, other conditions associated with IE included neoplasms in 9.5%, prematurity in 5.8%, connective tissue disease in 5.6%, and diabetes mellitus in 2.4%.

The aortic and mitral valves are the most commonly affected valves in children with IE with structurally normal hearts. Right-sided lesions are uncommon, which may in part reflect that illicit intravenous drug use is not a common predisposing condition in children.[8] Congenital or acquired immunodeficiency does not seem to be a risk factor for pediatric IE.

Day and colleagues[6] detailed the IE organisms accounting for admission in 632 of the 1588 hospitalizations. *S aureus* was the most common organism isolated by far, accounting for 57% of identified cases, followed by the viridans group of streptococci at 20%, and coagulase-negative staphylococci at 14%.

Newborns

In newborns, IE particularly occurs in normally formed hearts. Infants less than 30 days of age accounted for 108 out of 1480 cases (7.3%).[6] Among this group, CHD accounted for less than one-third of IE cases.

This shift in demographics is apparent in the age at IE diagnosis for different eras. For example, at a single institution, in the preantibiotic era (1930–1959) the mean age at diagnosis was 8 years; from 1977 to 1992 it was 8.2 years; but in the most recent period, between 1992 and 2004, it decreased significantly to 1.5 years.[8] This was likely caused by the increase in neonates affected by IE.

As care for premature neonates has evolved, invasive technologies such as central indwelling catheters for parenteral nutrition have become more common. In this population, compared with an older pediatric population, lesions involving the right-sided structures are more common.[30] Clinical manifestations are variable and nonspecific in neonates with IE, and may range from apparent sepsis or congestive heart failure. Septic emboli are more common in this population.

Although many of the gram-positive species continue to play a large role, other organisms, including gram-negative bacilli and *Candida* sp, have increased. Fungal infections have been reported: in one study of surgical therapy for IE, they accounted for 11% of cases that required surgical intervention and all were seen in infants.[30] Prevention of central line bloodstream infections can be achieved by adhering to evidence-based guidelines for central line care.[31] Mortality for IE in neonates is high. Diagnosis may be made at autopsy.

IMPROVEMENT IN DIAGNOSIS
Echocardiography

Echocardiography was a major new development in the diagnostic armamentarium for pediatric IE. Starting in the late 1970s, reports began to emerge showing the clinical utility of ultrasonography, initially with M-mode echocardiography and subsequently two-dimensional transthoracic echocardiography (TTE). In this early era, the sensitivity of pediatric TTE was estimated at between 59% and 82% of IE cases that were made by clinical diagnosis.[32,33] TTE was particularly useful in selected patients who remained culture negative but met clinical criteria for IE.[32] In many cases echocardiography was useful in guiding risk assessment of clinical events (eg, abscess, emboli) and outcomes because TTE could be readily obtained and followed serially.

Over time, imaging quality of echocardiography has improved significantly and been aided by the introduction of Doppler and color-Doppler echocardiography. In a recent study among pediatric patients weighing less than 60 kg, TTE had a sensitivity of 97% for detection of lesions.[34] When the patient size was greater than 60 kg, that sensitivity was only 70%.[34] In those cases, transesophageal echocardiogram remains an important tool and should be considered in all patients who meet the criteria listed earlier and in whom endocarditis is considered. Echocardiography is an essential component of the clinical evaluation in suspected cases and part of the modified Duke criteria used for diagnosis.[35]

Changing Techniques in Microbiology

During the periods covered by this article there have been many advances in diagnostic microbiology that have increased the sensitivity of blood culture, have shortened the time to identification of the organisms responsible for causing infective endocarditis, and are probably responsible for some changes in understanding of the organisms responsible for IE. In most hospitals, automated blood culture detection systems are used that are highly sensitive, and these systems frequently use blood-collection vials with antibiotic binding resins that allow organisms to grow even when the blood contains antibiotics. Continuous-monitoring blood culture systems such as Bactec and newer molecular identification methods are more rapid and more sensitive than more conventional methods were in the past. Thus the rate of so-called culture-negative endocarditis has decreased. However, even now blood cultures are persistently negative in 5% to 10% of patients who satisfy other diagnostic criteria for IE.[29]

It is now recognized that IE is frequently caused by fastidious organisms such as *Abiotrophia* and *Granulicatella* spp or HACEK organisms (*Haemophilus aphrophilus, Haemophilus paraphrophilus, Haemophilus influenzae, Haemophilus parainfluenzae, Actinobacillus actinomycetemcomitans, Cardiobacterium hominis, Eikenella corrodens,* and *Kingella* spp), which grow poorly *in vitro*. Other less common organisms can be diagnosed using nucleic acid amplification tests (ie, polymerase chain reaction), including *Bartonella* spp, *Tropheryma whipplei, Coxiella burnetti* (Q fever), and *Brucella* spp. Diagnosis is sometimes made by molecular confirmation of material removed at the time of surgery, including vegetations, thrombi, emboli, or valves.[36] In the future it is likely that molecular identification will be the standard for diagnosing IE based on testing samples of blood or tissue.

SUMMARY

This article traces the changes in the microbiology of pediatric IE over 80 years of publications from a variety of pediatric departments. The changes in age of presentation, microorganisms isolated, prognosis, and history of prior surgery seem to be related to the contemporary practices that have evolved at the time of infection. In particular, underlying CHD remains a significant risk, although the epidemiology has evolved to reflect contemporary CHD management. Survival from IE is related to the availability of experts in cardiology and cardiac imaging, cardiac surgeons, critical care specialists, and infectious disease consultants to aid in timely diagnosis and interventions.

REFERENCES

1. Johnson DH, Rosenthal A, Nadas AS. A forty-year review of bacterial endocarditis in infancy and childhood. Circulation 1975;51(4):581–8.
2. Blumenthal S. Bacterial endocarditis in children. Heart Bull 1962;11:8–11.
3. Van Hare GF, Ben-Shachar G, Liebman J, et al. Infective endocarditis in infants and children during the past 10 years: a decade of change. Am Heart J 1984; 107(6):1235–40.

4. Pasquali SK, He X, Mohamad Z, et al. Trends in endocarditis hospitalizations at us children's hospitals: impact of the 2007 American Heart Association antibiotic prophylaxis guidelines. Am Heart J 2012;163(5):894–9.

5. Rushani D, Kaufman JS, Ionescu-Ittu R, et al. Infective endocarditis in children with congenital heart disease: cumulative incidence and predictors. Circulation 2013;128(13):1412–9.

6. Day MD, Gauvreau K, Shulman S, et al. Characteristics of children hospitalized with infective endocarditis. Circulation 2009;119(6):865–70.

7. Paget J. On obstructions of the branches of the pulmonary artery. Med Chir Trans 1844;27:162–494.4.

8. Rosenthal LB, Feja KN, Levasseur SM, et al. The changing epidemiology of pediatric endocarditis at a children's hospital over seven decades. Pediatr Cardiol 2010;31(6):813–20.

9. Gelfman R, Levine SA. The incidence of acute and subacute bacterial endocarditis in congenital heart disease. Am J Med Sci 1942;204:324–33.

10. Cutler JG, Ongley PA, Shwachman H, et al. Bacterial endocarditis in children with heart disease. Pediatrics 1958;22(4 Part 1):706–14.

11. Zakrzewski T, Keith J. Bacterial endocarditis in infants and children. J Pediatr 1965;67:1179.

12. Stull TL, LiPuma J. Endocarditis in children. In: Kaye D, editor. Infective endocarditis. 2nd edition. New York: Raven Press; 1992. p. 313–27.

13. Vricella LA, Gott VL, Cameron DE. Milestones in congenital cardiac surgery. In: Yuh DD, Vricella LA, Yang SC, et al, editors. Johns Hopkins textbook of cardiothoracic surgery. 2nd edition. New York: McGraw-Hill Professional; 2014. p. 943–54.

14. Morris CD, Reller MD, Menashe VD. Thirty-year incidence of infective endocarditis after surgery for congenital heart defect. JAMA 1998;279(8):599–603.

15. Stanton BF, Baltimore RS, Clemens JD. Changing spectrum of infective endocarditis in children. Analysis of 26 cases, 1970–1979. Am J Dis Child 1984;138(8):720–5.

16. Caspi J, Zalstein E, Zucker N, et al. Surgical management of tetralogy of Fallot in the first year of life. Ann Thorac Surg 1999;68(4):1344–8 [discussion: 1348–9].

17. Wilson W, Taubert KA, Gewitz M, et al. Prevention of infective endocarditis: guidelines from the American Heart Association: a guideline from the American Heart Association Rheumatic Fever, Endocarditis, and Kawasaki Disease Committee, Council on Cardiovascular Disease in the Young, and the Council on Clinical Cardiology, Council on Cardiovascular Surgery and Anesthesia, and the Quality of Care and Outcomes Research Interdisciplinary Working Group. Circulation 2007;116(15):1736–54.

18. Saiman L, Prince A, Gersony WM. Pediatric infective endocarditis in the modern era. J Pediatr 1993;122(6):847–53.

19. Di Filippo S, Delahaye F, Semiond B, et al. Current patterns of infective endocarditis in congenital heart disease. Heart 2006;92(10):1490–5.

20. Kutty S, Hazeem AA, Brown K, et al. Long-term (5- to 20-year) outcomes after transcatheter or surgical treatment of hemodynamically significant isolated secundum atrial septal defect. Am J Cardiol 2012;109(9):1348–52.

21. Slesnick TC, Nugent AW, Fraser CD Jr, et al. Images in cardiovascular medicine. Incomplete endothelialization and late development of acute bacterial endocarditis after implantation of an Amplatzer septal occluder device. Circulation 2008;117(18):e326–7.

22. Zahr F, Katz WE, Toyoda Y, et al. Late bacterial endocarditis of an Amplatzer atrial septal defect occluder device. Am J Cardiol 2010;105(2):279–80.

23. Kassis I, Shachor-Meyouhas Y, Khatib I, et al. Kingella endocarditis after closure of ventricular septal defect with a transcatheter device. Pediatr Infect Dis J 2012; 31(1):105–6.

24. Scheuerman O, Bruckheimer E, Marcus N, et al. Endocarditis after closure of ventricular septal defect by transcatheter device. Pediatrics 2006;117(6):e1256–8.

25. Saint-Andre C, Iriart X, Ntsinjana H, et al. Residual shunt after ductus arteriosus occluder implantation complicated by late endocarditis. Circulation 2012;125(6): 840–2.

26. Zahn EM, Hellenbrand WE, Lock JE, et al. Implantation of the Melody transcatheter pulmonary valve in patients with a dysfunctional right ventricular outflow tract conduit early results from the U.S. clinical trial. J Am Coll Cardiol 2009;54(18): 1722–9.

27. Lurz P, Coats L, Khambadkone S, et al. Percutaneous pulmonary valve implantation: impact of evolving technology and learning curve on clinical outcome. Circulation 2008;117(15):1964–72.

28. Meadows JJ, Moore PM, Berman DP, et al. Use and performance of the melody transcatheter pulmonary valve in native and postsurgical, nonconduit right ventricular outflow tracts. Circ Cardiovasc Interv 2014;7(3):374–80.

29. Stockheim JA, Chadwick EG, Kessler S, et al. Are the Duke criteria superior to the Beth Israel criteria for the diagnosis of infective endocarditis in children? Clin Infect Dis 1998;27(6):1451–6.

30. Russell HM, Johnson SL, Wurlitzer KC, et al. Outcomes of surgical therapy for infective endocarditis in a pediatric population: a 21-year review. Ann Thorac Surg 2013;96(1):171–4 [discussion: 174–5].

31. Bizzarro MJ, Sabo B, Noonan M, et al. A quality improvement initiative to reduce central line-associated bloodstream infections in a neonatal intensive care unit. Infect Control Hosp Epidemiol 2010;31(3):241–8.

32. Kavey RE, Frank DM, Byrum CJ, et al. Two-dimensional echocardiographic assessment of infective endocarditis in children. Am J Dis Child 1983;137(9): 851–6.

33. Bricker JT, Latson LA, Huhta JC, et al. Echocardiographic evaluation of infective endocarditis in children. Clin Pediatr 1985;24(6):312–7.

34. Penk JS, Webb CL, Shulman ST, et al. Echocardiography in pediatric infective endocarditis. Pediatr Infect Dis J 2011;30(12):1109–11.

35. Li JS, Sexton DJ, Mick N, et al. Proposed modifications to the Duke criteria for the diagnosis of infective endocarditis. Clin Infect Dis 2000;30(4):633–8.

36. Lamas C da C, Ramos RG, Lopes GQ, et al. *Bartonella* and *Coxiella* infective endocarditis in Brazil: molecular evidence from excised valves from a cardiac surgery referral center in Rio de Janeiro, Brazil, 1998 to 2009. Int J Infect Dis 2013; 17(1):e65–6.

37. Martin JM, Neches WH, Wald ER. Infective endocarditis: 35 years of experience at a children's hospital. Clin Infect Dis 1997;24(4):669–75.

38. Coward K, Tucker N, Darville T. Infective endocarditis in Arkansan children from 1990 through 2002. Pediatr Infect Dis J 2003;22(12):1048–52.

The Complexities of the Diagnosis and Management of Kawasaki Disease

CrossMark

Anne H. Rowley, MD

KEYWORDS

- Coronary artery aneurysm • Prolonged fever • Systemic inflammation
- Myocardial infarction • Acquired pediatric heart disease

KEY POINTS

- The diagnosis of Kawasaki disease (KD) requires a high index of suspicion. Infants and children may present with "soft" or incomplete clinical features, yet still develop significant coronary artery abnormalities.
- Asian children have the highest incidence of KD of all ethnic/racial groups. Siblings and children of KD patients are at increased risk.
- Laboratory and echocardiographic findings can help establish the diagnosis in nonclassic cases. In particular, a child with prolonged fever, laboratory evidence of systemic inflammation, and a coronary artery z score of 2.5 or higher has a very high probability of having KD.
- Prompt treatment with intravenous gammaglobulin and aspirin can be life-saving. Children who do not have resolution of fever with this primary therapy are at increased risk of developing coronary artery abnormalities, and additional anti-inflammatory therapies should be administered.

INTRODUCTION

Although Kawasaki disease (KD) has been recognized in Japan and the United States for decades, the etiology and pathogenesis of the illness remain major pediatric mysteries. The abrupt onset of clinical signs such as fever, exanthem, and enanthem in previously healthy children, the rarity of recurrence, the very young age group affected, and the well-documented epidemics and outbreaks of illness are strongly suggestive of infectious etiology, as well described in a classic epidemiologic study from the 1980s.[1] The very high incidence of the illness in Japan, where approximately

Disclosure statement: The author has nothing to disclose.
Department of Pediatrics, Northwestern University Feinberg School of Medicine, 310 East Superior Street, Morton 4-685B, Chicago, IL 60611, USA
E-mail address: a-rowley@northwestern.edu

Infect Dis Clin N Am 29 (2015) 525–537
http://dx.doi.org/10.1016/j.idc.2015.05.006
0891-5520/15/$ – see front matter © 2015 Elsevier Inc. All rights reserved.
id.theclinics.com

1 in 90 children develop KD by age 5 years,[2] is highly suggestive of a ubiquitous infectious agent affecting young susceptible children who are genetically predisposed. Key features of KD are presented in **Box 1**. It is important to understand the major pathologic features of KD arteriopathy, briefly summarized in **Box 1**, because these features predict the adverse clinical outcomes observed in KD patients who develop coronary artery abnormalities.[3] Moreover, knowledge of the many organs and tissues involved in the systemic inflammation of KD assists in understanding the many possible clinical manifestations of the illness (**Box 2**).[4] Risk factors for KD and the development of coronary artery abnormalities are summarized in **Box 3**.

INCIDENCE AND MORTALITY RATES

The incidence of KD varies in different countries throughout the world (**Table 1**) and remains unknown in many regions, especially in those that continue to have a high prevalence of measles, which shares many clinical features with KD. In Japan, there is high recognition and early treatment of the condition, and mortality rates have fallen from 1.4% in 1970 to 0.01% in recent years; fatality rates began to decrease markedly after the introduction of intravenous gammaglobulin therapy in the late 1980s.[8] In the United States, fatality rates are also very low; fatal cases are often associated with delayed or missed diagnoses.[3] Peak months of KD incidence vary somewhat by country, but a consistent theme seems to be a peak during the winter in nontemperate climates.[9]

PATIENT HISTORY

The history is particularly important in KD, as some clinical features of the illness may begin and abate before the patient's presentation. It is recommended that the parent or guardian is asked nonleading questions about symptoms to avoid introducing recall bias. **Box 4** lists common features in the history of children with KD. Excessive irritability, refusal to bear weight, redness and swelling of the hands and feet, and an

---

Box 1
Key features of Kawasaki disease (KD)

An acute onset of prolonged febrile illness in previously healthy children.

The leading cause of acquired heart disease in children in developed nations.

A systemic inflammatory illness affecting many organs and tissues, but leading to long-term consequences almost exclusively confined to medium-sized muscular arteries, particularly the coronary arteries.

KD arteriopathy is characterized by 3 linked pathologic processes: necrotizing arteritis, subacute/chronic arteritis, and luminal myofibroblastic proliferation. Necrotizing arteritis occurs in the first 2 weeks after onset and can result in necrosis of the coronary arteries; if the necrosis is extensive, giant coronary artery aneurysms can form, which are associated with severe outcomes. Subacute/chronic arteritis begins in the first 2 weeks and can continue for months to years after onset. It is closely associated with luminal myofibroblastic proliferation, an active proliferative process of smooth muscle cell–derived myofibroblasts and their matrix products, which can lead to progressive arterial stenosis.

The etiology remains unknown, but clinical and epidemiologic features support an infectious cause.

Genetic factors play a role in susceptibility, with Asian children at highest risk. However, children of all racial and ethnic groups can develop KD.

Box 2
Systemic pathologic abnormalities reported in KD

- Cardiovascular: vasculitis, endocarditis, myocarditis, pericarditis
- Gastrointestinal: sialoductitis, enteritis, hepatitis, cholangitis, pancreatitis, pancreatic ductitis
- Respiratory: bronchitis, segmental interstitial pneumonia
- Genitourinary: cystitis, focal interstitial nephritis, prostatitis
- Nervous system: aseptic leptomeningitis, choriomeningitis, ganglionitis, neuritis
- Hematopoietic: lymphadenitis, splenitis, thymitis

Data from Amano S, Hazama F, Kubagawa H, et al. General pathology of Kawasaki disease. On the morphological alterations corresponding to the clinical manifestations. Acta Pathol Jpn 1980;30(5):681–94.

---

erythematous, peeling groin rash may be helpful in establishing the diagnosis, as these are not common features of most other diseases in the differential diagnosis. In a child who has received Bacillus Calmette-Guérin vaccine, redness at the site should prompt consideration of KD[21]; the mechanism of this response is unknown.

PHYSICAL EXAMINATION

Physical findings in KD can be very striking in classic cases (**Box 5**, **Figs. 1** and **2**). However, young infants in particular can present with incomplete clinical signs (fever with fewer than 4 of the other findings) or signs that are relatively mild. The findings of classic KD are listed in **Box 5**. Although some clinicians refer to incomplete KD as atypical KD, it is important to recognize that these terms indicate a lack of full clinical features, not to the presence of unexpected signs not listed in **Box 5**. An alternative diagnosis should be strongly considered in a child who has signs or symptoms not generally associated with KD. Because hydrops of the gallbladder occurs commonly in KD, right upper quadrant pain may be present on abdominal examination. Marked irritability, greater than that observed in other routine childhood febrile illnesses, is also characteristic and commonly observed during physical examination.

Box 3
Risk factors for KD

Factors associated with an increased risk of KD

- Asian ethnicity
- Age less than 5 years
- Parent or sibling with prior history of KD[5,6]

Factors associated with higher risk of coronary artery abnormalities in children with KD[7]

- Age less than or equal to 12 months or greater than or equal to 8 years
- Male gender
- Longer interval from disease onset to treatment with intravenous gammaglobulin
- Failure to respond to initial intravenous gammaglobulin therapy
- Laboratory features (albumin <3.0 mg/dL, anemia for age, elevated alanine aminotransferase, hyponatremia, thrombocytopenia)

Table 1
Incidence of KD in various countries, as reported in the last decade

Country	Approximate Risk of Child Developing KD by Age 5 y[a]	Authors,[Ref.] Year
Japan	1 in 90	Nakamura et al,[2] 2012
Korea	1 in 150	Kim et al,[10] 2014
China	1 in 400	Du et al,[11] 2007
Taiwan	1 in 300	Huang et al,[12] 2013
Continental USA	1 in 1000	Holman et al,[13] 2010
Hawaii—Japanese American	1 in 95	Holman et al,[14] 2010
Hawaii—Native Hawaiian	1 in 230	Holman et al,[14] 2010
Hawaii—Chinese American	1 in 240	Holman et al,[14] 2010
Hawaii—Other Asian	1 in 235	Holman et al,[14] 2010
Hawaii—Caucasian	1 in 1000	Holman et al,[14] 2010
Canada	1 in 770	Lin et al,[15] 2010
France	1 in 2200	Heuclin et al,[16] 2009
Australia	1 in 2200	Saundankar et al,[17] 2014
Finland	1 in 1750	Salo et al,[18] 2012
Norway	1 in 3700	Salo et al,[18] 2012
Sweden	1 in 2700	Salo et al,[18] 2012
Chile	1 in 2600	Borzutzky et al,[19] 2012
Israel	1 in 1680	Bar-Meir et al,[20] 2011

[a] Based on yearly incidence per 100,000 children younger than 5 years in each country.

Box 4
Common features in the history of children with KD

- Prolonged intermittent high-spiking fevers (ask parent how temperatures are taken; oral or rectal temperatures are most accurate)
- Excessive irritability when compared with other previous febrile illnesses
- Refusal to bear weight or hold objects in hands
- Redness and swelling of hands and feet
- Redness and peeling of the skin in the groin area
- Red eyes
- Red lips and tongue
- Red rash on body, primarily on trunk, arms, and legs
- Swollen glands in neck
- Vomiting
- Diarrhea
- Cough
- Redness at site of bacillus Calmette-Guérin injection (children born in countries where this vaccine is routinely administered)

Box 5
Physical examination findings (classic diagnostic criteria)

- Intermittent high fever
- Plus 4 of the following 5 features:
  - Bulbar conjunctival injection, generally without exudate and often with limbal sparing (see **Fig. 1**)
  - Oral changes: redness of the throat, strawberry tongue, redness of the lips, sometimes with bleeding or peeling of the lips (see **Fig. 1**)
  - Rash: erythematous maculopapular (see **Fig. 2**), scarlatiniform, or erythema multiforme, sometimes with marked groin erythema and desquamation
  - Extremity changes: redness and swelling of the hands and feet during the first week; typical periungual desquamation occurs in the second or third week (**Fig. 3**)
  - Cervical lymphadenopathy 1.5 cm or more in diameter
- Illness not explained by other known disease process

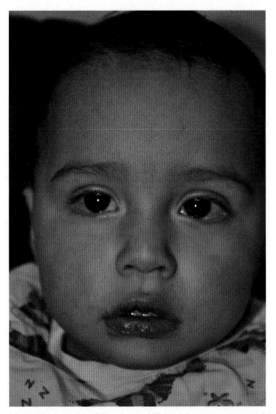

Fig. 1. Conjunctival injection and red lips in a child with acute Kawasaki disease (KD).

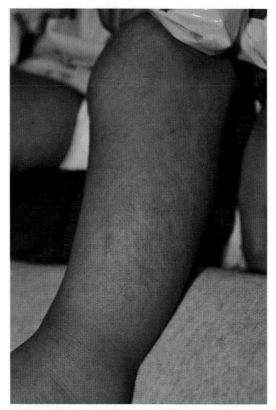

Fig. 2. Maculopapular rash on the extremities in a child with acute KD.

OTHER CLINICAL MANIFESTATIONS OF KAWASAKI DISEASE

Children with KD can present with shock syndrome; such patients are at higher risk of intravenous gammaglobulin (IVIG) resistance and of developing coronary artery abnormalities.[22–26] Although cervical lymphadenopathy is the least commonly observed clinical feature among the classic diagnostic criteria for KD, it can be the dominant clinical feature, and some of these patients also have retropharyngeal phlegmon (without abscess) documented by neck imaging studies.[27–29] KD should be considered in the differential diagnosis of any infant with prolonged fever and aseptic meningitis.[30]

IMAGING AND ADDITIONAL TESTING

Laboratory findings in KD are nondiagnostic, but can support the diagnosis (**Box 6**). In particular, a child with a low or normal peripheral white blood cell count with a lymphocyte predominance does not have a compatible laboratory profile of KD. In nontemperate climates KD is most prevalent in the winter, when many respiratory viruses are circulating. Therefore, some children with KD will concurrently have infection with one of these viruses; this should not preclude the diagnosis in cases with clinical and laboratory features of KD. Echocardiography can be very useful in assessing a child for possible KD, as a right or left anterior descending coronary artery z score

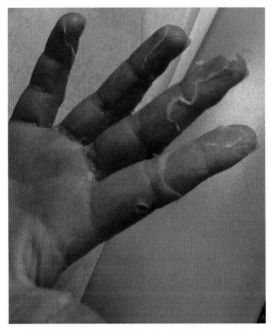

Fig. 3. Periungual desquamation of the fingers 2 weeks after fever onset in a child with KD.

greater than 2.5 is highly supportive of the diagnosis,[31,32] and 30% of KD patients have abnormal coronary artery z scores at the time of initial diagnosis, in the first 10 days of illness.[33,34] The presence of 3 of the following echocardiographic findings should also increase clinical suspicion of KD: pericardial effusion, lack of tapering of the coronary arteries, a coronary artery z score of 2 to 2.5 of the right or left anterior descending coronary arteries, decreased left ventricular function, and mitral regurgitation.[7]

Box 6
Laboratory findings

Normal peripheral white blood cell count with left shift, or elevated white blood cell count with predominance of neutrophils

Elevated erythrocyte sedimentation rate ($\geq$40 mm/h) and/or C-reactive protein ($\geq$3.0 mg/dL)

Anemia for age

Albumin less than 3.0 mg/dL

Hyponatremia

Thrombocytosis in second to third week

Sterile pyuria ($\geq$10 white blood cells/high-powered field)

Elevated serum transaminases with or without elevated serum gamma glutamyl transpeptidase or bilirubin

Cerebrospinal fluid pleocytosis, usually with normal glucose and protein levels

Leukocytosis in synovial fluid

DIAGNOSIS OF INCOMPLETE (ATYPICAL) KAWASAKI DISEASE

Although the classic diagnostic criteria are the mainstay of diagnosis, some children with KD, particularly infants, manifest fever with fewer than 4 of the 5 clinical signs described in **Box 5**; these children are considered to have incomplete KD. In some infants, the clinical findings are mild, and may not be noted unless there is a high index of suspicion for KD. Unfortunately, coronary artery abnormalities in incomplete cases can be as severe as in classic cases. Because incomplete KD can be difficult to diagnose and has potentially severe consequences that may be prevented by early treatment, the American Heart Association Committee on Endocarditis, Rheumatic Fever, and Kawasaki Disease developed a treatment algorithm combining laboratory and echocardiographic findings with clinical signs and symptoms to identify patients who may benefit from therapy for incomplete KD (**Fig. 4**).[7]

PRIMARY THERAPY

All patients diagnosed with KD should be treated with 2 g/kg IVIG with oral high-dose aspirin (80–100 mg/kg/d divided every 6 hours) as soon as possible after diagnosis.[35] IVIG significantly reduces the prevalence of coronary artery abnormalities when given within the first 10 days of illness,[35,36] and improves myocardial function.[37] However, improved echocardiographic imaging and use of body surface area-adjusted z scores to identify coronary artery dilation has led to the realization that coronary artery injury

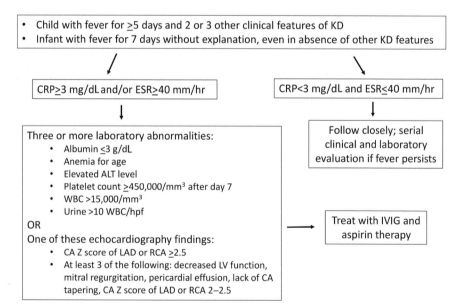

Fig. 4. Treatment algorithm for children with suspected incomplete KD. ALT, alanine aminotransferase; CA, coronary artery; CRP, C-reactive protein; ESR, erythrocyte sedimentation rate; hpf, high-power field; IVIG, intravenous gammaglobulin; LAD, left anterior descending artery; RCA, right coronary artery; WBC, white blood cells. (*Adapted from* Newburger JW, Takahashi M, Gerber MA, et al. Diagnosis, treatment, and long-term management of Kawasaki disease: a statement for health professionals from the Committee on Rheumatic Fever, Endocarditis and Kawasaki Disease, Council on Cardiovascular Disease in the Young, American Heart Association. Circulation 2004;110(17):2748.)

likely occurs in many patients in the first week of illness,[33,34] and that coronary artery z scores greater than 2 can be observed in 18% of KD children at about 6 weeks after onset even with treatment within the first 10 days.[34] This finding emphasizes the need for early diagnosis and treatment. At least 80% of KD patients respond to initial therapy with IVIG and aspirin with resolution of fever, improvement in clinical signs and symptoms, and decreased laboratory markers of inflammation. Aspirin is maintained at high doses for anti-inflammatory effect until the patient is afebrile for 2 to 3 days; at some centers, it is continued until the 14th day of illness. Aspirin is then reduced to antiplatelet doses of 3 to 5 mg/kg/d in a single daily dose, and continued until echocardiography at 6 to 8 weeks after the onset remains normal and acute-phase reactants have normalized. In patients who develop coronary artery abnormalities, low-dose aspirin is continued indefinitely. In patients with severe coronary artery abnormalities, clopidogrel and/or anticoagulation therapy with warfarin or low molecular weight heparin may be indicated, and consultation with a pediatric cardiologist is advised.[7]

RESEARCH STUDIES ON ADJUNCTIVE PRIMARY THERAPY

Unfortunately, approximately 15% to 20% of children with KD do not respond to initial IVIG therapy, with persistence of fever 36 hours after completion of IVIG infusion, and these patients are at increased risk of developing coronary artery abnormalities. Some KD patients, especially infants, can develop coronary artery abnormalities despite apparent clinical response to IVIG treatment given in the first 10 days of illness. Therefore, recent research has focused on the study of combination immunomodulatory therapies given with IVIG as primary therapy for KD. A randomized study of a single 30 mg/kg dose of methylprednisolone administered with IVIG did not reveal a significant improvement in outcomes.[38] A randomized, double-blind, placebo-controlled trial of infliximab (a tumor necrosis factor α inhibitor) for intensification of primary therapy for KD did not show a reduction in treatment resistance nor a reduction in the overall prevalence of coronary artery abnormalities when infliximab was administered with IVIG, although the addition of infliximab did result in lower levels of C-reactive protein and absolute neutrophil counts 24 hours after the infusion.[39] More promising was the Randomized controlled trial to Assess Immunoglobulin plus Steroid Efficacy for Kawasaki disease (RAISE study), which demonstrated improvement in coronary artery outcomes in Japanese patients with high-risk KD when prednisolone was given with IVIG and continued for 15 days after normalization of the C-reactive protein level.[40] A randomized trial of cyclosporin with IVIG for Japanese children with high-risk KD is presently under way in Japan, and the results of this study will also be of interest. Because the identification of risk scoring systems with high sensitivity for the prediction of coronary artery abnormalities in mixed ethnic populations has proved elusive, application of the RAISE study protocol or other high-risk protocols to KD children in countries such as the United States and Canada is not presently feasible.[41]

REFRACTORY KAWASAKI DISEASE

Refractory KD generally refers to the persistence of fever for 36 hours or longer after completion of initial IVIG infusion. Patients with IVIG resistance have a higher prevalence of coronary artery abnormalities.[42] Most of these patients respond to a second 2 g/kg dose of IVIG. For those patients who do not respond to a second dose of IVIG, several options for treatment exist, although controlled data are lacking (**Box 7**).

Box 7
Options for treatment of refractory KD

- Additional dose(s) of 2 g/kg of intravenous gammaglobulin[43]
- Intravenous methylprednisolone 30 mg/kg/d for 1 to 3 days[44]
- Infliximab 5 mg/kg × 1[45]
- Other possible therapies: cyclosporine,[46,47] methotrexate[48]
  - Therapies sometimes used in Japan: plasmapheresis, neutrophil elastase inhibitor
- Possible future therapies: statins, interleukin-1 inhibitors

---

CLINICAL OUTCOMES AND COMPLICATIONS

Most children with KD respond to IVIG, and those who do not develop coronary artery abnormalities by 4 to 6 weeks after the onset of fever have no known adverse outcomes. In patients who develop coronary artery dilation or aneurysm formation, outcomes depend on the severity of coronary artery disease. In severe cases giant coronary artery aneurysms can form, which can rarely rupture, and virtually always thrombose to a varying extent. Patients with this severe complication of KD are generally maintained on antiplatelet and anticoagulation therapy, and are at the highest risk for thrombotic occlusion and myocardial infarction, in some cases requiring catheter interventions or coronary artery bypass surgery. However, coronary artery stenosis in KD patients can also be caused by luminal myofibroblastic proliferation (LMP) with or without thromboses. LMP is an active proliferative process of smooth muscle cell–derived myofibroblasts and their matrix products that can result in progressive arterial stenosis.[3] In rare cases, LMP or thrombosis can result in such significant stenoses of multiple coronary arteries that heart transplantation is required.[3,49] KD can affect all medium-sized muscular arteries outside of the central nervous system, but peripheral arterial aneurysms seem to occur only in children with severe coronary artery disease. The most commonly affected arteries are the axillary, brachial, and inguinal arteries; aneurysms in these arteries rarely result in morbidity or mortality.[3,50]

REFERENCES

1. Yanagawa H, Nakamura Y, Yashiro M, et al. A nationwide incidence survey of Kawasaki disease in 1985-1986 in Japan. J Infect Dis 1988;158(6):1296–301.
2. Nakamura Y, Yashiro M, Uehara R, et al. Epidemiologic features of Kawasaki disease in Japan: results of the 2009-2010 nationwide survey. J Epidemiol 2012; 22(3):216–21.
3. Orenstein JM, Shulman ST, Fox LM, et al. Three linked vasculopathic processes characterize Kawasaki disease: a light and transmission electron microscopic study. PLoS One 2012;7(6):e38998.
4. Amano S, Hazama F, Kubagawa H, et al. General pathology of Kawasaki disease. On the morphological alterations corresponding to the clinical manifestations. Acta Pathol Jpn 1980;30(5):681–94.
5. Fujita Y, Nakamura Y, Sakata K, et al. Kawasaki disease in families. Pediatrics 1989;84(4):666–9.
6. Uehara R, Yashiro M, Nakamura Y, et al. Kawasaki disease in parents and children. Acta Paediatr 2003;92(6):694–7.
7. Newburger JW, Takahashi M, Gerber MA, et al. Diagnosis, treatment, and long-term management of Kawasaki disease: a statement for health professionals

from the Committee on Rheumatic Fever, Endocarditis and Kawasaki Disease, Council on Cardiovascular Disease in the Young, American Heart Association. Circulation 2004;110(17):2747–71.

8. Takahashi K, Oharaseki T, Yokouchi Y, et al. A half-century of autopsy results–incidence of pediatric vasculitis syndromes, especially Kawasaki disease. Circ J 2012;76(4):964–70.

9. Uehara R, Belay ED. Epidemiology of Kawasaki disease in Asia, Europe, and the United States. J Epidemiol 2012;22(2):79–85.

10. Kim GB, Han JW, Park YW, et al. Epidemiologic features of Kawasaki disease in South Korea: data from nationwide survey, 2009-2011. Pediatr Infect Dis J 2014; 33(1):24–7.

11. Du ZD, Zhao D, Du J, et al. Epidemiologic study on Kawasaki disease in Beijing from 2000 through 2004. Pediatr Infect Dis J 2007;26(5):449–51.

12. Huang SK, Lin MT, Chen HC, et al. Epidemiology of Kawasaki disease: prevalence from national database and future trends projection by system dynamics modeling. J Pediatr 2013;163(1):126–31.e1.

13. Holman RC, Belay ED, Christensen KY, et al. Hospitalizations for Kawasaki syndrome among children in the United States, 1997-2007. Pediatr Infect Dis J 2010;29(6):483–8.

14. Holman RC, Christensen KY, Belay ED, et al. Racial/ethnic differences in the incidence of Kawasaki syndrome among children in Hawaii. Hawaii Med J 2010; 69(8):194–7.

15. Lin YT, Manlhiot C, Ching JC, et al. Repeated systematic surveillance of Kawasaki disease in Ontario from 1995 to 2006. Pediatr Int 2010;52(5):699–706.

16. Heuclin T, Dubos F, Hue V, et al. Increased detection rate of Kawasaki disease using new diagnostic algorithm, including early use of echocardiography. J Pediatr 2009;155(5):695–699 e1.

17. Saundankar J, Yim D, Itotoh B, et al. The epidemiology and clinical features of Kawasaki disease in Australia. Pediatrics 2014;133(4):e1009–14.

18. Salo E, Griffiths EP, Farstad T, et al. Incidence of Kawasaki disease in northern European countries. Pediatr Int 2012;54(6):770–2.

19. Borzutzky A, Hoyos-Bachiloglu R, Cerda J, et al. Rising hospitalization rates of Kawasaki disease in Chile between 2001 and 2007. Rheumatol Int 2012;32(8): 2491–5.

20. Bar-Meir M, Haklai Z, Dor M. Kawasaki disease in Israel. Pediatr Infect Dis J 2011; 30(7):589–92.

21. Lai CC, Lee PC, Wang CC, et al. Reaction at the Bacillus Calmette-Guerin inoculation site in patients with Kawasaki disease. Pediatr Neonatol 2013;54(1): 43–8.

22. Gatterre P, Oualha M, Dupic L, et al. Kawasaki disease: an unexpected etiology of shock and multiple organ dysfunction syndrome. Intensive Care Med 2012; 38(5):872–8.

23. Gamez-Gonzalez LB, Murata C, Munoz-Ramirez M, et al. Clinical manifestations associated with Kawasaki disease shock syndrome in Mexican children. Eur J Pediatr 2013;172(3):337–42.

24. Kanegaye JT, Wilder MS, Molkara D, et al. Recognition of a Kawasaki disease shock syndrome. Pediatrics 2009;123(5):e783–9.

25. Lin MT, Fu CM, Huang SK, et al. Population-based study of Kawasaki disease shock syndrome in Taiwan. Pediatr Infect Dis J 2013;32(12):1384–6

26. Dominguez SR, Friedman K, Seewald R, et al. Kawasaki disease in a pediatric intensive care unit: a case-control study. Pediatrics 2008;122(4):e786–90.

27. Kanegaye JT, Van Cott E, Tremoulet AH, et al. Lymph-node-first presentation of Kawasaki disease compared with bacterial cervical adenitis and typical Kawasaki disease. J Pediatr 2013;162(6):1259–63, 1263.e1–2.

28. Stamos JK, Corydon K, Donaldson J, et al. Lymphadenitis as the dominant manifestation of Kawasaki disease. Pediatrics 1994;93(3):525–8.

29. Nomura O, Hashimoto N, Ishiguro A, et al. Comparison of patients with Kawasaki disease with retropharyngeal edema and patients with retropharyngeal abscess. Eur J Pediatr 2014;173(3):381–6.

30. Yeom JS, Park JS, Seo JH, et al. Initial characteristics of Kawasaki disease with cerebrospinal fluid pleocytosis in febrile infants. Pediatr Neurol 2012;47(4): 259–62.

31. Bratincsak A, Reddy VD, Purohit PJ, et al. Coronary artery dilation in acute Kawasaki disease and acute illnesses associated with fever. Pediatr Infect Dis J 2012; 31(9):924–6.

32. Muniz JC, Dummer K, Gauvreau K, et al. Coronary artery dimensions in febrile children without Kawasaki disease. Circ Cardiovasc Imaging 2013;6(2):239–44.

33. Dominguez SR, Anderson MS, Eladawy M, et al. Preventing coronary artery abnormalities: a need for earlier diagnosis and treatment of Kawasaki disease. Pediatr Infect Dis J 2012;31(12):1217–20.

34. Printz BF, Sleeper LA, Newburger JW, et al. Noncoronary cardiac abnormalities are associated with coronary artery dilation and with laboratory inflammatory markers in acute Kawasaki disease. J Am Coll Cardiol 2011;57(1):86–92.

35. Newburger JW, Takahashi M, Beiser AS, et al. A single intravenous infusion of gamma globulin as compared with four infusions in the treatment of acute Kawasaki syndrome. N Engl J Med 1991;324(23):1633–9.

36. Newburger JW, Takahashi M, Burns JC, et al. The treatment of Kawasaki syndrome with intravenous gamma globulin. N Engl J Med 1986;315(6):341–7.

37. Newburger JW, Sanders SP, Burns JC, et al. Left ventricular contractility and function in Kawasaki syndrome. Effect of intravenous gamma-globulin. Circulation 1989;79(6):1237–46.

38. Newburger JW, Sleeper LA, McCrindle BW, et al. Randomized trial of pulsed corticosteroid therapy for primary treatment of Kawasaki disease. N Engl J Med 2007;356(7):663–75.

39. Tremoulet AH, Jain S, Jaggi P, et al. Infliximab for intensification of primary therapy for Kawasaki disease: a phase 3 randomised, double-blind, placebo-controlled trial. Lancet 2014;383(9930):1731–8.

40. Kobayashi T, Saji T, Otani T, et al. Efficacy of immunoglobulin plus prednisolone for prevention of coronary artery abnormalities in severe Kawasaki disease (RAISE study): a randomised, open-label, blinded-endpoint trial. Lancet 2012; 379(9826):1613–20.

41. Son MB, Newburger JW. Management of Kawasaki disease: corticosteroids revisited. Lancet 2012;379(9826):1571–2.

42. Wallace CA, French JW, Kahn SJ, et al. Initial intravenous gammaglobulin treatment failure in Kawasaki disease. Pediatrics 2000;105(6):E78.

43. Sundel RP, Burns JC, Baker A, et al. Gamma globulin re-treatment in Kawasaki disease. J Pediatr 1993;123(4):657–9.

44. Wright DA, Newburger JW, Baker A, et al. Treatment of immune globulin-resistant Kawasaki disease with pulsed doses of corticosteroids. J Pediatr 1996;128(1): 146–9.

45. Burns JC, Best BM, Mejias A, et al. Infliximab treatment of intravenous immunoglobulin-resistant Kawasaki disease. J Pediatr 2008;153(6):833–8.

46. Tremoulet AH, Pancoast P, Franco A, et al. Calcineurin inhibitor treatment of intravenous immunoglobulin-resistant Kawasaki disease. J Pediatr 2012;161(3): 506–512 e1.
47. Suzuki H, Terai M, Hamada H, et al. Cyclosporin a treatment for Kawasaki disease refractory to initial and additional intravenous immunoglobulin. Pediatr Infect Dis J 2011;30(10):871–6.
48. Lee TJ, Kim KH, Chun JK, et al. Low-dose methotrexate therapy for intravenous immunoglobulin-resistant Kawasaki disease. Yonsei Med J 2008;49(5):714–8.
49. Checchia PA, Pahl E, Shaddy RE, et al. Cardiac transplantation for Kawasaki disease. Pediatrics 1997;100(4):695–9.
50. Suda K, Tahara N, Honda A, et al. Persistent peripheral arteritis long after Kawasaki disease - another documentation of ongoing vascular inflammation. Int J Cardiol 2015;180:88–90.

Recognition of and Prompt Treatment for Tick-Borne Infections in Children

Sheena Mukkada, MD[a,b], Steven C. Buckingham, MD, MA[a,*]

KEYWORDS

- Tick-borne infections • Rocky Mountain spotted fever • Ehrlichiosis • Anaplasmosis
- Lyme disease • Tularemia • Babesiosis • Doxycycline

KEY POINTS

- Tick-borne infections occur more often that is generally recognized, and they frequently present with nonspecific clinical findings.
- In cases of suspected tick-borne rickettsial infections, specific antimicrobial therapy should be initiated promptly, without depending on results of confirmatory laboratory tests.
- Doxycycline is the drug of choice for treatment of tick-borne rickettsial infections, even in young children.
- Prevention of tick-borne infections depends on decreasing the likelihood of tick attachments and promptly removing attached ticks.

INTRODUCTION

A variety of tick-borne infections are endemic in North America. This review focuses on widely prevalent diseases for which specific antimicrobial treatment is available—namely, Rocky Mountain spotted fever (RMSF), ehrlichiosis, anaplasmosis, Lyme disease, tularemia, and babesiosis. Other regionally important tick-associated illnesses on this and other continents are not emphasized. Our aim is not to provide exhaustive reviews of these diseases, but rather to highlight concepts that apply broadly to the care of patients with suspected tick-borne illnesses. Although children are the focus of this review, the principles underscored are largely applicable to adults as well.

Dr S. Mukkada and Dr S.C. Buckingham have nothing to disclose.
[a] Department of Pediatrics, Le Bonheur Children's Hospital, University of Tennessee College of Medicine, 50 North Dunlap Street, Memphis, TN 38103, USA; [b] Department of Infectious Diseases, St. Jude Children's Research Hospital, 262 Danny Thomas Place, Memphis, TN 38105, USA
* Corresponding author.
E-mail address: sbucking@uthsc.edu

Infect Dis Clin N Am 29 (2015) 539–555
http://dx.doi.org/10.1016/j.idc.2015.05.002
0891-5520/15/$ – see front matter © 2015 Elsevier Inc. All rights reserved.

ETIOLOGIC AGENTS AND VECTORS

Etiologic agents of North American tick-borne diseases include rickettsiae (intracellular gram-negative coccobacilli, including *Rickettsia*, *Ehrlichia*, and *Anaplasma* spp.), spirochetes (*Borrelia* spp.), other bacteria (eg, *Francisella tularensis*), protozoa (*Babesia* spp.) and viruses. The causative organisms, vectors, geography, and prominent clinical findings of the diseases emphasized in this review are summarized in **Table 1**.[1–4] Similar data are provided for selected additional North American tick-borne infections in **Table 2**.

Tick-borne diseases occur across vast areas of North America, although not all diseases occur in all regions. Although it was first described in the northern Rocky Mountains, RMSF cases are most heavily concentrated in the southeastern, south-central, and mid-Atlantic regions of the United States (**Fig. 1**). RMSF has been reported in all US states except Alaska and Hawaii, as well as in Mexico and throughout Central and South America (where it is also known as Brazilian spotted fever). Ehrlichiosis cases are also most frequent in the southern and mid-Atlantic regions. Unlike RMSF, however, ehrlichiosis only occurs within the geographic range of the Lone Star tick, which runs eastward from the Great Plains (**Fig. 2**).[1,2]

By contrast, Lyme disease occurs most frequently in northeastern and upper Midwestern states, with scattered endemic cases in the Pacific Northwest (**Fig. 3**). Reports of Lyme disease from nonendemic regions generally represent either acquired illnesses in travelers returning from Lyme-endemic areas or false-positive serologic results in patients inappropriately tested for Lyme disease. In the southern United States, a disease has emerged—named, fittingly enough, the Southern tick-associated rash illness (STARI)—that mimics the early localized rash of Lyme disease (see **Table 2**). Anaplasmosis and babesiosis follow geographic distributions similar to Lyme disease.[2,3]

Unlike the aforementioned diseases, tularemia is associated not only with multiple tick vectors, but also with numerous other arthropods and mammals (most notoriously, rabbits). Tularemia is widely distributed across North America, although cases are relatively concentrated in the south-central United States (**Fig. 4**).[2,5]

EPIDEMIOLOGY

Tick-borne infections occur more frequently than is generally recognized. For example, data from the southeast and south-central United States indicate that more than 10% of children have serologic evidence of prior rickettsial infections.[6,7] The gap between seroprevalence and reported cases may be related to missed diagnoses as well as cross-reactions to other rickettsiae of uncertain pathogenicity.

Seasonality

Most tick-borne infections occur between April and October, when both tick and outdoor human activity are at their peaks; however, these infections do occur all year, even in regions with cold winters. Ixodid ticks live for 2 years, and although they are less active during winter months, they are not necessarily killed by cold weather.[8] Underscoring this point, 4% of RMSF cases, 3% of ehrlichiosis cases, and 3% of anaplasmosis cases reported to US Centers for Disease Control and Prevention (CDC) from 2000 to 2007 occurred during the months of December, January, or February.[9,10] Indeed, 9% of all RMSF cases from New York, New Jersey, and Pennsylvania were reported during these months.[9]

Table 1
Principal tick-borne infections of North America

Disease	Organism	Geographic Distribution and Vector	Selected Clinical Findings[a]
Rocky Mountain spotted fever (RMSF)	Rickettsia rickettsii	Eastern United States: Dermacentor variabilis (dog tick); Mountain West: Dermacentor andersoni (wood tick); Southwestern US deserts: Rhipicephalus sanguineus (brown dog tick); Mexico, Central America, Texas: Amblyomma cajennense (Cayenne tick)	Fever, headache, nausea, vomiting, rash (frequently petechial), hyponatremia, thrombocytopenia
Ehrlichiosis[b]	Ehrlichia chaffeensis	Southeastern and south-central United States: Amblyomma americanum (Lone Star tick)	Similar to RMSF, but rash is less common; leukopenia, thrombocytopenia, elevated transaminases
Anaplasmosis[c]	Anaplasma phagocytophilum	Northeastern and upper Midwestern United States: Ixodes scapularis (blacklegged tick); Pacific Coast: Ixodes pacificus (Western blacklegged tick)	Similar to ehrlichiosis, but rash is rarely present
Lyme disease	Borrelia burgdorferi	Northeastern and upper Midwestern United States: I scapularis; Pacific Coast: I pacificus	Early localized stage: erythema migrans rash, lymphadenopathy, flulike symptoms (malaise, headache, fever, myalgia, arthralgia) Early disseminated stage: multiple erythema migrans lesions, flulike symptoms, carditis (heart block), cranial nerve palsies, meningitis, peripheral neuropathy Late stage: arthritis (large joints), encephalopathy, encephalomyelitis
Tularemia	Francisella tularensis	Eastern United States: D variabilis; Mountain West: D andersoni; Southeastern and south-central United States: A americanum	Fever, chills, malaise, vomiting, diarrhea; ulceroglandular disease presents with cutaneous eschar and regional lymphadenopathy
Babesiosis[d]	Babesia microti[d]	Northeastern and upper Midwestern United States: I scapularis	Fever, malaise, headache, hepatosplenomegaly, thrombocytopenia, hemolytic anemia

Abbreviation: RMSF, Rock Mountain spotted fever.
[a] The listed clinical findings are not an exhaustive summary, but those considered "typical" for each disease. Some patients may present without all of these findings, whereas others may have additional features not listed here.
[b] Also known as human monocytotropic ehrlichiosis.
[c] Also known as human granulocytotropic anaplasmosis; previously termed human granulocytic ehrlichiosis.
[d] Besides B microti, other Babesia species, transmitted by uncertain vectors, have been linked to cases of babesiosis in Pacific Coast states and Missouri.
Data from Refs.[1–4]

Table 2
Selected additional North American tick-borne infections

Disease	Organism	Geographic Distribution and Vector	Prominent Clinical Findings[a]
Rickettsia parkeri infection[b]	Rickettsia parkeri	Southeastern United States: Amblyomma maculatum (Gulf Coast tick)	Similar to RMSF, but with eschar at inoculation site; rash may be vesicular or pustular; vomiting, abdominal pain less prominent than in RMSF
Rickettsia spp. 364D infection[b]	Rickettsia spp. 364D	California: Dermacentor occidentalis (Pacific Coast tick)	Fever, headache, myalgias, ± rash, cutaneous eschar
Ehrlichia ewingii infection	E ewingii	Southeastern and south-central United States: Amblyomma americanum	Similar to anaplasmosis (see **Table 1**)
STARI	Borrelia lonestari[c]	Southeastern and south-central United States: A americanum	Rash similar to erythema migrans, ± mild constitutional symptoms[d]
Endemic relapsing fever	Borrelia hermsii B turicatae B parkeri	Western mountains and deserts of the United States: Ornithodoros species (soft ticks)	Fever, chills, relapsing course
Colorado tick fever	Colorado tick fever virus (genus: Coltivirus)	Western mountains of United States and southern Canada: Dermacentor andersoni	Fever, headache, leukopenia, thrombocytopenia; biphasic course
Powassan encephalitis	Powassan virus (genus: Flavivirus)	Northeastern and north-central United States, Canada: Ixodes species, D andersoni	Headache, seizures, altered sensorium, focal neurologic signs, meningismus
Heartland virus infection	Heartland virus (genus: Phlebovirus)	South-central United States: A americanum	Fever, headache, fatigue, nausea, myalgia, leukopenia, thrombocytopenia

Abbreviations: RMSF, Rock Mountain spotted fever; STARI, southern tick-associated rash illness.

[a] The listed clinical findings are not an exhaustive summary, but those considered "typical" for each disease. Some patients may present without all of these findings, whereas others may have additional features not listed here. For many of these diseases, the full spectrum of clinical illness has yet to be defined.

[b] Besides R parkeri and Rickettsia species 364D, many other rickettsial species have been identified in North America, but their roles as human pathogens are still under investigation.

[c] Limited data implicates B lonestari as the cause of STARI. Some would argue that the cause of this disease awaits confirmation.

[d] Patients with STARI present with clinical findings suggestive of early localized Lyme disease. Manifestations of disseminated Lyme disease (eg, arthritis, neuropathy) have not been seen in these patients.

Data from Refs.[1–4,42–44]

Exposure History

Tick-borne infections are underrecognized, in part, because individuals bitten by ticks are often unaware of their exposure. Three factors account for why tick bites may pass unnoticed: ticks are small, especially in their pre-adult stages (eg, nymphs are only 1–2 mm long); they frequently attach at body sites that escape detection; and their

SPOTTED FEVER RICKETTSIOSIS. Number of reported cases, by county — United States, 2012

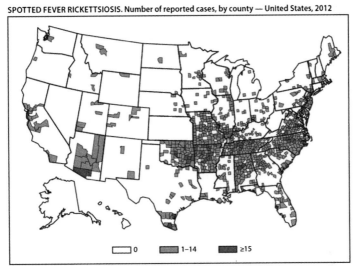

Fig. 1. Geographic distribution of spotted fever rickettsial infections (mostly Rocky Mountain spotted fever) in the United States in 2012. Counties that reported 1 to 14 cases to the US Centers for Disease Control and Prevention are shaded lightly, whereas those that reported more than 15 cases are shaded darkly. Cases are widely dispersed, but are especially concentrated in the southeastern, south-central, and mid-Atlantic portions of the country. (*From* the Centers for Disease Control and Prevention. Summary of Notifiable Diseases, 2012. Morb Mortal Wkly Rep 2014;61(53):89.)

EHRLICHIOSIS, *EHRLICHIA CHAFFEENSIS*. Number of reported cases, by county — United States, 2012

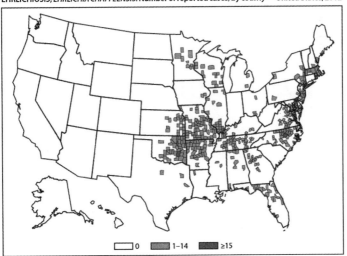

Fig. 2. Geographic distribution of ehrlichiosis in the United States in 2012. Counties that reported 1 to 14 cases to the US Centers for Disease Control and Prevention are shaded lightly, whereas those that reported more than 15 cases are shaded darkly. Cases occur across much of the eastern United States, but incidence is greatest in the southeastern, south-central, and mid-Atlantic portions of the country. (*From* the Centers for Disease Control and Prevention. Summary of Notifiable Diseases, 2012. Morb Mortal Wkly Rep 2014;61(53):64.)

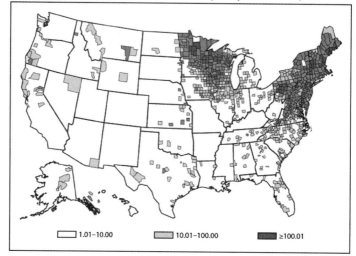

Fig. 3. Geographic distribution of reported Lyme disease cases in the United States in 2012. Counties with a disease incidence of 10.01 to 100 cases per 100,000 population are shaded lightly, whereas those with an incidence of greater than 100.01 cases per 100,000 population are shaded darkly. The vast majority of cases are reported from counties in the Northeast, mid-Atlantic, and upper Midwest regions. [a] Per 100, 000 population. (*From* the Centers for Disease Control and Prevention. Summary of Notifiable Diseases, 2012. Morb Mortal Wkly Rep 2014;61(53):80.)

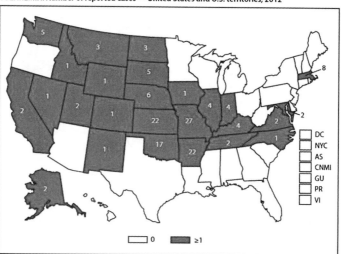

Fig. 4. Geographic distribution of reported cases of tularemia in the United States in 2012. States with reported cases are shaded, and the number of cases is shown. Cases are widely dispersed, but especially concentrated in the south-central states of Oklahoma, Arkansas, Missouri, and Kansas. (*From* the Centers for Disease Control and Prevention. Summary of Notifiable Diseases, 2012. Morb Mortal Wkly Rep 2014;61(53):96.)

attachments are usually painless. Although a history of a known tick bite can be a helpful diagnostic clue, the absence of such a history never precludes the diagnosis of a tick-borne disease. At least one-third of all patients with serologically diagnosed RMSF or ehrlichiosis do not recall a preceding tick bite.[1,11–13]

Risk Factors

Many patients with tick-borne infections lack supposed epidemiologic risk factors for tick-borne infections. Historically, male sex has been considered a risk factor; however, in a recent multicenter study of 92 children with laboratory-diagnosed RMSF in the southeastern United States, 53% of patients were female.[11] Similarly, although outdoor activities such as hiking and camping in wooded areas are recognized risk factors, tick-borne infections also occur in urban areas and in patients whose only outdoor exposures take place in their own yards.[1,14] Recent studies identified a history of exposure to a wooded area in only 34% of children with RMSF, and in 31% of children with ehrlichiosis.[11,12] Such epidemiologic clues are thus only helpful to clinicians when they are present.

CLINICAL FEATURES

In most cases, children with tick-borne illnesses present with nonspecific symptoms such as fever, malaise, headache, nausea, vomiting, and myalgias. Although some tick-borne infections are associated with certain "classic" findings (such as the petechial rash of RMSF), the absence of such findings early in the disease course often leads clinicians to initially suspect other, more common childhood illnesses, such as viral infections or streptococcal pharyngitis. Thus, although clinicians should be aware of the "typical" clinical findings associated with tick-borne diseases (see **Table 1**), they must also realize that these are not always present.

Rocky Mountain Spotted Fever

RMSF manifests as a multisystem vasculitis that can affect any organ. The most characteristic clinical finding is the rash, which typically begins as a macular or maculopapular eruption and becomes purpuric or petechial in 50% of cases. It begins on the ankles and wrists, often involving palms and soles before spreading centrally. The rash may not be apparent initially, and it may be difficult to ascertain in dark-skinned individuals, but it ultimately appears in more than 90% of children with RMSF.[1,11] The oft-cited clinical triad of fever, rash, and history of tick bite is present in fewer than 60% of children with RMSF. Likewise, the alternative triad of fever, rash, and headache is present in only about one-half of such cases. Many other clinical findings are possible, the most prominent of which are conjunctival injection and mental status impairment. Meningismus, seizures, coma, and shock are reported uncommonly.[11]

Routine laboratory tests often reveal nonspecific abnormalities. The total leukocyte count may be increased or decreased, but is usually normal. About 60% of children have platelet counts below 150,000/mm^3, but profound thrombocytopenia is unusual. Serum sodium concentrations lower than 135 mEq/dL occur in about 50% of patients, and a similar percentage have modest elevations of hepatic transaminases. Other abnormalities can include increases in serum urea nitrogen or creatinine concentrations, hyperbilirubinemia, hypoalbuminemia, and prolonged prothrombin or partial thromboplastin times. Cerebrospinal fluid examination may reveal a mononuclear cell pleocytosis and an increased protein concentration.[1,11]

Ehrlichiosis

Overall, the clinical syndrome of ehrlichiosis is highly similar to that of RMSF. In children with ehrlichiosis, compared with those with RMSF, the rash occurs less often (present in about two-thirds of children and in one-third of adults), appears later in the disease course (median 4 days into illness in ehrlichiosis vs 1 day in RMSF), is less frequently petechial, and less commonly involves the palms and soles. Laboratory abnormalities, however, are more pronounced in children with ehrlichiosis: thrombocytopenia is present in more than 90%, as are elevations of hepatic transaminases; leukopenia (<4000/mm^3) occurs in about 60% of patients.[1,11,12,15]

Anaplasmosis

Patients with anaplasmosis present with signs, symptoms, and laboratory findings similar to those observed in ehrlichiosis, with the notable exception that rash is present in fewer than 10% of patients with anaplasmosis.[1,3]

Lyme Disease

The clinical progression of Lyme disease is traditionally classified into 3 stages. The early localized stage is characterized by erythema migrans, which presents at the site of a preceding tick bite as an erythematous expansile patch that may have central clearing. The rash is typically nonpruritic and nontender, and it may have purpuric, vesicular, or pustular characteristics. Patients who do not receive appropriate antibiotic therapy can progress to experience the early disseminated and late stages of disease (see **Table 1**). Fever and other nonspecific constitutional symptoms frequently accompany the early stages of disease. However, patients with Lyme disease almost always present with characteristic signs and symptoms such as erythema migrans, facial nerve palsy, or large joint arthritis. In the absence of such findings, nonspecific complaints such as fever, fatigue, or weakness are not suggestive of Lyme disease.[3,16]

Tularemia

Multiple forms of tularemia are described, all of which are marked by abrupt onset of fever and other constitutional symptoms. Patients with tick-borne tularemia usually present with either ulceroglandular or glandular disease, which are typified by painful regional lymphadenopathy with or without an inoculation ulcer at the site of a recent tick bite. Typhoidal and pneumonic tularemia, the forms most associated with fatal outcomes, are rare in children.[2,5,15]

Babesiosis

Asymptomatic infections with *Babesia microti* are common, occurring in approximately 50% of infected children and 25% of adults. Symptomatic patients present with the gradual onset of fever and other nonspecific symptoms. Physical examination may reveal hepatosplenomegaly. Characteristic laboratory findings include anemia, thrombocytopenia, and evidence of hemolysis (eg, reticulocytosis, decreased haptoglobin, and increased lactate dehydrogenase). The disease usually runs a mild course, especially in children. Nonetheless, babesiosis can be life threatening, especially in asplenic or otherwise immunocompromised patients.[2,15,17,18]

DIAGNOSIS

Although routine laboratory testing has limited value in diagnosing tick-borne illnesses, specific confirmatory tests are available for the principal North American tick-borne infections (**Table 3**). For most of these illnesses, confirmation relies on

Table 3
Diagnostic tests and antimicrobial therapies for principal North American tick-borne infections

Disease	Confirmatory Diagnostic Tests[a]	Antimicrobial Therapy[a]
RMSF	Serology: 4-fold increase in antibody titer[b]; PCR of skin biopsy specimen; IHC staining of skin or other tissue specimen	Doxycycline (4.4 mg/kg/d, divided into 2 doses, maximum 200 mg/d), continued until ≥3 d after fever resolution; minimum treatment course, 5–7 d
Ehrlichiosis	Serology: 4-fold increase in antibody titer[b]; PCR of whole blood specimen; visualization of morulae in cytoplasm of blood monocytes; IHC staining of bone marrow or other tissue specimen	Doxycycline (dosed as for RMSF)
Anaplasmosis	Serology: 4-fold increase in antibody titer[b]; PCR of whole blood specimen; visualization of morulae in cytoplasm of blood granulocytes; IHC staining of bone marrow or other tissue specimen	Doxycycline (dosed as for RMSF, but continued for 10–14 d)
Lyme disease	Serology: positive EIA or IFA confirmed by positive Western immunoblot[c]	Localized erythema migrans: oral regimen[d] (14 d) Multiple erythema migrans: oral regimen[d] (21 d) Cranial nerve palsy: oral regimen[d] (14–21 d) Meningitis: parenteral regimen[e] (14–28 d) or oral doxycycline[f] Carditis: oral or parenteral regimen[d,e] (14–21 d) Arthritis: oral regimen[d] (28 d) Recurrent arthritis: oral regimen[d] (28 d) or parenteral regimen[e] (14–28 d) Late neurologic disease: parenteral regimen[e] (14–28 d)
Tularemia	Detection of *F tularensis* in clinical specimens by culture,[g] PCR, or IHC staining; serology: 4-fold increase in antibody titer[b]	Parenteral regimens: gentamicin (7.5 mg/kg/d, divided into 3 doses) or streptomycin (30 mg/kg/d, divided into 2 doses, maximum 2 g/d), for minimum of 10 d Oral regimens: doxycycline (dosed as for RMSF) for 14–21 d; or ciprofloxacin (30 mg/kg/d divided into 2 doses, maximum 1.5 g/d) for 10–14 d

(continued on next page)

Table 3 (continued)		
Disease	Confirmatory Diagnostic Tests[a]	Antimicrobial Therapy[a]
Babesiosis	Visualization of intraerythrocytic parasites in peripheral blood smear; PCR of whole blood specimen[h]	Clindamycin (20–40 mg/kg/d divided into 3 or 4 doses, maximum 600 mg/dose), orally or intravenously, plus quinine (orally, 25–30 mg/kg/d divided into 3 doses; adult dose, 650 mg every 8 h) for 7–10 d[i]; or Atovaquone (40 mg/kg/d divided into 2 doses, maximum 750 mg/dose) orally for 7–10 d, plus azithromycin (10 mg/kg once, maximum 500 mg,[j] on day 1; then 5 mg/kg once daily, maximum 250 mg/dose[j]) orally for 10 d

Abbreviations: EIA, enzyme immunoassay; IFA, indirect immunofluorescent antibody; IHC, immunohistochemical; PCR, polymerase chain reaction; RMSF, Rocky Mountain spotted fever.

[a] Summary data are provided here. For additional details, see the appropriate references for each disease.

[b] Four-fold increase in antibody titer between acute and convalescent serum specimens, obtained ≥2 weeks apart.

[c] If serologic testing is performed to confirm early disease, both immunoglobulin (Ig)M and IgG immunoblots should be performed. For patients with ≥1 month of symptoms, only an IgG immunoblot should be performed.

[d] Oral regimens for Lyme disease: doxycycline (4 mg/kg/d, divided into 2 doses; maximum 200 mg/d), amoxicillin (50 mg/kg/d, divided into 3 doses; maximum 1.5 g/d), or cefuroxime (30 mg/kg/d, divided into 2 doses, maximum 1 g/d).

[e] Parenteral regimens for Lyme disease: ceftriaxone (50–75 mg/kg, once daily; maximum 2 g/d), penicillin (200,000–400,000 U/kg/d, given every 4 hours; maximum 24 million U/d), or cefotaxime (150–200 mg/kg/d, divided into 3 or 4 doses; maximum, 6 g/d).

[f] Doxycycline (4–8 mg/kg/d in 2 divided doses; maximum 200–400 mg), administered orally for 14 days (range, 10–28 days) is an alternative therapy for Lyme meningitis in patients ≥8 years of age.

[g] Culture of *F tularensis* requires appropriate media and biosafety precautions. Laboratory personnel should be notified when sending specimens for culture from patients with suspected tularemia.

[h] Serologic testing can provide supportive evidence of babesiosis, but high rates of background positivity in endemic areas limit its usefulness for confirming the diagnosis.

[i] For patients with severe babesiosis (see text), the combination of clindamycin and quinine is preferred, and in such patients the clindamycin should be administered intravenously.

[j] In immunocompromised patients with babesiosis, the maximum daily dose of azithromycin may be increased to 600–1000 mg.

Data from Refs.[1–3,5,13,16,18,22]

either demonstration of an increase in antibody titer between acute and convalescent sera or identification of the etiologic agent in host tissue (eg, through culture, microscopic visualization, or nucleic acid amplification).

The key point, for purposes of this review, is that clinicians must suspect and diagnose tick-borne illnesses on clinical grounds, without depending on results of confirmatory laboratory tests. This is especially important in patients with rickettsial infections, in whom the risk of mortality increases substantially if treatment is delayed. Serologic testing during the acute phase of any of these illnesses is of little value, because antibody responses will not be detectable until several days into the disease course. Serologic tests establish a baseline for subsequent comparison, but as a rule the decision to send such tests is tantamount to the decision to prescribe appropriate antimicrobial therapy.

One significant drawback to diagnostic testing for Lyme disease is the poor specificity of available serologic tests. Even with "2-step" testing (ie, Western immunoblot confirmation of positive enzyme immunoassay results), this lack of specificity means that positive tests usually represent false positives in areas where Lyme disease is not endemic. Thus, serologic testing for Lyme disease should only be performed in patients in whom clinical and epidemiologic findings are compatible with that diagnosis.[16,19]

ANTIBIOTIC THERAPY

Appropriate antibiotic therapies for the principal North American tick-borne illnesses are listed in **Table 3**. Details regarding therapy for certain diseases are discussed in this section.

Rocky Mountain Spotted Fever, Ehrlichiosis, and Anaplasmosis

Doxycycline is the drug of choice for all patients with suspected tick-borne rickettsial infections in North America, regardless of age. Unfortunately, many clinicians remain unaware of this recommendation, because misinformation persists about the supposed risk of doxycycline to stain the permanent teeth of young children.[20] At one time, chloramphenicol was recommended for treatment of suspected RMSF in children younger than 8 years of age. Today, however, several lines of reasoning support the use of doxycycline for treatment of tick-borne rickettsial infections, even in children.

- Compared with chloramphenicol, doxycycline provides more effective therapy against RMSF. Patients with RMSF who receive chloramphenicol alone have an increased risk of death compared with those who receive tetracycline or doxycycline.[21]
- Doxycycline provides effective therapy for ehrlichiosis, and chloramphenicol does not. This is important because the 2 diseases cannot be distinguished reliably on clinical grounds.[22]
- Doxycycline has never been shown to stain permanent teeth. Although this side effect was seen in children who received repeated courses of tetracycline, published studies have not found evidence of dental staining among children treated with doxycycline.[23–26]
- Unlike doxycycline, chloramphenicol is linked to serious toxicities, including life-threatening aplastic anemia, and it requires monitoring of serum levels owing to its unpredictable pharmacokinetics. The oral formulation of chloramphenicol was withdrawn from the US market in 1995 and is no longer available.[21]

In addition to doxycycline, clinicians should consider providing an antibiotic active against *Neisseria meningitidis*, such as a parenteral third-generation cephalosporin, to children treated for suspected RMSF, at least until blood culture results rule out meningococcemia. For patients with RMSF or ehrlichiosis, inappropriate treatment with sulfa-containing antibiotics (eg, trimethoprim–sulfamethoxazole) has been associated with an increased risk of severe disease; thus, such agents should be avoided strictly in patients with possible rickettsial infections.[1,11,12]

Lyme Disease

Antibiotic therapy is indicated for patients in all stages of Lyme disease. Treatment of patients with early localized disease helps to speed the resolution of the skin rash and prevents progression to subsequent stages. Recommended therapeutic regimens vary depending on patient age and clinical manifestations (see **Table 3**). Doxycycline is appropriate therapy for most adults and children 8 years of age and older, and amoxicillin is the preferred oral agent for younger children. Macrolide antibiotics (eg, erythromycin and azithromycin) are less effective than tetracyclines, penicillins, and cephalosporins, and should only be used in patients who are unable to tolerate the recommended regimens. The administration of prolonged antibiotic courses (ie, exceeding 4 weeks) has not been found to be beneficial and is not recommended.[3,16]

Tularemia

The aminoglycosides streptomycin and gentamicin are considered drugs of choice for treatment of tularemia. Gentamicin is generally preferred because it is inexpensive, can be administered intravenously, and is less toxic and more readily available than streptomycin. For patients with relatively mild disease, oral therapy with doxycycline or ciprofloxacin can be considered. If doxycycline is used, therapy should be continued for 14 days to decrease the risk of relapse (see **Table 3**).[2,5,15] Because fluoroquinolones are generally not recommended in children, clinicians should consider their associated benefits and risks, as compared with those of other options, before prescribing ciprofloxacin for this indication.[27]

Babesiosis

Combination therapy with either atovaquone plus azithromycin or clindamycin plus quinine is recommended for symptomatic patients with babesiosis. The atovaquone–azithromycin combination is associated with substantially fewer side effects. In patients with severe illness (defined by parasitemia levels of $\geq$10%, significant hemolysis, or end-organ compromise), therapy with clindamycin (intravenously) and quinine is recommended, and exchange transfusion should be considered.[2,3,18]

CLINICAL OUTCOMES
Rocky Mountain Spotted Fever

Before effective antibiotics were developed, 25% to 30% of patients with RMSF died.[8] Even today, with appropriate therapy, the prognosis for children with RMSF remains guarded. In 1 study, most children improved promptly after starting doxycycline, with defervescence usually occurring within 72 hours. Still, 3% of children died, and 15% of survivors had significant neurologic deficits at the time of hospital discharge.[11] Among RMSF cases reported to CDC between 2000 and 2007, fatality rates were highest among children 5 to 9 years of age (2.6%) and among Native Americans (2.2%).[9] The chief modifiable risk factor for mortality from RMSF, identified repeatedly in published reports, is delayed initiation of antirickettsial therapy.[28–30] Indeed, the risk of mortality increases by more than 3-fold in patients for whom therapy is delayed until the fifth day of illness or later.[31,32]

Ehrlichiosis and Anaplasmosis

Like RMSF, ehrlichiosis can cause severe and even fatal disease in children. From 2000 to 2007, 1.9% of patients reported to CDC with ehrlichiosis died, and the highest case fatality rate, at 3.7%, was seen in children 5 to 9 years of age. The prognosis is generally better with anaplasmosis, which carries an overall case fatality rate of less than 1%. For both diseases, the risk of adverse outcomes is increased among immunocompromised patients.[10] As with RMSF, delays in the initiation of therapy have been linked with worse outcomes in patients with these diseases.[33,34]

Lyme Disease

Lyme disease is rarely, if ever, fatal, and its prognosis is almost uniformly good, especially for children treated in early disease stages. As in adults, nonspecific complaints may persist in some children after therapy, but these are no more common in those with Lyme disease than in the general population. There is no convincing evidence that *Borrelia burgdorferi* infections persist after appropriate therapy, and randomized controlled trials have not found any benefit to prolonged or repeated courses of antibiotics in patients with persistent post-Lyme symptoms.[3,35,36]

Tularemia

Children with tick-borne tularemia usually present with glandular or ulceroglandular disease and respond well to therapy. Relapses can occur after treatment, requiring additional courses of therapy. Although the pneumonic and typhoidal forms of tularemia are associated with mortality rates of 30% to 60%, these forms are rare in children and are not typically associated with tick-borne disease.[2,5,15,37]

Babesiosis

Patients with mild-to-moderate babesiosis begin to improve within 48 hours of starting therapy, and recovery should be complete within 3 months. In some patients, parasitemia can persist for months after treatment. Evaluation for immunodeficiency (eg, human immunodeficiency virus infection, asplenia) should be considered in patients with severe, protracted, or relapsing episodes of babesiosis.[3] Fatality rates of 6% to 9% have been reported for hospitalized patients with babesiosis, and rates of up to 21% have been reported in immunosuppressed patients.[17] These numbers likely overstate the risk of poor outcome among children, however.

PREVENTION

Vaccines to prevent North American tick-borne infections do not exist. Thus, prevention rests on avoidance of tick bites and prompt removal of attached ticks (**Box 1**).

Insect repellants containing N, N-diethyl-meta-toluamide (DEET) in concentrations of 10% to 30% are highly effective in preventing tick and insect bites. Other repellants have been developed, but none has the proven track record of DEET, which has been in use since the 1950s. Although concerns over their potential neurotoxicity have been voiced, substantial evidence indicates that DEET-containing products are quite safe when used appropriately. The US Environmental Protection Agency has concluded that "normal use of DEET does not present a health concern to the general US population, including children," and the American Academy of Pediatrics has stated that concerns over DEET's potential toxicity are "unfounded." DEET-containing products should be used according to manufacturers' directions, and care should be taken to avoid their ingestion or exposure to mucous membranes.[1,38–41]

Chemoprophylaxis against Lyme disease with a single dose of oral doxycycline may be offered to selected adults and older children after recognized *Ixodes scapularis* attachments in hyperendemic regions.[3,16] Data are insufficient to recommend amoxicillin for this indication, or to recommend chemoprophylaxis for the prevention of other tick-borne diseases. In general, children with known tick exposures should be monitored closely and only receive therapy if symptoms develop.

Box 1
Keys to prevention of tick-borne infections

- Avoid potentially tick-infested areas[a] when possible.
- When entering potentially infested areas:
  - Wear light colored clothes with long sleeves and pants;
  - Tuck pants into socks;
  - Wear clothing sprayed or impregnated with 0.5% permethrin; and
  - Apply insect repellants (preferably containing DEET) to exposed skin and clothing.[b]
- Examine persons and pets who have spent time outdoors for attached ticks.
  - Pay special attention to body regions where ticks can hide (eg, the head, neck, axillae, and groin).
- Remove any attached ticks, preferably with tweezers, by grasping close to the skin and gently pulling straight out.
- Wash skin surface with soap and water after removal of an attached tick.
- Do not apply foreign substances (eg, fingernail polish, gasoline, isopropyl alcohol, petroleum jelly) or a hot kitchen match to an attached tick.[c]

Abbreviation: DEET, N, N-diethyl-meta-toluamide.
   [a] Ticks may be encountered in many types of outdoor settings, but they are especially prevalent in and around wooded areas with heavy growth of shrubs and small trees.
   [b] Avoid ingestion of or exposure of mucous membranes to DEET. Repellants containing DEET should be applied away from food and should not be sprayed on the hands of young children. Use products according to manufacturers' directions. DEET is not recommended for use in infants less than 2 months of age.
   [c] Such methods are not only ineffective for dislodging ticks, but may actually increase the risk of pathogen transmission.
   Data from Refs.[1,38,39]

SUMMARY

The clinical challenges created by tick-borne infections are 2-fold. On one hand, they frequently present with nonspecific findings, leading clinicians to initially suspect viral or other common childhood illnesses. At the same time, delays in their diagnosis—and hence, in starting therapy—are linked to an increased risk of adverse outcomes, including death. For these reasons, clinicians must maintain an index of suspicion for tick-borne infections, especially during the warmer months of the year, and promptly prescribe therapy when such infections are suspected. Of note, such a prompt initiation of therapy requires clinicians to make diagnoses presumptively—that is, without depending on the results of confirmatory laboratory tests, which are likely to be falsely negative early in the disease course.

Once the decision is made to prescribe therapy, the choice of therapy is usually straightforward. Doxycycline is the clearly the antibiotic of choice for all patients with suspected RMSF, ehrlichiosis, and anaplasmosis. These are not only the tick-borne illnesses most likely to result in adverse outcomes, but also those for which delayed therapy has been clearly linked to an increased risk of morbidity and mortality. Concerns over doxycycline's potential to stain the permanent teeth of young children are unfounded; and even if they were valid, such concerns would still have to be weighed against the potentially devastating consequences of leaving rickettsial infections untreated. Of course, for some other tick-borne infections, alternative therapies might be more appropriate (eg, amoxicillin for young children with Lyme disease). But clinicians should not shrink from prescribing doxycycline, even to young children, when tick-borne rickettsial infections are suspected.

REFERENCES

1. Chapman AS, Bakken JS, Folk SM, et al. Diagnosis and management of tick-borne rickettsial diseases: Rocky Mountain spotted fever, ehrlichioses, and anaplasmosis—United States. Morb Mortal Wkly Rep 2006;55(RR-4):1–28.
2. Centers for Disease Control and Prevention. Tickborne diseases of the United States: a reference manual for health care providers. 2nd edition. 2014. Available at: http://www.cdc.gov/lyme/resources/TickborneDiseases.pdf. Accessed March 27, 2015.
3. Wormser GP, Dattwyler RJ, Shapiro ED, et al. The clinical assessment, treatment, and prevention of Lyme disease, human granulocytic anaplasmosis, and babesiosis: clinical practice guidelines by the Infectious Diseases Society of America. Clin Infect Dis 2006;43:1089–134.
4. Woods CR. Rocky Mountain spotted fever in children. Pediatr Clin North Am 2013;60:455–70.
5. American Academy of Pediatrics. Tularemia. In: Pickering LK, Baker CJ, Kimberlin DW, et al, editors. Red Book: 2012 report of the Committee on Infectious Diseases. 29th edition. Elk Grove Village (IL): American Academy of Pediatrics; 2012. p. 768–9.
6. Marshall GS, Jacobs RF, Schutze GE, et al. Ehrlichia chaffeensis seroprevalence among children in the southeast and south-central regions of the United States. Arch Pediatr Adolesc Med 2002;156:166–70.
7. Marshall GS, Stout GG, Jacobs RF, et al. Antibodies reactive to Rickettsia rickettsii among children living in the southeast and south central regions of the United States. Arch Pediatr Adolesc Med 2003;157:443–8.
8. Harrell GT. Rocky Mountain spotted fever. Medicine 1949;28:333–70.
9. Openshaw JJ, Swerdlow DL, Krebs JW, et al. Rocky Mountain spotted fever in the United States, 2000–2007: interpreting contemporary increases in incidence. Am J Trop Med Hyg 2010;83:174–82.
10. Dahlgren FS, Mandel EJ, Krebs JW, et al. Increasing incidence of Ehrlichia chaffeensis and Anaplasma phagocytophilum in the United States, 2000–2007. Am J Trop Med Hyg 2011;85:124–31.
11. Buckingham SC, Marshall GS, Schutze GE, et al. Clinical and laboratory features of Rocky Mountain spotted fever in children. J Pediatr 2007;150:180–4.
12. Schutze GE, Buckingham SC, Marshall GS, et al. Human monocytic ehrlichiosis in children. Pediatr Infect Dis J 2007;26:475–9.
13. American Academy of Pediatrics. Rocky Mountain spotted fever. In: Pickering LK, Baker CJ, Kimberlin DW, et al, editors. Red Book: 2012 report of the Committee on Infectious Diseases. 29th edition. Elk Grove Village (IL): American Academy of Pediatrics; 2012. p. 623–5.
14. Salgo MP, Telzak EE, Currie B, et al. A focus of Rocky Mountain spotted fever within New York City. N Engl J Med 1988;318:1345–8.
15. Buckingham SC. Tick-borne diseases in children: epidemiology, clinical manifestations and optimal treatment strategies. Paediatr Drugs 2005;7:163–76.
16. American Academy of Pediatrics. Lyme disease. In: Pickering LK, Baker CJ, Kimberlin DW, et al, editors. Red Book: 2012 report of the committee on infectious

diseases. 29th edition. Elk Grove Village (IL): American Academy of Pediatrics; 2012. p. 474–9.

17. Vannier E, Krause PJ. Human babesiosis. N Engl J Med 2012;366:2397–407.

18. American Academy of Pediatrics. Babesiosis. In: Pickering LK, Baker CJ, Kimberlin DW, et al, editors. Red Book: 2012 report of the Committee on Infectious Diseases. 29th edition. Elk Grove Village (IL): American Academy of Pediatrics; 2012. p. 244–5.

19. Seltzer EG, Shapiro ED. Misdiagnosis of Lyme disease: when not to order serologic tests. Pediatr Infect Dis J 1996;15:762–3.

20. Mosites E, Carpenter LR, McElroy K, et al. Knowledge, attitudes, and practices regarding Rocky Mountain spotted fever among healthcare providers, Tennessee, 2009. Am J Trop Med Hyg 2013;88:162–6.

21. Holman RC, Paddock CD, Curns AT, et al. Analysis of risk factors for fatal Rocky Mountain spotted fever: evidence for superiority of tetracyclines for therapy. J Infect Dis 2001;184:1437–44.

22. American Academy of Pediatrics. Ehrlichia and anaplasma infections. In: Pickering LK, Baker CJ, Kimberlin DW, et al, editors. Red Book: 2012 report of the Committee on Infectious Diseases. 29th edition. Elk Grove Village (IL): American Academy of Pediatrics; 2012. p. 312–5.

23. Forti G, Benincori C. Doxycycline and the teeth. Lancet 1969;1(7598):782–3.

24. Lochary ME, Lockhart PB, Williams WT. Doxycycline and staining of permanent teeth. Pediatr Infect Dis J 1998;17:429–31.

25. Volovitz B, Shkap R, Amir J, et al. Absence of tooth staining with doxycycline treatment in young children. Clin Pediatr 2007;46:121–6.

26. Todd SR, Dahlgren FS, Traeger MS, et al. No visible dental staining in children treated with doxycycline for suspected Rocky Mountain spotted fever. J Pediatr 2015;166:1246–51.

27. American Academy of Pediatrics. Fluoroquinolones. In: Pickering LK, Baker CJ, Kimberlin DW, et al, editors. Red Book: 2012 report of the Committee on Infectious Diseases. 29th edition. Elk Grove Village (IL): American Academy of Pediatrics; 2012. p. 800–1.

28. Hattwick MAW, Retailliau H, O'Brien RJ, et al. Fatal Rocky Mountain spotted fever. JAMA 1978;240:1499–503.

29. Helmick CG, Bernard KW, D'Angelo LJ. Rocky Mountain spotted fever: clinical, laboratory, and epidemiological features of 262 cases. J Infect Dis 1984;150:480–8.

30. Dahlgren FS, Holman RC, Paddock CD, et al. Fatal Rocky Mountain spotted fever in the United States, 1999–2007. Am J Trop Med Hyg 2012;86:713–9.

31. Dalton MJ, Clarke MJ, Holman RC, et al. National surveillance for Rocky Mountain spotted fever, 1981–1992: epidemiologic summary and evaluation of risk factors for fatal outcome. Am J Trop Med Hyg 1995;52:405–13.

32. Kirkland KB, Wilkinson WE, Sexton DJ. Therapeutic delay and mortality in cases of Rocky Mountain spotted fever. Clin Infect Dis 1995;20:1118–21.

33. Fishbein DB, Dawson JE, Robinson LE. Human ehrlichiosis in the United States, 1985 to 1990. Ann Intern Med 1994;120:736–43.

34. Hamburg BJ, Storch GA, Micek ST, et al. The importance of early treatment with doxycycline in human ehrlichiosis. Medicine 2008;87:53–60.

35. Halperin JJ, Baker P, Wormser GP. Common misconceptions about Lyme disease. Am J Med 2013;126:264.e1–7.

36. Skogman BH, Croner S, Nordwall M, et al. Lyme neuroborreliosis in children: a prospective study of clinical features, prognosis, and outcome. Pediatr Infect Dis J 2008;27:1089–94.

37. Ellis J, Oyston PCF, Green M, et al. Tularemia. Clin Microbiol Rev 2002;15: 631–46.
38. American Academy of Pediatrics. Prevention of tickborne infections. In: Pickering LK, Baker CJ, Kimberlin DW, et al, editors. Red Book: 2012 report of the Committee on Infectious Diseases. 29th edition. Elk Grove Village (IL): American Academy of Pediatrics; 2012. p. 207–9.
39. Due C, Fox W, Medlock JM, et al. Tick bite prevention and tick removal. BMJ 2013;347:f7123.
40. Environmental Protection Agency web site. DEET: 2014 review. Available at: www.epa.gov/pesticides/factsheets/chemicals/deet.htm?src=QHA099. Accessed March 27, 2015.
41. American Academy of Pediatrics. Prevention of mosquitoborne infections. In: Pickering LK, Baker CJ, Kimberlin DW, et al, editors. Red Book: 2012 report of the Committee on Infectious Diseases. 29th edition. Elk Grove Village (IL): American Academy of Pediatrics; 2012. p. 209–11.
42. Johnston SH, Glaser CA, Padgett K, et al. Rickettsia spp. 364D causing a cluster of eschar-associated illness, California. Pediatr Infect Dis J 2013;32:1036–9.
43. Salinas LJ, Greenfield RA, Little SE, et al. Tickborne infections in the southern United States. Am J Med Sci 2010;340:194–201.
44. Pastula DM, Turabelidze G, Yates KF, et al. Heartland virus disease—United States, 2012–2013. Morb Mortal Wkly Rep 2014;63:270–1.

Osteoarticular Infections in Children

John C. Arnold, MD[a],*, John S. Bradley, MD[b]

KEYWORDS

- Pediatric • Osteoarticular infection • Acute bacterial osteomyelitis
- Acute bacterial arthritis • Septic arthritis • Hematogenous • C-reactive protein (CRP)

KEY POINTS

- Pediatric bone and joint infections peak at a rate of 80 per 100,000.
- Osteomyelitis and septic arthritis have a distinct profile of pathogens, age group affected, and duration of therapy, so consideration as separate entities is reasonable.
- Early diagnosis and treatment of osteoarticular infections is important to minimize complications.
- A thorough history and physical examination is critical to diagnose bone and joint infections.
- Laboratory evaluation should include, at a minimum, a complete blood count, blood culture, erythrocyte sedimentation rate (ESR), and C-reactive protein (CRP).
- Empiric therapy should target *Staphylococcus aureus* (methicillin susceptible and resistant) as the most common pathogen.
- Initial intravenous courses of antibiotic therapy are usually short: 3 to 7 days in most cases.
- Clinical examination, fever, and CRP dictate the duration of therapy and need for additional debridement surgery.

INTRODUCTION
Disease Description

Acute bacterial osteomyelitis (ABO) and acute bacterial arthritis (ABA) occur when a bacterial infection of the bone or joint occurs and are manifested most often by fever and pain or inability to use the affected limb. Although traumatic infections do occur,

Disclosure: The authors of this article do not have any conflicts of interest to disclose. The views expressed herein are those of the authors and do not reflect the official policy or position of the Department of the Navy, Department of Defense, or the United States Government.
[a] Pediatrics and Infectious Diseases, Naval Medical Center, San Diego, 34800 Bob Wilson Drive, San Diego, CA 92134, USA; [b] Division of Infectious Diseases, Department of Pediatrics, Rady Children's Hospital San Diego, University of California San Diego School of Medicine, San Diego, CA, USA
* Corresponding author.
E-mail address: john.c.arnold.mil@mail.mil

Infect Dis Clin N Am 29 (2015) 557–574
http://dx.doi.org/10.1016/j.idc.2015.05.012
0891-5520/15/$ – see front matter Published by Elsevier Inc.

id.theclinics.com

hematogenous ABA/ABO are much more common. The likely pathogenesis of acute hematogenous osteomyelitis in children is the simultaneous occurrence of occult bacteremia and an anatomic susceptibility to bacterial invasion of the well-vascularized metaphysis (most often of the long-bones) in children.[1–4] Between 15% and 50% of osteoarticular infections involved both the joint and the bone (**Fig. 1**).[5–7] Transphyseal vessels may allow direct invasion of the joint, and the joint may become infected as a result of infection of the adjacent metaphysis, which is intra-articular in young children.[7] These combined ABO + ABA infections tend to be more serious, with higher levels of inflammatory markers, more sequelae, and longer treatment courses.[5,7,8]

In 2015, the organisms for which a child is most likely to be bacteremic are also the most common organisms that cause ABO and ABA. Specifically, S aureus, methicillin susceptible (MSSA) and methicillin resistant (MRSA), have been the most commonly cultured organisms during the past 4 decades.[9,10] Before an effective vaccine, *Haemophilus influenzae*, type B, was the second most common cause of ABA,[10] although it is now rarely reported in well-immunized populations. *Kingella kingae* is an oral gram-negative bacterium, and descriptions of this fastidious organism causing ABO and ABA have been increasingly common because of better culture techniques, inoculating sterile body fluids into blood culture bottles, and advancing molecular techniques. A study suggested that by using molecular diagnostic methods, *K kingae* actually supplanted S aureus as the most common pathogen in ABO/ABA,[11] especially in children aged 1 to 2 years (**Fig. 2**). The list of pathogens is rounded out by less frequent but consistent isolation of *Streptococcus pyogenes, Streptococcus pneumoniae*, and even less commonly gram-negative enteric organisms such as *Salmonella* species and *Escherichia coli*. **Table 1** lists less common infections and possible exposures associated with them.

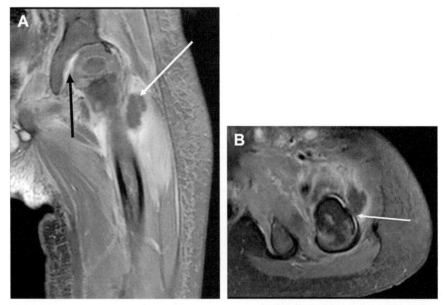

Fig. 1. (*A*) Coronal MRI of the hip. T1-weighted image of a child with osteomyelitis, arthritis (*black arrow* directed at joint effusion), and pyomyositis (*white arrow*) of the hip, caused by MRSA. (*B*) Axial MRI of the hip. T1-weighted image of the same child. In the axial image, the continuity of the proximal femur metaphysis and the adjacent abscess is appreciated (*white arrow*).

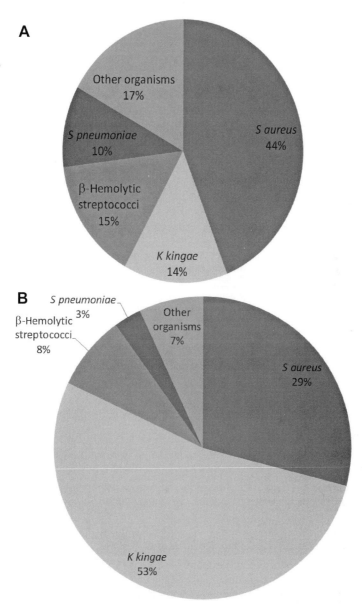

Fig. 2. Most common bacteria identified in osteoarticular infections either by (A) culture alone or (B) culture + polymerase chain reaction.

Prevalence/Incidence

- ABO and ABA occur worldwide and reflect the circulating microbial patterns and immunization rates.
- In well-resourced countries, the incidence of ABA is 4 to 10 per 100,000 children and ABO is estimated at 10 to 80 per 100,000 children.
- The incidence is higher in boys than in girls: a 2012 French study of 2592 children younger than 18 years with ABO or ABA had a male/female ratio of 1.4:1.[12]

Table 1
Important aspects of the patient history and associated pathogens or syndromes

Historical Finding	Associated Diagnosis
Travel	
International	Tuberculosis
Western United States	Coccidioidomycosis
Midwest United States	Histoplasmosis
Eastern United States	Lyme arthritis
Hunting/forest	Blastomycosis
Animal exposures	
Cat/kitten scratch	*Bartonella henselae*
Cat bite	*Pasteurella multocida*
Cat or livestock birth	*Coxiella burnetti* (Q-fever)
Reptiles/amphibians	*Salmonella* spp
Ingestions	
Unpasteurized dairy	Brucellosis Tuberculosis (*Mycobacteria tuberculosis*)
Not fully immunized	*Haemophilus influenza* *Streptococcus pneumoniae*
Sickle cell disease	*Salmonella* spp
Recent pharyngitis	*Streptococcus pyogenes* (invasive infection or postinfectious arthritis) *Fusobacterium necrophorum* (Lemierre disease)
Recent diarrheal illness	Postgastrointestinal infection arthritis (reactive arthritis) *Salmonella* spp

- Depending on the study, peak age of infection ranges from less than 2 years to 6 years, with isolated septic arthritis and *K kingae* infections occurring at younger ages, and osteomyelitis and *S aureus* occurring at older ages.[5,9,12–14]

Clinical correlation (**Fig. 3**) – Distribution of osteoarticular infections.[6,7,13–17] Overall, more than 80% of osteoarticular infections occur in the lower extremities.

Patient History

Most infections occur in the major weight-bearing joints or long bones of the extremities, for which the history most frequently encountered is that of a fever coinciding with the decreased use of the affected extremity. Older children may be able to identify the specific site of the infection; however, younger verbal children often simply say the extremity hurts. The diagnosis is even more challenging in nonverbal children. Fever and refusal to bear weight should be considered a lower extremity bacterial osteoarticular infection until proven otherwise.

Much more challenging is the vague history that occurs with the less common sites of osteoarticular infections, such as pelvic, sacroiliac, or vertebral infections. In these cases, there may be nonspecific discomfort or abdominal or flank pain, which is initially thought to be an intra-abdominal process.

Around 20% of children have a history of injury to the affected extremity or a nonspecific fall in the days or weeks before presentation; however, the frequency of falls and injuries in this age group is high, so the presence or lack of a history of falls should not affect the decision to consider an acute bacterial infection.[18]

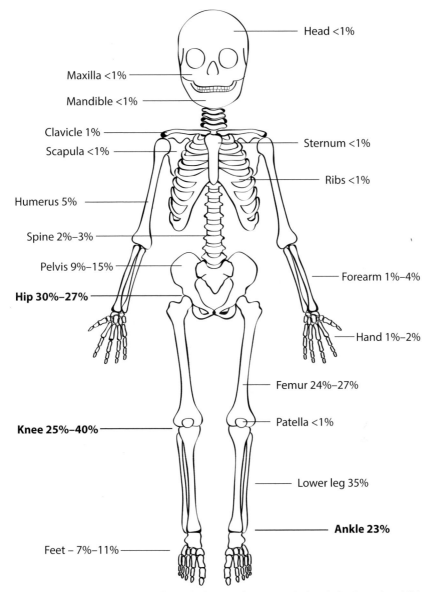

Fig. 3. Anatomic distribution of acute bacterial osteoarticular infections in children. Locations in bold face represent acute bacterial arthritis. All others represent acute bacterial osteomyelitis.

Supporting history is critical to ruling out uncommon infections (see **Table 1**). Travel history, sick contacts, and ingestion of unpasteurized dairy products should be queried to assess the risk of tuberculosis, brucellosis, and salmonellosis. *Bartonella henselae* and *Pasteurella multocida* infections are well described with exposure to cats and kittens.[19,20] The immunization status should be verified, especially when considering risk for *H influenzae* and pneumococcus. A family or medical history suggestive of sickle cell anemia or immunodeficiency could alter the empiric antibiotic choices. The history of a recent pneumonia or persistent cough could suggest tuberculosis or dimorphic fungal infections, such as histoplasmosis, coccidioidomycosis, or blastomycosis.

Physical Examination

The physical examination of a child with suspected ABO or ABA can be a challenge. A wide range of clinical presentations exist based primarily on the pathogen and toxins that may be produced to create local or systemic disease (**Table 2**). A child with an acute osteoarticular infection may be well appearing with mild local tenderness or have an overwhelming sepsis syndrome. For uncomplicated ABO, there is often point tenderness at the metaphyseal site of infection, accompanied by warmth and swelling. The degree of pain, swelling, and tenderness depends on (1) the duration

Table 2		
Pediatric osteoarticular infections: important aspects of the physical examination and associated pathogens or syndromes		
System	**Finding/Red Flag**	**Associated Diagnosis**
Vital signs	Fever, tachycardia, tachypnea, hypotension	Sepsis
Appearance	Ill appearing, fussy, in pain	Sepsis, meningitis
Neck	Nuchal rigidity or neck stiffness	Meningitis, cervical or deep neck infection
	Adenopathy/swelling	Cervical or deep neck infection
Mucous membranes	Dry, tacky	Dehydration
	Erythematous	Staphylococcal/streptococcal toxin or Kawasaki disease
Eyes	Conjunctival injection	Staphylococcal/streptococcal toxin or Kawasaki disease
Heart	Murmur	Endocarditis
	Rub	Pericarditis from atypical organism (tuberculosis) or rheumatologic disorder
Lungs	Abnormal breath sounds, retractions	Associated pneumonia (especially *Staphylococcus aureus* or *Streptococcus pyogenes*) or adjacent rib infection
	—	Atypical infection such as tuberculosis, histoplasmosis, coccidioidomycosis, or blastomycosis
Abdomen	Pain, guarding	Pelvic osteomyelitis or nonosteoarticular infection (appendicitis, psoas abscess)
	Organomegaly	Atypical pathogen (*Brucella*, Q-fever) or non-infectious (rheumatologic or oncologic)
Musculoskeletal	Refusal to bear weight	Leg, pelvic, or vertebral infection
	Refusal to use extremity	Localized infection
	Hip flexed/externally rotated	Hip joint infection
	Pain/redness/swelling	Localized infection
Skin	Skin trauma	Traumatic infection or invasion of pathogen through the skin (*Streptococcus pyogenes* or *Staphylococcus aureus*)
	Diffuse rash	Staphylococcal/streptococcal toxin or Kawasaki disease
Neurologic	Weakness, abnormal reflexes	Spinal epidural abscess, transverse myelitis

of symptoms before presentation for medical evaluation, (2) the location of the infection, (3) the age of the child, and (4) the pathogen. Erosion through the cortex of the bone to create a subperiosteal abscess and subsequent rupture through the periosteum into the soft tissues of the extremity may lead to marked swelling and tenderness (see **Fig. 1**). With swelling and tenderness around a joint, it is not always possible to discern a primary osteomyelitis that has decompressed into the joint, from a primary joint infection.

It is important to assess vital signs to ensure the child is admitted to the appropriate unit. Tachycardia could be due to pain, fever, dehydration, or septic/toxic shock. Tachypnea may suggest a concomitant pneumonia. The child with a serious osteoarticular infection is often ill appearing, so examination for nuchal rigidity or other signs of central nervous system infection is important. A thorough examination includes auscultation of the heart for murmurs and the lungs for effusions or pneumonia. Palpation of the liver and spleen size could be important as clues for unusual infections as well as noninfectious causes of bone pain, such as lymphoma. A history of a chronic rash associated with joint pain could suggest a rheumatologic process.

The most important part of the musculoskeletal examination of a child with a suspected osteoarticular infection of an unknown location is to make the child comfortable. Generally, having the child sitting or lying on the mother's lap is recommended, so pain can be differentiated from the crying of fear or anxiety. Observation for reluctance to move an extremity or visible swelling can be helpful. Passive range of motion, starting with the unaffected extremities is a critical aspect of the examination. Palpation along the spine and gentle compression of the pelvis can help detect vertebral and pelvic infections.

A close examination of the skin and lymph nodes is needed to detect the redness, tenderness, warmth, and swelling associated with the primary infection, as well as adenopathy, rashes, abrasions, or scratches that might be important to the differential diagnosis. Assessment of the reflexes and strength is important to differentiate decreased movement of an extremity between osteoarticular infection and neurologic causes such as spinal epidural abscesses.

IMAGING AND ADDITIONAL TESTING
Laboratory Testing

The initial laboratory testing for a patient with suspected osteoarticular infection should, at a minimum, consist of complete blood count including a leukocyte differential, ESR, CRP, and a blood culture, with the culture obtained before antibiotic administration. In an analysis of 265 patients enrolled in a prospective study, the sensitivity of using elevated ESR and CRP level to diagnose acute osteoarticular infections was 98%.[8] Although validated only for ABA, in 1999, Kocher and colleagues[21] developed a clinical prediction scale that consisted of the following 4 criteria: fever, refusal to bear weight, leukocyte count greater than 12,000, and ESR greater than 40. The diagnostic sensitivity for ABO was 93% and 99%, respectively, for the presence of 3 or 4 criteria. A blood culture is recommended because of the presence of bacteremia in as many as 59% of patients.[22] Additional testing, such as serologic testing for various pathogens (eg, *Bartonella*, *Histoplasma*, or *Brucella* antibody), tuberculin skin testing, or an interferon-gamma release assay test for tuberculosis, may be useful depending on the clinical scenario. The need for a stool culture would be determined by risk factors in the patient's history. If surgical specimens are obtained, they should be submitted for bacterial, fungal, and mycobacterial cultures and staining, and joint fluid should be inoculated into a blood culture bottle to enhance the growth of fastidious organisms.

The future of testing for osteoarticular infections may include several methodologies that are either recently available or currently in the testing phases. Molecular detection of nucleic acid using pathogen-directed (*S aureus*) or broad bacterial (16S ribosomal DNA) polymerase chain reaction methodology will likely become a mainstay at many larger institutions, because of rapid turnaround times and the ability to detect pathogens in cases in which cultures are negative.[23,24] Table-top devices designed to analyze finger-stick blood samples for CRP are commercially available but are not used at most institutions currently. Newer tests that are nonspecific for inflammation are more sensitive in detecting inflammation from a bacterial infection earlier in the disease process. One such marker is procalcitonin, which has been studied for ABO and ABA and found to be sensitive[25]; however, it is not yet available at this time to most clinicians in the United States.

Radiologic Imaging

Although a conventional radiograph of the affected site is certainly recommended in all cases, its sensitivity in acute infection is extremely low because 50% bone mineral loss must occur to see an abnormality[26] and abnormalities usually appear 10 or more days after the onset of the infection. A radiograph is important to exclude other processes such as an acute fracture.

MRI is the mainstay of imaging methodologies for suspected osteoarticular infections when an anatomic site is identifiable. MRI is sensitive in detecting cortical and bone marrow edema and inflammation. It is occasionally difficult to differentiate a bone infection from adjacent soft-tissue infection creating sympathetic edema in the bone. The major advantage of MRI is that it provides high-quality images of the bone, joint, and surrounding tissue, which is critical to guide the decision on whether surgery might be necessary for a subperiosteal abscess or associated pyomyositis.

Bone scans have been used for decades and consist of injection of a radiotracer (usually technetium 99) followed by a series of images immediately after and hours after injection. The tracer is retained in areas of increased blood flow, and the presence of increased tracer (or in some cases absent tracer where it is expected) is considered abnormal. Although the bone scan is sensitive for osteoarticular infections,[27,28] it generally gives abnormal results in bone-related cancers and fractures and is more difficult to interpret in children because of normal uptake into the growth plate. Despite these complicating issues, bone scan remains an important test when multifocal disease is suspected, when osteoarticular disease of an unknown anatomic site is suspected, and when MRI is not readily available. Bone scans also have the advantage of lower cost and less often requires anesthesia for young children, and the radiation risk is considered very low.

Ultrasound imaging of suspected joint infections is a rapid, noninvasive test with no radiation risk and is particularly helpful for suspected hip infections in which case palpation is not sensitive to detect effusions and rapid drainage of the joint is often desired. Although a negative result on ultrasound imaging of the hip is sensitive and the absence of fluid in the hip generally rules out a septic arthritis,[29] similar symptoms can be caused by a nearby osteomyelitis or pyogenic myositis. Therefore, a negative result on ultrasound imaging may need to be followed by an MRI if symptoms are severe or persistent.

The most practical approach to imaging, then, is to obtain a plain radiograph and an ultrasound image for suspected deep joint infections and then proceed to MRI, based on the presentation, focal examination findings (or lack thereof), and availability of the technology and sedation capabilities. For the ill-appearing child, because of the high probability of bacteremia, therapy should not usually be withheld while awaiting imaging and/or surgery, especially if the child demonstrates any signs or symptoms consistent with sepsis.

SURGICAL TREATMENT

Although the initial choices of antimicrobials are discussed later, one of the first questions to be answered when treating a child with an osteoarticular infection is "does the child need surgery?" There are 3 basic reasons for surgical intervention in ABA and ABO: microbiologic diagnosis, source control, and preservation of maximal function. As with many areas of bone and joint infections, there are few studies on which to make an evidence-based decision.

Starting with preservation of function, it has often been assumed that lack of drainage or delayed drainage of a major joint such as the hip would increase the chance of complications such as avascular necrosis or permanent cartilaginous damage. Limited data are available to support this conclusion, in part because many physicians have been uncomfortable studying immediate versus delayed incision and drainage of the hip. Immediate drainage and irrigation of all major joints (eg, hips and shoulders) suspected of having a bacterial infection is still considered the standard of care in many settings. A 2009 publication describing a series of prospectively enrolled children in Finland with ABA reported good outcomes, with 84% having needle aspiration of the joint and only 12% undergoing a full arthrotomy; none of the children had MRSA infection.[15] Given that surgical treatment was at the discretion of the physician, the benefit of surgery in more severe cases still cannot be excluded.

Source control is probably one of the most important reasons for surgical intervention. In the 30% to 56% of patients with bacteremia, drainage of the source is important, especially with persistent bacteremia. Furthermore, in the case of subperiosteal abscess, the effective antimicrobial therapy requires the drug to reach the source of the infection and the success of early therapy largely depends on removal of purulent fluid, debridement of necrotic tissue, and restoration of blood flow to the site. Based on published experience, one of the most important indicators of adequate source control is a sustained and rapid decrease in the CRP level.[5] For cases in which the CRP level does not decrease within the first 48 hours or initially decreases and then plateaus more than 5, an undrained, persistent purulent collection requiring surgery or possibly an occult sequestered focus initially missed by history, examination, or imaging is likely.[5,30]

Finally, confirmation of a pathogen is critical to selecting the best, most narrow-spectrum antimicrobial for definitive therapy. National guidelines being written for the diagnosis and management of pediatric bone and joint infections, cosponsored by the Pediatric Infectious Diseases Society and Infectious Diseases Society of America, stress the importance of cultures when an orthopedic surgeon decides to aspirate or formally open the suspected site of infection (Bradley, personal communication, 2015). However, wide variation in the surgical approach exists in North America with respect to indications for bone aspiration and formal debridement, including the creation of a bone window for ongoing drainage following the procedure. However, for mild or moderate infections involving the midshaft of a long bone, and without evidence of an abscess, some experts believe that the risks of surgery may outweigh the benefits. Using objective measures such as the CRP level to trend the success of therapy can be helpful in reassessing the need for surgical intervention. Having a good working relationship between medical and surgical care providers is critical to making the right risk to benefit decision.

MEDICAL TREATMENT
Antibiotic Choice

The decision of which antibiotic to use empirically and as definitive therapy has also been an area of debate, especially since the early 2000s with the emergence of community-associated (CA)-MRSA. Based on the historical pathogens, the mainstay of therapy until the emergence of MRSA was β-lactams, including the first-generation cephalosporins (cefazolin/cephalexin) and the penicillinase-stable penicillins (dicloxacillin and oxacillin). K kingae is also susceptible to first-generation cephalosporins and oxacillin (with resistance to clindamycin and vancomycin). Therefore, these early empiric treatment regimens, before the introduction of CA-MRSA, addressed all the top pathogens even when cultures could not be obtained or were negative. When an organism is identified and is known to be susceptible, β-lactam antibiotics are still the preferred therapy for osteoarticular infections.

However, as CA-MRSA emerged and became a significant contributor to osteoarticular infections, the empiric and definitive therapy strategies had to be adjusted. The obvious first choice of therapy was the glycopeptide vancomycin, for which resistance in S aureus continues to be extremely unusual and there is no resistance among group A streptococcus or S pneumoniae. Although the advantage of vancomycin is the likelihood that any of the gram-positive pathogens will be adequately treated, there are disadvantages that must be considered when using this antimicrobial for the initial treatment of bone and joint infections. The first and foremost is that vancomycin has no activity against the potential gram-negative organisms that can cause osteoarticular infections. In a highly immunized population, K kingae is the leading gram-negative pathogen, but based on immunization status and other risk factors, consideration might be given to H influenzae and Salmonella species. A second consideration is the decreased effectiveness of vancomycin in comparison with the β-lactam class when treating otherwise susceptible S aureus. Multiple investigators have described worse outcomes when vancomycin monotherapy is used in place of β-lactams for a β-lactam–susceptible organism. One such example was a 37% versus 18% mortality in patients with MSSA bacteremia treated with vancomycin or a β-lactam, respectively.[31] Finally, vancomycin is a medication that can be given only intravenously (IV) and must have blood level monitoring to minimize toxicity and maximize effectiveness, particularly with the higher dosages that seem to be needed to treat invasive CA-MRSA infections.

One of the most common alternative therapies is clindamycin, which has a successful record in the treatment of ABA and ABO. Clindamycin belongs to the lincosamide class and is a protein synthesis inhibitor that has traditionally been used as an alternative for gram-positive organisms causing bone and joint infections in a patient allergic to β-lactam or when the organism is resistant to first-line β-lactam therapy. Several studies have documented effectiveness in osteoarticular infections, including prospective, comparative evaluations.[32,33] The emergence of CA-MRSA across the country has highlighted the weakness of clindamycin, which is resistance. Resistance to clindamycin is variable, ranging from 7% to 50% among CA-MRSA.[34,35] The erm gene encodes the methylase protein that is responsible for methylation of the 23S rRNA-binding site, ultimately causing resistance to clindamycin as well as macrolides and streptogramins (dalfopristin/quinopristin), and is referred to as the MLS-B (macrolide, lincosamide, streptogramin-B) mechanism.[36] This methylase may be inducible or, in a subset of any population of S aureus that contain the gene, be constitutively producing the enzyme such that this subpopulation of organisms is always resistant to clindamycin, even before exposure. This subpopulation is likely to be selected during therapy with clindamycin, leading to treatment failure in high-density infections. The microbiological manifestation of inducible MLS-B (iMLS-B) is demonstrated by the induction of clindamycin resistance in the presence of erythromycin, which approximates a D instead of a perfect circle and is thus called the D-test (**Fig. 4**). In addition to selection of constitutive methylase-producing organisms, there is clinical concern for induction of the *erm* resistance while on therapy, so most treatment guidelines suggest that clinicians avoid the use of clindamycin altogether with D-test-positive organisms. However, there have only been rare reports of actual treatment failure and the development of resistance on therapy,[36–38] and many patients have undoubtedly been successfully treated with clindamycin despite having an inducible MLS-B genotype pathogen. There are few data to inform on whether it is reasonable to use clindamycin for a D-test-positive organism in mild skin and skin structure infections (SSTI) or for convalescent therapy in mild osteoarticular infections. Logic would suggest that for a mild, low-density infection or for an infection in which good source control has occurred, and is responding to therapy, it could be appropriate to continue therapy with clindamycin despite the presence of a positive result on D-test, avoiding the need to use more toxic or less well-studied antibiotics. An important and often overlooked detail is that clindamycin resistance among group

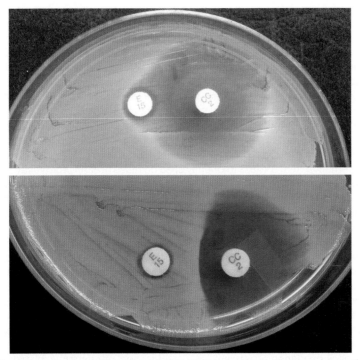

Fig. 4. The D-test result is determined by the pattern of growth when an erythromycin and clindamycin disc are placed in proximity. D-test negative (*top*) indicates no inducible clindamycin resistance. D-test positive (*bottom*), which approximates the shape of the letter D indicates inducible clindamycin resistance.

A streptococcus is around 15% in many communities and inducible MLS-B resistance was described in the 1980s in S pyogenes,[39] so it is not exclusively present in S aureus. In the right setting (ie, organism that is not susceptible to β-lactams or in a penicillin-allergic patient), clindamycin is still a mainstay of oral therapy for osteoarticular infections. The main limitations of clindamycin are diarrhea (including a low rate of Clostridium difficile enteritis) and poor compliance for children to take it, given the unpalatable taste of the suspension.

With the dramatic increase in CA-MRSA, trimethoprim-sulfamethoxasole (TMP-SMX, Septra, Bactrim), has come into favor in the treatment of skin and skin structure infections and to some extent osteoarticular infections. TMP-SMX, with a mechanism of action of inhibiting 2 different steps in intrinsic folic acid synthesis, has a history as an effective antimicrobial mainly in the treatment of gram-negative organisms such as the common causes of urinary tract infections. Initial enthusiasm as an effective therapy for respiratory tract infections caused by gram-positive organisms quickly faded as it became clear that resistance developed rapidly in streptococci. However, CA-MRSA is generally susceptible to TMP-SMX, so a resurgence of its use has occurred, especially for SSTI, for which data support its general effectiveness.[40] Although use of TMP-SMX in ABO/ABA has increased, there are no high-quality retrospective studies evaluating its outcomes in bone or joint infections caused by CA-MRSA or prospective comparisons with any of the other traditional antimicrobials in osteoarticular infections. Conversely, there have been no reports of treatment failures with sulfonamide therapy, so the use of this class might be considered, especially where clindamycin is not an appropriate alternative. The main concerns with TMP-SMX are the rare side effects of temporary bone marrow suppression and Stevens-Johnson syndrome.

The last 2 decades have established a place for linezolid in the treatment of bone and joint infections. The oxazolidinone shares a similar mechanism of action (ribosomal protein synthesis inhibition) with clindamycin, although it has a broader spectrum of activity among gram-positive organisms. Well-designed studies established appropriate dosing for neonates, infants, and children early following its approval in the United States, and the anecdotal successful use of linezolid for ABA and ABO has been described.[41] One major advantage of linezolid is the almost 100% gastrointestinal absorption compared with IV dosing. However, cost remains prohibitively high to recommend its frequent use and serious side effects include thrombocytopenia and neutropenia occurring after 10 or more days of use.

Other alternatives that are less frequently used because of either age limitations or lack of data on dosing or effectiveness include doxycycline, fluoroquinolones, and daptomycin. The addition of rifampin for certain infections such as bloodstream infections and device-related infections is occasionally recommended[42] but there are no published data to support routine use of rifampin combination therapy in pediatric osteoarticular infections. Daptomycin is currently being investigated in a prospective comparative trial for ABO, as documented on ClinicalTrials.gov (NCT01922011). Other glycolipopeptides and oxazolidinones may be studied for pediatric osteoarticular infections in the future.

Given all of the presented information on the pros and cons of different antimicrobials, there are several different strategies used in the empiric and definitive choice of antibiotic therapy for bone and joint infections. Some of the decisions are dictated by the clinical presentation and others by local resistance patterns. For example, a critically ill child with a suspected osteoarticular source would be likely to have S aureus or S pyogenes. Therefore, the combination of vancomycin and a broad-spectrum β-lactam would be appropriate with the possible addition of clindamycin if toxic shock is suspected (based on the ability of clindamycin to decrease ribosomal production of bacterial toxins). A similar combination might be considered for an obvious septic arthritis of the hip, in which preserving maximal function is paramount. On the other hand, for the nontoxic child with a bone or joint infection in regions where the resistance to clindamycin is 10% or less, empiric clindamycin therapy with close observation is reasonable, given the greater safety of clindamycin compared with vancomycin. No prospective data for TMP-SMX monotherapy of bone or joint infection exist; therefore, use of the TMP-SMX should be reserved for children for whom well-established antibiotic options are not available.

The final consideration is whether *K kingae* should be treated empirically. Some clinicians ensure that adequate gram-negative therapy is initiated for all patients, whereas others would be comfortable with initial therapy targeting gram-positive organisms (eg, clindamycin or vancomycin) and adding therapy for *K kingae* if resolution is not rapid (within 48–72 hours, particularly in situations in which cultures are negative). There is some aspect of the art of medicine when choosing antimicrobial therapy for the treatment of ABA and ABO.

Route and Duration of Therapy

The route and duration of treatment of osteoarticular infections has been an area of debate for decades. Until the 1980s, the best treatment route and duration was thought to be long intravenous courses of antimicrobials to prevent a relapse or complications. Outpatient intravenous antibiotic therapy was not feasible at that time, and therefore, children with bone and joint infections were required to spend 4 to 6 weeks in the hospital while receiving therapy. Thirty-five years ago, it was suggested that a transition to oral therapy could be safe and equally effective. Syrogiannopoulos and Nelson[10] published data that described the duration of IV and oral antimicrobial therapy and the outcomes and found that combined courses of IV and oral therapy were safe and effective in the range of 4 to 6 weeks. However, the initial duration of IV therapy was not precisely defined, and for decades to follow the original dogma of long IV courses of therapy remained the rule for many physicians. Recent reviews on route of therapy, based on retrospective review of national pediatric hospital databases, have documented that transition to oral therapy produces equivalent outcomes, with fewer therapy-associated adverse events.[43,44] However, the factors involved in considerations for time to switch to oral therapy and the duration of therapy have not been well addressed.

In the past 2 decades, there has been a keen interest in minimizing the duration of antimicrobial therapy. Reasons for this include health care costs, antimicrobial resistance, nosocomial infections and other hospital-related risks, risks of central venous access, and most importantly patient comfort and lifestyle.

In 2012, Arnold and colleagues[5] published an article describing 194 patients who had ABO, ABA, or both. During the 7-year review period, the group of Pediatric Infectious Diseases and Pediatric Orthopedic Physicians used a strategy of transitioning to oral therapy when the patient was afebrile, able to use the affected extremity with minimal pain, and the CRP level was less than 3 μg/dL. The care of 113 patients with ABO, 32 patients with ABA, and 49 with both was reviewed. This study described a total IV duration of 1.4 weeks for ABO and ABA and 2.7 weeks for ABO + ABA, with variability by the pathogen, whereby the duration of IV therapy tended to be longer for MRSA and much shorter for *S pneumoniae*. The total duration of therapy was 7.3 weeks for ABO, 4.7 weeks for ABA, and 7.9 weeks for ABO + ABA. The most important point from this article, however, is that using the strategy of transitioning to oral therapy when the 3 criteria are met (CRP<3, afebrile, and decreased pain), only 1 of 194 patients had a treatment failure, and this was thought to be due to a retained infected bone fragment in the hip joint where the initial infection occurred. In addition, those patients who were defined as having a complicated course actually had a lower CRP level at the transition to oral therapy than those who had an uncomplicated course, which implied that the physicians had an understanding of the more serious nature of that specific infection, so more conservative criteria were used to decide when oral therapy could be started. Therefore, as opposed to setting a standard duration of IV and oral therapy, this 2012 article suggests that using subjective and objective findings, including CRP level less than 3, patients may safely be switched to oral therapy.

A 2013 publication by Copley and colleagues[45] described the impact of implementation of a clinical guideline that standardized diagnosis and treatment of osteomyelitis at their hospital. The duration of therapy was based on the clinical response and CRP level, for which a CRP level of less than 2 mg/L was considered one of the criteria for switching over to oral therapy and discharging home. In a preintervention and postintervention retrospective design, the records of 210 children were reviewed. Although no specific complications were mentioned, the readmission rate was 11.4% for the preguideline cohort and 6.6% in the postguideline cohort ($P = .34$). The preguideline cohort also had a longer length of stay (12.8 vs 9.7 days, $P = .54$).

A series of articles have also been published by Peltola and colleagues[15] which advocate for an even earlier switch to oral antimicrobial therapy and shorter total durations.[16,46–49] These publications have focused on a multisite cohort of children who were enrolled in a series of prospective studies that began in 1983. The first publication in 1997 included 50 patients infected with S aureus (all MSSA) who were treated IV for an average of 4 days, with a total duration of IV + oral therapy of 3 weeks.[49] No adverse outcomes were reported at a 12-month follow-up, and it was suggested that shorter treatment durations were safe and effective. Following this initial publication, children with ABA were enrolled and randomized to either a first-generation cephalosporin (which changed during the course of the study) or clindamycin for a total duration of 10 or 30 days, and those with ABO were randomized to the same antimicrobials for a duration of 20 or 30 days.[15,16] The IV course was generally 2 to 4 days, followed by oral medication; however, treating physician discretion allowed for protocol deviation and prolongation of either IV or oral antimicrobial therapy. The outcomes of shorter-course therapy were overall favorable, with only 1 of 235 patients reported to have truly failed shorter-duration therapy; a 10-year old boy had 2 separate recurrences (one with the original S aureus and the other with a coagulase-negative staphylococcus) in the same location as the original infection. This patient was in the longer-course group at randomization. Some caution must be used when generalizing these results. First, particularly for the ABA series, 17% of the patients had H influenzae type B, and of the S aureus, all were MSSA, so it is unclear whether in an era when 50% or more of the invasive isolates are CA-MRSA, the same short-course therapy would be as successful. In addition, 7% of the ABA and 5% of the ABO cases deviated from the short-course therapy for either slow clinical response or a persistently elevated CRP level. Therefore, a single short-course protocol should be adopted with caution and should never override the clinical judgment if a slow response is observed.

Using the information detailed earlier, it is reasonable to presume that a shorter course of IV therapy followed by oral therapy is safe and effective for most patients with hematogenous osteoarticular infections. Using objective measures to guide the duration of therapy is the more conservative route but will still lead to short IV courses. There are data to support shorter oral courses of therapy as well, although in an era of frequent CA-MRSA infections more data may be needed to adopt this universally, and clinical judgment is always an important aspect when deciding the duration of therapy.

Complications and Concerns

Although antimicrobial therapy is now successful in achieving a complete cure for most patients, there are still adverse outcomes related to severe disease, delayed therapy, and the location of the infection. The most severe outcome would be death due to the infection, which most often is related to sepsis from the initial infection. In environments of easily accessed and early medical care, death as a complication of osteomyelitis is rare, with no deaths in any of the large series described earlier. Persistent bacteremia without sepsis is most likely due to an undrained abscess, a septic thrombophlebitis adjacent to the infection, or, rarely, an associated bacterial endocarditis. MRSA osteomyelitis in particular has been associated with deep venous thrombosis and infected pulmonary emboli.[50,51]

Less serious but more frequent are the complications related to the site of infection. For example, with infections frequently occurring at the end of the long bones, damage to the growth plate with subsequent growth plate arrest and limb length discrepancy is a common concern. Similarly, femoral head damage with resultant avascular necrosis is a rare complication. However, each of these complications was only documented in 0% and 2% of the modern era studies discussed earlier.[5,15] Similarly, pathologic fractures and loss of function may rarely occur in any weight-bearing locations, such as the vertebral body.

Relapse of infection is also extremely uncommon with current therapeutic strategies, with only 1 relapse in each of the large series described previously. Chronic osteomyelitis, a common complication in the preantibiotic era, is virtually unknown with present management strategies.

SUMMARY

Pediatric hematogenous osteoarticular infections are uncommon, although given the consequences of a missed or late diagnosis, providers of pediatric acute care should be familiar with the presentation, diagnosis, and initial therapy. The history of fever and refusal to walk or use an extremity should prompt an immediate evaluation for a bacterial bone or joint infection. A thorough history and physical examination can help to diagnose less common pathogens and identify the site of infection for difficult-to-localize regions such as the spine or pelvis. Laboratory evaluation should include a complete blood count, blood culture, and markers of inflammation (ESR and CRP). Initial empiric therapy should include agents active against *S aureus* (including CA-MRSA), streptococci, and ideally *K kingae*. Although a short IV course with a rapid transition to oral therapy is now the rule for an uncomplicated case, the ideal time to switch to oral therapy, the total duration of therapy, and the need for surgery are still in need of systematic, prospective study and should be individualized based on the patient.

REFERENCES

1. Alderson M, Speers D, Emslie K, et al. Acute haematogenous osteomyelitis and septic arthritis–a single disease. A hypothesis based upon the presence of trans-physeal blood vessels. J Bone Joint Surg Br 1986;68(2):268–74.
2. Emslie KR, Nade S. Acute hematogenous staphylococcal osteomyelitis. A description of the natural history in an avian model. Am J Pathol 1983;110(3): 333–45.
3. Emslie KR, Nade S. Pathogenesis and treatment of acute hematogenous osteo-myelitis: evaluation of current views with reference to an animal model. Rev Infect Dis 1986;8(6):841–9.

4. Stephen RF, Benson MK, Nade S. Misconceptions about childhood acute osteo-myelitis. J Child Orthop 2012;6(5):353–6.

5. Arnold JC, Cannavino CR, Ross MK, et al. Acute bacterial osteoarticular infections: eight-year analysis of C-reactive protein for oral step-down therapy. Pediatrics 2012;130(4):e821–8.

6. Chen WL, Chang WN, Chen YS, et al. Acute community-acquired osteoarticular infections in children: high incidence of concomitant bone and joint involvement. J Microbiol Immunol Infect 2010;43(4):332–8.

7. Jackson MA, Burry VF, Olson LC. Pyogenic arthritis associated with adjacent osteomyelitis: identification of the sequela-prone child. Pediatr Infect Dis J 1992;11(1):9–13.

8. Paakkonen M, Kallio MJ, Kallio PE, et al. Sensitivity of erythrocyte sedimentation rate and C-reactive protein in childhood bone and joint infections. Clin Orthop Relat Res 2010;468(3):861–6.

9. Moumile K, Merckx J, Glorion C, et al. Bacterial aetiology of acute osteoarticular infections in children. Acta Paediatr 2005;94(4):419–22.

10. Syrogiannopoulos GA, Nelson JD. Duration of antimicrobial therapy for acute suppurative osteoarticular infections. Lancet 1988;1(8575–6):37–40.

11. Chometon S, Benito Y, Chaker M, et al. Specific real-time polymerase chain reaction places Kingella kingae as the most common cause of osteoarticular infections in young children. Pediatr Infect Dis J 2007;26(5):377–81.

12. Grammatico-Guillon L, Maakaroun Vermesse Z, Baron S, et al. Paediatric bone and joint infections are more common in boys and toddlers: a national epidemiology study. Acta Paediatr 2013;102(3):e120–5.

13. Mitha A, Boutry N, Nectoux E, et al. Community-acquired bone and joint infections in children: a 1-year prospective epidemiological study. Arch Dis Child 2015;100(2):126–9.

14. Trifa M, Bouchoucha S, Smaoui H, et al. Microbiological profile of haematogenous osteoarticular infections in children. Orthop Traumatol Surg Res 2011;97(2):186–90.

15. Peltola H, Paakkonen M, Kallio P, et al. Prospective, randomized trial of 10 days versus 30 days of antimicrobial treatment, including a short-term course of parenteral therapy, for childhood septic arthritis. Clin Infect Dis 2009;48(9):1201–10.

16. Peltola H, Paakkonen M, Kallio P, et al. Short- versus long-term antimicrobial treatment for acute hematogenous osteomyelitis of childhood: prospective, randomized trial on 131 culture-positive cases. Pediatr Infect Dis J 2010;29(12):1123–8.

17. Dartnell J, Ramachandran M, Katchburian M. Haematogenous acute and subacute paediatric osteomyelitis: a systematic review of the literature. J Bone Joint Surg Br 2012;94(5):584–95.

18. Paakkonen M, Kallio MJ, Lankinen P, et al. Preceding trauma in childhood hematogenous bone and joint infections. J Pediatr Orthop B 2014;23(2):196–9.

19. Kodama Y, Maeno N, Nishi J, et al. Multifocal osteomyelitis due to Bartonella henselae in a child without focal pain. J Infect Chemother 2007;13(5):350–2.

20. Weber DJ, Wolfson JS, Swartz MN, et al. Pasteurella multocida infections. Report of 34 cases and review of the literature. Medicine 1984;63(3):133–54.

21. Kocher MS, Zurakowski D, Kasser JR. Differentiating between septic arthritis and transient synovitis of the hip in children: an evidence-based clinical prediction algorithm. J Bone Joint Surg Am 1999;81(12):1662–70.

22. Paakkonen M, Kallio MJ, Kallio PE, et al. C-reactive protein versus erythrocyte sedimentation rate, white blood cell count and alkaline phosphatase in diagnosing

bacteraemia in bone and joint infections. J Paediatr Child Health 2013;49(3): E189–92.

23. Alraddadi B, Al-Azri S, Forward K. Influence of 16S ribosomal RNA gene polymerase chain reaction and sequencing on antibiotic management of bone and joint infections. Can J Infect Dis Med Microbiol 2013;24(2):85–8.

24. Valour F, Blanc-Pattin V, Freydiere AM, et al. Rapid detection of *Staphylococcus aureus* and methicillin resistance in bone and joint infection samples: evaluation of the GeneXpert MRSA/SA SSTI assay. Diagn Microbiol Infect Dis 2014;78(3): 313–5.

25. Maharajan K, Patro DK, Menon J, et al. Serum procalcitonin is a sensitive and specific marker in the diagnosis of septic arthritis and acute osteomyelitis. J Orthop Surg Res 2013;8:19.

26. Tumeh SS, Aliabadi P, Weissman BN, et al. Disease activity in osteomyelitis: role of radiography. Radiology 1987;165(3):781–4.

27. Lee BF, Chiu NT, Chang JK, et al. Technetium-99m(V)-DMSA and gallium-67 in the assessment of bone and joint infection. J Nucl Med 1998;39(12):2128–31.

28. Machens HG, Pallua N, Becker M, et al. Technetium-99m human immunoglobulin (HIG): a new substance for scintigraphic detection of bone and joint infections. Microsurgery 1996;17(5):272–7.

29. Eich GF, Superti-Furga A, Umbricht FS, et al. The painful hip: evaluation of criteria for clinical decision-making. Eur J Pediatr 1999;158(11):923–8.

30. Paakkonen M, Peltola H. Acute osteomyelitis in children. N Engl J Med 2014; 370(14):1365–6.

31. Kim SH, Kim KH, Kim HB, et al. Outcome of vancomycin treatment in patients with methicillin-susceptible *Staphylococcus aureus* bacteremia. Antimicrob Agents Chemother 2008;52(1):192–7.

32. Feigin RD, Pickering LK, Anderson D, et al. Clindamycin treatment of osteomyelitis and septic arthritis in children. Pediatrics 1975;55(2):213–23.

33. Kaplan SL, Mason EO Jr, Feigin RD. Clindamycin versus nafcillin or methicillin in the treatment of *Staphylococcus aureus* osteomyelitis in children. South Med J 1982;75(2):138–42.

34. Buckingham SC, McDougal LK, Cathey LD, et al. Emergence of community-associated methicillin-resistant *Staphylococcus aureus* at a Memphis, Tennessee Children's Hospital. Pediatr Infect Dis J 2004;23(7):619–24.

35. Leifso KR, Gravel D, Mounchili A, et al. Clinical characteristics of pediatric patients hospitalized with methicillin-resistant *Staphylococcus aureus* in Canadian hospitals from 2008 to 2010. Can J Infect Dis Med Microbiol 2013;24(3): e53–6.

36. Lewis JS 2nd, Jorgensen JH. Inducible clindamycin resistance in staphylococci: should clinicians and microbiologists be concerned? Clin Infect Dis 2005;40(2): 280–5.

37. Siberry GK, Tekle T, Carroll K, et al. Failure of clindamycin treatment of methicillin-resistant *Staphylococcus aureus* expressing inducible clindamycin resistance in vitro. Clin Infect Dis 2003;37(9):1257–60.

38. Patra KP, Vanchiere JA, Bocchini JA Jr. Adherence to CLSI recommendations for testing of *Staphylococcus aureus* isolates in Louisiana hospitals: report of a clinical failure and results of a questionnaire study. J Clin Microbiol 2011;49(8): 3019–20.

39. Golubkov VI, Reichardt W, Boitsov AS, et al. Sequence relationships between plasmids associated with conventional MLS resistance and zonal lincomycin resistance in *Streptococcus pyogenes*. Mol Gen Genet 1982;187(2):310–5.

40. Cenizal MJ, Skiest D, Luber S, et al. Prospective randomized trial of empiric therapy with trimethoprim-sulfamethoxazole or doxycycline for outpatient skin and soft tissue infections in an area of high prevalence of methicillin-resistant *Staphylococcus aureus*. Antimicrob Agents Chemother 2007;51(7):2628–30.

41. Chen CJ, Chiu CH, Lin TY, et al. Experience with linezolid therapy in children with osteoarticular infections. Pediatr Infect Dis J 2007;26(11):985–8.

42. Czekaj J, Dinh A, Moldovan A, et al. Efficacy of a combined oral clindamycin/rifampicin regimen for therapy of staphylococcal osteoarticular infections. Scand J Infect Dis 2011;43(11–12):962–7.

43. Keren R, Shah SS, Srivastava R, et al. Comparative effectiveness of intravenous vs oral antibiotics for postdischarge treatment of acute osteomyelitis in children. JAMA Pediatr 2015;169(2):120–8.

44. Zaoutis T, Localio AR, Leckerman K, et al. Prolonged intravenous therapy versus early transition to oral antimicrobial therapy for acute osteomyelitis in children. Pediatrics 2009;123(2):636–42.

45. Copley LA, Kinsler MA, Gheen T, et al. The impact of evidence-based clinical practice guidelines applied by a multidisciplinary team for the care of children with osteomyelitis. J Bone Joint Surg Am 2013;95(8):686–93.

46. Paakkonen M, Kallio MJ, Kallio PE, et al. Shortened hospital stay for childhood bone and joint infections: analysis of 265 prospectively collected culture-positive cases in 1983-2005. Scand J Infect Dis 2012;44(9):683–8.

47. Paakkonen M, Peltola H. Simplifying the treatment of acute bacterial bone and joint infections in children. Expert Rev Anti Infect Ther 2011;9(12):1125–31.

48. Peltola H, Paakkonen M, Kallio P, et al. Clindamycin vs. first-generation cephalosporins for acute osteoarticular infections of childhood–a prospective quasi-randomized controlled trial. Clin Microbiol Infect 2012;18(6):582–9.

49. Peltola H, Unkila-Kallio L, Kallio MJ. Simplified treatment of acute staphylococcal osteomyelitis of childhood. The Finnish Study Group. Pediatrics 1997;99(6):846–50.

50. Gonzalez BE, Hulten KG, Dishop MK, et al. Pulmonary manifestations in children with invasive community-acquired *Staphylococcus aureus* infection. Clin Infect Dis 2005;41(5):583–90.

51. Gonzalez BE, Teruya J, Mahoney DH Jr, et al. Venous thrombosis associated with staphylococcal osteomyelitis in children. Pediatrics 2006;117(5):1673–9.

Evaluation and Management of Febrile, Well-appearing Young Infants

Eric A. Biondi, MD, MS[a],*, Carrie L. Byington, MD[b]

KEYWORDS

- Fever • Infant • Serious bacterial infection • Viral illness • Management

KEY POINTS

- Urinary tract infection is the most common bacterial infection in young infants.
- Infants with certain viral infections are at lower risk for bacterial infection and can therefore be managed differently.
- Hospital admission and antimicrobial therapy should be avoided if possible for low-risk infants.
- When hospitalization occurs, length of stay and duration of antimicrobial therapy can be safely shortened to 24 to 36 hours.
- Adherence to a care process model can decrease the substantial variation in care of well-appearing febrile infants, can improve infant outcomes, and can reduce costs.

INTRODUCTION

The diagnosis and management of well-appearing, febrile infants younger than 90 days represents a common clinical conundrum encountered by child health care providers in ambulatory and hospital settings. Many febrile infants have no obvious focus of infection on physical examination. However, serious bacterial infection (SBI), including urinary tract infection (UTI), bacteremia, and/or meningitis, occurs in nearly 10% of febrile infants in this age range.[1–3] Fever may be the only sign of these infections, which, if unrecognized, can result in severe illness or even death. Therefore, febrile infants often undergo invasive evaluations that include laboratory testing,

Disclosures: CLB is supported through the HA and Edna Benning Presidential Endowment and the National Center for Advancing Translational Sciences of the National Institutes of Health (1ULTR001067) and has received National Institutes of Health funding with BioFire Diagnostics through the National Institute of Allergy and Infectious Diseases (5U01AI082482; 5U01AI074419; and U01A1061611).
[a] Department of Pediatrics, University of Rochester Medical Center, 601 Elmwood Avenue, Box #667, Rochester, NY 14642, USA; [b] Department of Pediatrics, University of Utah, HSEB Suite 5515, 26 South 2000 East, Salt Lake City, UT 84112, USA
* Corresponding author.
E-mail address: eric_biondi@urmc.rochester.edu

Infect Dis Clin N Am 29 (2015) 575–585
http://dx.doi.org/10.1016/j.idc.2015.05.008
0891-5520/15/$ – see front matter © 2015 Elsevier Inc. All rights reserved.

lumbar puncture, and empiric antimicrobial therapy, often in the hospital setting while awaiting the results of bacterial cultures.

In the United States, there are no nationally accepted guidelines for the management of febrile infants. This omission has resulted in significant and unwarranted variation in the management of these infants, which may lead to overtreatment, undertreatment, and suboptimal outcomes for infants.[1,2,4]

Multiple screening methods have been developed to identify infants who have low risk of SBI and do not require hospitalization or empiric antibiotics.[5,6] However, without evidence-based guidance, the management of febrile infants may result in unnecessary hospitalizations and health care overuse in emergency departments,[4,7] inpatient settings,[8] and outpatient settings for low-risk infants.[2] There is also risk of inappropriate underuse and failure to recognize treatable bacterial infections in high-risk infants. The unwarranted variation in care is so great that similar febrile infants seen at 2 different hospitals may receive a minimal outpatient evaluation at one and invasive testing, antibiotics, and hospitalization at the other.[4]

Before 1985, it was recommended that febrile infants be hospitalized and treated with empiric antibiotics pending results of an evaluation for sepsis that most often included cultures of blood, cerebrospinal fluid (CSF), and urine. Predictably, this practice resulted in unnecessary hospitalizations and nosocomial infections.[9] In an effort to improve care, the following decades saw numerous attempts to identify febrile infants who were at low risk for SBI and thus did not require antimicrobial therapy or hospitalization. The first, and arguably most well known, of these classification systems, colloquially termed the Rochester criteria, has been shown to identify febrile infants with a less than 2% chance of SBI.[9,10] Following the publication of the Rochester criteria, other low-risk criteria were published (**Fig. 1**, **Table 1**),[3,5,10–17] most with a similar ability to reliably identify low-risk infants.[5,6]

PREVALENCE/INCIDENCE

Evaluation for fever (defined here as $\geq 38^\circ$C) in well-appearing infants less than 90 days old and without a focal source of infection is common and results in a large number of ambulatory and emergency department visits.[6]

Although all febrile infants are at risk for bacterial infection, SBI is ultimately diagnosed in the minority of these infants and mortality is extremely rare.[1,2,4] Infants

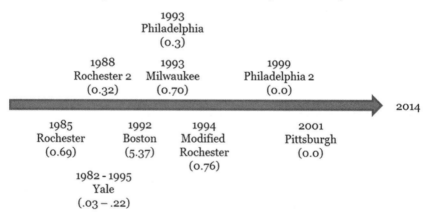

Fig. 1. Timeline showing publication of commonly used low-risk criteria for febrile infants. Values in parentheses represent the risk of SBI in febrile infants meeting the criteria. (*Data from* Refs.[3,5,11–18])

Table 1
Summary of commonly used low-risk criteria

	Rochester	Boston	Philadelphia
Age (d)	≤60	28–89	29–60
History[a]	Term birth No prior antibiotics Uncomplicated history	No antibiotics or IMZ in prior 48 h	Not defined
Physical[a]	Well appearing No focal findings	Well appearing No focal findings	Well appearing Unremarkable
Testing[a]	WBC 5000–15,000/mm^3 UA<10 WBC/hpf	WBC<20,000 mm^3 UA<10 WBC/hpf CSF<10 WBC/mm^3	WBC<15,000 mm^3 UA<10 WBC/hpf CSF<8 WBC/mm^3
NPV (%)	99[10]	95[11]	98[12]

Abbreviations: hpf, high powered field; IMZ, immunizations; NPV, negative predictive value for SBI in low-risk infants; UA, urinalysis; WBC, white blood cell count.
[a] Descriptors are examples within each criteria rather than an exhaustive list.
Data from Hui C, Neto G, Tsertsvadze A, et al. Diagnosis and management of febrile infants (0–3 months). Evid Rep Technol Assess (Full Rep) 2012(205):1–297.

with bacterial infection often have a similar appearance to infants with viral infections. Clinical appearance alone has been shown to be insensitive at identifying febrile infants with bacteremia or bacterial meningitis. In one of the largest studies to date, with all infants examined by experienced pediatricians, only 58% appeared clinically ill at the time of the first medical evaluation.[2]

The overall risk of SBI in this population is approximately 7% to 11% (**Table 2**). A few themes are worth mentioning with regard to risk of SBI in febrile infants: (1) neonates

Table 2
Percentage prevalence of SBI in febrile infants aged less than 90 days

	SBI	Meningitis	Bacteremia	UTI
All Infants	7–11	<0.5	1–2	7–9
Age				
≤28 d	11–25	Limited data	5–7	8–17
29–90 d	4–14	Limited data	0–2	12
Risk[a]				
Not low	11–24	<0.5	2	8
Low	0–3	<0.5	<0.5	0.5–1
Viral Status				
Viral Positive[b]	4–7	0[c]	0–1	2–6
Viral Negative	12–13	0–1	2–3	10
Setting				
Primary Care	8–10	0.5	2–4	5
Emergency Room	4–25	<1	4	8–19

Abbreviation: SBI, serious bacterial infection.
[a] Risk stratification based on several commonly used low-risk criteria.
[b] Includes positive viral testing or clinical bronchiolitis.
[c] No events noted in the included studies.
Data from Refs.[1–3,5,6,9,13,17,19,20,22–36]

($\leq$28 days old) are at higher risk of SBI than older infants[2,18]; (2) SBI, especially meningitis, in infants deemed to be at low-risk per published criteria is rare[5,9,19]; (3) infants who test positive for viruses, especially enteroviruses, parechovirus, influenza viruses, and respiratory syncytial virus, or who have clinical bronchiolitis, are at lower risk for SBI[20–22]; (4) infants presenting with fever to the emergency room are likely to be at higher risk for SBI than those who present to outpatient clinics; and (5) UTI is the most common form of SBI in almost all subgroups of febrile infants.[1,2,10]

Infectious Causes

Viral illness is far more common than bacterial illness in febrile, well-appearing infants, because up to 40% of infants who have viral testing performed have a positive viral test; most commonly respiratory syncytial virus, enterovirus, or influenza.[20] With the increased availability of polymerase chain reaction (PCR) testing for viruses, the diagnosis of rhinovirus in febrile infants has become more common. Rhinovirus RNA can be detected in the nasopharynx by PCR for up to 91 days following acute infection.[37] The clinical significance of a positive rhinovirus test in a well-appearing febrile infant is therefore unknown and alternative sources for fever should be investigated because bacterial infections have been reported in febrile infants with rhinovirus.[38]

Herpes simplex virus (HSV) is a rare (<0.3%)[27] but serious viral infection that occurs in febrile infants, particularly in the neonatal period, and has a mortality approaching 15%.[6] However, fever by itself is not useful in discerning neonates with HSV infection and it is commonly absent at the time of neonatal HSV infection.[39,40] Skin–eye–mucous membrane disease is the most common presentation of HSV in healthy-appearing febrile infants. Thus careful examination of the skin, including the scalp, is an important aspect of the physical examination.

The most common bacterial pathogen causing SBI in febrile infants is *Escherichia coli*, followed by Group B *Streptococcus* (GBS). Other gram-negative pathogens such as *Klebsiella* spp and *Salmonella* spp, along with gram-positive pathogens, including *Streptococcus pneumoniae* and *Enterococcus* spp, are less common but may be detected in well-appearing, febrile infants. *Neisseria meningitidis* is a rare cause of bacterial infection in this age group and may signal an underlying complement deficiency or, rarely, asplenia. *Staphylococcus aureus* is an increasing cause of bacterial infection in this age group and often presents with concomitant skin infection. *Listeria monocytogenes*, once considered an important neonatal pathogen, has become exceedingly rare in the last 2 decades, perhaps because of improvements in food safety.[6,41–43]

CLINICAL CORRELATION, PATIENT HISTORY, AND PHYSICAL EXAMINATION

In this age group, bacterial and viral infections can present with fever in the absence of other signs or symptoms. Therefore, the first step in the evaluation of an otherwise well-appearing, febrile infant less than 90 days of age should be to perform a thorough evaluation of risk factors. This evaluation can be accomplished by using any of the published low-risk criteria.[5,6] These criteria aid clinicians in obtaining pertinent information regarding the infant's birth history, past medical history, prior antibiotic use, history of current illness, physical examination, and relevant laboratory values.

Although the published criteria vary in their definition of low risk (eg, Boston criteria require <10 cells/mm^3 in the CSF, whereas Rochester criteria do not require CSF fluid analysis), the negative predictive value of the low-risk designation of any of these criteria ranged from 93.7% to 100%.[6]

Given the increased risk of SBI and conflicting data regarding the performance of risk stratification in neonates,[44,45] infants less than or equal to 28 days of age should not be classified as low risk regardless of other clinical factors.[46]

It is a salient point that infants categorized as non–low risk are at higher risk of SBI than infants categorized as low risk, but even in the non–low-risk group, SBI occurs in only a minority of infants (<20%).

ADDITIONAL TESTING

The most basic diagnostic screening evaluation for SBI in febrile, well-appearing infants less than or equal to 90 days of age includes a complete blood count (CBC) with differential, urinalysis (UA), blood culture, and urine culture. The CBC and UA have rapid turnaround times and provide sufficient data to classify an infant as either low risk or non–low risk per the original low-risk criteria (the Rochester criteria).[5] Specifically, UA should not be deferred because UTI is, by far, the most common bacterial infection in these infants.[6,41]

Other screening criteria require CSF analysis in order to perform risk stratification, and several require additional studies such as stool white blood cell (WBC) analysis and/or inflammatory markers in certain settings.[5] The low-risk criteria selected by the provider should guide the standard diagnostic testing obtained and the emphasis does not rest on the selection of the specific set of criteria, because they perform similarly, but in the consistent use of the selected set of criteria.

Infants classified as low risk do not require further testing, antimicrobial administration, or hospitalization; however, these infants do require close observation and repeat evaluation by a medical provider 12 to 24 hours after initial evaluation.

In addition to the basic work-up (CBC; UA; blood, urine, and CSF cultures), infants classified as non–low risk for SBI may benefit from additional diagnostic testing. These tests may identify the source of fever and may help guide the selection of antimicrobial therapy (**Table 3**) and, in the case of viral testing, if positive may be used to decrease the duration of antimicrobial therapy and shorten hospital length of stay.

THERAPEUTIC OPTIONS

Variability in care results in undertreatment and overtreatment, and the risks and harms associated with these. Variation can be decreased, infant outcomes improved, and costs reduced if a provider, practice, or hospital system adopts and uses consistently an evidence-based care process.[1] This consistent use includes selecting a single low-risk set of screening criteria and adopting a standard diagnostic practice.

Once an infant has been stratified as low risk or non–low risk, the treatment paths diverge. Infants who meet low-risk criteria can be safely managed at home with follow-up by a medical provider in 12 to 24 hours, provided that (1) the infant will be monitored at home by a parent or caregiver, (2) the medical provider has obtained reliable contact information for the infant, and (3) in-process cultures will be monitored.

For non–low-risk infants, hospitalization pending culture results is the preferred option. During hospitalization, management should focus on avoiding unnecessary testing, facilitating breastfeeding, and involving parents in decision making. Discharge planning should begin at the time of admission. Inpatient practice should focus on the identification or exclusion of bacterial infection by 24 hours. Efforts can then be made to discontinue antimicrobials and, if other discharge criteria are met, to release the infant from the hospital by 24 to 36 hours.

Antimicrobial therapy should be directed toward *E coli*, which is the most common pathogen in this age group, and, for patients with suspected meningitis, should

Table 3
Diagnostic tests of potential benefit in well-appearing, febrile infants less than 90 days old

Study	Potential Benefit	Comments
EV and Parechovirus CSF PCR	Positive testing modifies risk for SBI. May shorten length of stay, useful in summer/fall[47]	Infants may not show CSF pleocytosis with EV or Parechovirus meningitis
HSV blood or CSF PCR	Consider in neonates with or without fever who have any of the following: vesicular skin lesions, seizures, or CSF pleocytosis given increased risk of HSV infection in these infants (~1%)[27]	Not recommended for all well-appearing, febrile infants because testing is associated with increased length of stay and hospital charges[48]
Respiratory viral testing	Positive testing, especially for RSV and influenza virus, can be used to modify SBI risk and shorten length of stay[1,23]	Availability varies; certain viruses, particularly bocavirus and rhinovirus, are of unclear significance; PCR testing for these viruses may remain positive for weeks after acute infection
Procalcitonin	May provide better sensitivity and specificity than CBC[49]	Availability varies; test is expensive and turnaround time may prohibit routine use
Chest radiograph	May provide value if there is concern for bacterial pneumonia in an infant with respiratory distress	Not needed to diagnose bronchiolitis or as part of the routine SBI evaluation

Abbreviations: EV, enterovirus; RSV, respiratory syncytial virus.

include coverage for other common pathogens, especially GBS. Regional epidemiology and antimicrobial resistance patterns should also be taken into account when selecting antimicrobial therapy. Common antimicrobial regimens in this age group include:

- Ampicillin and an aminoglycoside
- A third-generation cephalosporin and ampicillin
- A third-generation cephalosporin alone

Ampicillin is the preferred treatment of GBS infection. The addition of ampicillin to a third-generation cephalosporin provides coverage against *Enterococcus faecalis* and *L monocytogenes*. These two bacteria are rarely identified (comprising <6% of all SBI in this population) and ampicillin resistance of more commonly identified bacteria is an increasing concern.[18,41,50] Providers should incorporate local epidemiologic and antimicrobial resistance data and clinical data such as Gram stain of UA or CSF to inform their antimicrobial selections, particularly balancing the potential benefits and harms of the routine addition of ampicillin.

At present in the United States, the standard inpatient evaluation length of time for febrile infants admitted for SBI is 48 hours, with individual provider variation from 24 to greater than 72 hours of inpatient observation.[8] National and regional studies suggest that an inpatient observation period of 24 to 36 hours is safe, whereas greater than 36 hours provides little benefit relative to the prolonged length of stay.[1,43] One large hospital system has developed an evidence-based, integrated care pathway that has been shown to safely decrease length of stay and decrease health care costs associated with the evaluation of febrile infants.[1] After evaluating more than 8000 infants, this pathway can be considered to be a safe and efficient way of providing high-value care (**Fig. 2**).[1]

CLINICAL OUTCOMES

Most febrile but otherwise well-appearing infants less than 90 days of age return to baseline quickly, with morbidity and mortality largely limited to rare cases of bacterial meningitis or HSV disseminated disease or meningitis.[6]

Physician concern over missing SBI in this patient population may help to explain the variation in care and the fact that infants who meet low-risk classification are often unnecessarily admitted to the hospital for inpatient observation.[4] It is true that occasionally a low-risk infant is ultimately diagnosed with SBI based on microbiologic culture, and the question then becomes, does delayed treatment in these cases result in harm to the infant? There are limited data describing outcomes relating to harms associated with delayed SBI management; however, the available data suggest that low-risk infants less than 90 days old who have delayed treatment of SBI have similar outcomes to infants hospitalized on presentation, particularly those with UTI.[2,9,14]

COMPLICATIONS AND CONCERNS

In the United States, the absence of a standard for evaluation of well-appearing, febrile infants less than 90 days of age results in significant variation in care; missed opportunities to identify the highest risk infants; and, for low-risk infants, unnecessary hospitalizations, excessive antibiotic use, and poor allocation of health care resources.[1,4] In addition, a growing volume of primary literature suggests that infants who warrant hospitalization can be safely discharged at 24 to 36 hours, but 48-hour inpatient observation periods remain common, if not the norm.[8]

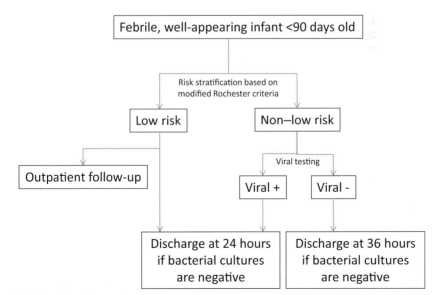

Fig. 2. Sample evidence-based, integrated care pathway for febrile, well-appearing infants less than 90 days of age. (*Adapted from* Byington CL, Reynolds CC, Korgenski K, et al. Costs and infant outcomes after implementation of a care process model for febrile infants. Pediatrics 2012;130(1):e16–24.)

In calculating the potential benefit of hospitalization, empiric antibiotics, and longer inpatient stays for febrile infants, clinicians must also consider the harms of such management decisions. The harms and costs of different management strategies have rarely been quantified,[6] but it is known that unnecessary testing, excessive antibiotic use, and prolonged lengths of stay in this population can have unintended consequences. These evaluations can result in iatrogenic complications (33%), financial stress (43%), parental belief that the infant might die (30%), and disruption of breast-feeding (36%).[51,52] Furthermore, excessive diagnostic testing increases the potential for false-positive results (eg a contaminated blood culture), which then may lead to additional evaluation and increases the potential for harm.

SUMMARY/DISCUSSION

Because bacterial infection often results in nonspecific signs and symptoms in febrile but otherwise well-appearing infants, this patient population presents a unique conundrum for providers. SBI in febrile infants less than 90 days of age is uncommon and, when it does occur, UTI is far more likely than bacteremia or meningitis. Appropriate use of a set of risk stratification criteria can aid providers in predicting whether a particular infant is at low risk of SBI.

Because low-risk infants do not require hospitalization or antimicrobial therapy, adherence to a care process model that uses a given set of risk stratification criteria can decrease unnecessary hospitalizations, iatrogenic and emotional harm, variability in care, and health care overuse. Such a care process model may also include rapid viral diagnostic testing, particularly for admitted infants. In addition to confirmation of a viral cause for fever, infants may benefit from avoidance of antibiotics, early hospital discharge, and those with influenza may also benefit from antiviral treatment. Viral testing also allows hospitals to cohort infants with the same infection, thereby allowing for the potential to increase bed capacity. When hospitalization does occur for febrile infants, efforts should be made to decrease length of stay and limit the duration of antimicrobial therapy to 24 to 36 hours if no bacterial infection is identified.

REFERENCES

1. Byington CL, Reynolds CC, Korgenski K, et al. Costs and infant outcomes after implementation of a care process model for febrile infants. Pediatrics 2012; 130(1):e16–24.
2. Pantell RH, Newman TB, Bernzweig J, et al. Management and outcomes of care of fever in early infancy. JAMA 2004;291(10):1203–12.
3. Herr SM, Wald ER, Pitetti RD, et al. Enhanced urinalysis improves identification of febrile infants ages 60 days and younger at low risk for serious bacterial illness. Pediatrics 2001;108(4):866–71.
4. Aronson PL, Thurm C, Alpern ER, et al. Variation in care of the febrile young infant <90 days in US pediatric emergency departments. Pediatrics 2014;134(4): 667–77.
5. Huppler AR, Eickhoff JC, Wald ER. Performance of low-risk criteria in the evaluation of young infants with fever: review of the literature. Pediatrics 2010;125(2): 228–33.
6. Hui C, Neto G, Tsertsvadze A, et al. Diagnosis and management of febrile infants (0–3 months). Evid Rep Technol Assess (Full Rep) 2012;(205):1–297.
7. Yarden-Bilavsky H, Ashkenazi S, Amir J, et al. Fever survey highlights significant variations in how infants aged ≤60 days are evaluated and underline the need for guidelines. Acta Paediatr 2014;103(4):379–85.

8. Biondi E, Murzycki J, Ralston S, et al. Fever and bacteremia. Pediatr Rev 2013; 34(3):134–6.

9. Jaskiewicz JA, McCarthy CA, Richardson AC, et al. Febrile infants at low risk for serious bacterial infection–an appraisal of the Rochester criteria and implications for management. Febrile Infant Collaborative Study Group. Pediatrics 1994;94(3): 390–6.

10. Dagan R, Powell KR, Hall CB, et al. Identification of infants unlikely to have serious bacterial infection although hospitalized for suspected sepsis. J Pediatr 1985;107(6):855–60.

11. Baskin MN, O'Rourke EJ, Fleisher GR. Outpatient treatment of febrile infants 28 to 89 days of age with intramuscular administration of ceftriaxone. J Pediatr 1992; 120(1):22–7.

12. Baker MD, Bell LM, Avner JR. Outpatient management without antibiotics of fever in selected infants. N Engl J Med 1993;329(20):1437–41.

13. Dagan R, Sofer S, Phillip M, et al. Ambulatory care of febrile infants younger than 2 months of age classified as being at low risk for having serious bacterial infections. J Pediatr 1988;112(3):355–60.

14. Bonadio WA, Hagen E, Rucka J, et al. Efficacy of a protocol to distinguish risk of serious bacterial infection in the outpatient evaluation of febrile young infants. Clin Pediatr 1993;32(7):401–4.

15. Chiu CH, Lin TY, Bullard MJ. Application of criteria identifying febrile outpatient neonates at low risk for bacterial infections. Pediatr Infect Dis J 1994;13(11): 946–9.

16. Baker MD, Bell LM, Avner JR. The efficacy of routine outpatient management without antibiotics of fever in selected infants. Pediatrics 1999;103(3):627–31.

17. McCarthy PL, Sharpe MR, Spiesel SZ, et al. Observation scales to identify serious illness in febrile children. Pediatrics 1982;70(5):802–9.

18. Byington CL, Rittichier KK, Bassett KE, et al. Serious bacterial infections in febrile infants younger than 90 days of age: the importance of ampicillin-resistant pathogens. Pediatrics 2003;111(5 Pt 1):964–8.

19. Dagan R, Jenista JA, Menegus MA. Association of clinical presentation, laboratory findings, and virus serotypes with the presence of meningitis in hospitalized infants with enterovirus infection. J Pediatr 1988;113(6):975–8.

20. Byington CL, Enriquez FR, Hoff C, et al. Serious bacterial infections in febrile infants 1 to 90 days old with and without viral infections. Pediatrics 2004;113(6): 1662–6.

21. Rittichier KR, Bryan PA, Bassett KE, et al. Diagnosis and outcomes of enterovirus infections in young infants. Pediatr Infect Dis J 2005;24(6):546–50.

22. Bender JM, Ampofo K, Gesteland P, et al. Influenza virus infection in infants less than three months of age. Pediatr Infect Dis J 2010;29(1):6–9.

23. Levine DA, Platt SL, Dayan PS, et al. Risk of serious bacterial infection in young febrile infants with respiratory syncytial virus infections. Pediatrics 2004;113(6): 1728–34.

24. Bachur RG, Harper MB. Predictive model for serious bacterial infections among infants younger than 3 months of age. Pediatrics 2001;108(2):311–6.

25. Andreola B, Bressan S, Callegaro S, et al. Procalcitonin and C-reactive protein as diagnostic markers of severe bacterial infections in febrile infants and children in the emergency department. Pediatr Infect Dis J 2007;26(8):672–7.

26. Bressan S, Andreola B, Cattelan F, et al. Predicting severe bacterial infections in well-appearing febrile neonates: laboratory markers accuracy and duration of fever. Pediatr Infect Dis J 2010;29(3):227–32.

27. Caviness AC, Demmler GJ, Almendarez Y, et al. The prevalence of neonatal herpes simplex virus infection compared with serious bacterial illness in hospitalized neonates. J Pediatr 2008;153(2):164–9.
28. Schwartz S, Raveh D, Toker O, et al. A week-by-week analysis of the low-risk criteria for serious bacterial infection in febrile neonates. Arch Dis Child 2009; 94(4):287–92.
29. Chiu CH, Lin TY, Bullard MJ. Identification of febrile neonates unlikely to have bacterial infections. Pediatr Infect Dis J 1997;16(1):59–63.
30. Caspe WB, Chamudes O, Louie B. The evaluation and treatment of the febrile infant. Pediatr Infect Dis 1983;2(2):131–5.
31. Rudinsky SL, Carstairs KL, Reardon JM, et al. Serious bacterial infections in febrile infants in the post-pneumococcal conjugate vaccine era. Acad Emerg Med 2009;16(7):585–90.
32. Wasserman GM, White CB. Evaluation of the necessity for hospitalization of the febrile infant less than three months of age. Pediatr Infect Dis J 1990;9(3):163–9.
33. Ralston S, Hill V, Waters A. Occult serious bacterial infection in infants younger than 60 to 90 days with bronchiolitis: a systematic review. Arch Pediatr Adolesc Med 2011;165(10):951–6.
34. Kuppermann N, Bank DE, Walton EA, et al. Risks for bacteremia and urinary tract infections in young febrile children with bronchiolitis. Arch Pediatr Adolesc Med 1997;151(12):1207–14.
35. Bilavsky E, Shouval DS, Yarden-Bilavsky H, et al. A prospective study of the risk for serious bacterial infections in hospitalized febrile infants with or without bronchiolitis. Pediatr Infect Dis J 2008;27(3):269–70.
36. Garra G, Cunningham SJ, Crain EF. Reappraisal of criteria used to predict serious bacterial illness in febrile infants less than 8 weeks of age. Acad Emerg Med 2005;12(10):921–5.
37. Loeffelholz MJ, Trujillo R, Pyles RB, et al. Duration of rhinovirus shedding in the upper respiratory tract in the first year of life. Pediatrics 2014;134(6):1144–50.
38. Bender JM, Taylor CS, Cumpio J, et al. Infants 1–90 days old hospitalized with human rhinovirus infection. J Clin Lab Anal 2014;28(5):349–52.
39. Kimberlin DW, Lin CY, Jacobs RF, et al. Natural history of neonatal herpes simplex virus infections in the acyclovir era. Pediatrics 2001;108(2):223–9.
40. Caviness AC, Demmler GJ, Selwyn BJ. Clinical and laboratory features of neonatal herpes simplex virus infection: a case-control study. Pediatr Infect Dis J 2008;27(5):425–30.
41. Greenhow TL, Hung YY, Herz AM, et al. The changing epidemiology of serious bacterial infections in young infants. Pediatr Infect Dis J 2014;33(6):595–9.
42. Biondi E, Evans R, Mischler M, et al. Epidemiology of bacteremia in febrile infants in the United States. Pediatrics 2013;132(6):990–6.
43. Biondi EA, Mischler M, Jerardi KE, et al. Blood culture time to positivity in febrile infants with bacteremia. JAMA Pediatr 2014;168(9):844–9.
44. Kadish HA, Loveridge B, Tobey J, et al. Applying outpatient protocols in febrile infants 1–28 days of age: can the threshold be lowered? Clin Pediatr 2000; 39(2):81–8.
45. Ferrera PC, Bartfield JM, Snyder HS. Neonatal fever: utility of the Rochester criteria in determining low risk for serious bacterial infections. Am J Emerg Med 1997;15(3):299–302.
46. Baraff LJ, Bass JW, Fleisher GR, et al. Practice guideline for the management of infants and children 0 to 36 months of age with fever without source. Agency for Health Care Policy and Research. Ann Emerg Med 1993;22(7):1198–210.

47. King RL, Lorch SA, Cohen DM, et al. Routine cerebrospinal fluid enterovirus polymerase chain reaction testing reduces hospitalization and antibiotic use for infants 90 days of age or younger. Pediatrics 2007;120(3):489–96.
48. Shah SS, Volk J, Mohamad Z, et al. Herpes simplex virus testing and hospital length of stay in neonates and young infants. J Pediatr 2010;156(5):738–43.
49. Olaciregui I, Hernandez U, Munoz JA, et al. Markers that predict serious bacterial infection in infants under 3 months of age presenting with fever of unknown origin. Arch Dis Child 2009;94(7):501–5.
50. Greenhow TL, Hung YY, Herz AM. Changing epidemiology of bacteremia in infants aged 1 week to 3 months. Pediatrics 2012;129(3):e590–6.
51. Paxton RD, Byington CL. An examination of the unintended consequences of the rule-out sepsis evaluation: a parental perspective. Clin Pediatr 2001;40(2):71–7.
52. De S, Tong A, Isaacs D, et al. Parental perspectives on evaluation and management of fever in young infants: an interview study. Arch Dis Child 2014;99(8): 717–23.

Index

Note: Page numbers of article titles are in **boldface** type.

Infect Dis Clin N Am 29 (2015) 587 596
http://dx.doi.org/10.1016/S0891-5520(15)00078-1
0891-5520/15/$ – see front matter © 2015 Elsevier Inc. All rights reserved.

id.theclinics.com

Moving?

Make sure your subscription moves with you!

To notify us of your new address, find your **Clinics Account Number** (located on your mailing label above your name), and contact customer service at:

Email: journalscustomerservice-usa@elsevier.com

800-654-2452 (subscribers in the U.S. & Canada)
314-447-8871 (subscribers outside of the U.S. & Canada)

Fax number: 314-447-8029

Elsevier Health Sciences Division
Subscription Customer Service
3251 Riverport Lane
Maryland Heights, MO 63043

*To ensure uninterrupted delivery of your subscription, please notify us at least 4 weeks in advance of move.